Artificial Immune Systems:
A New Computational Intelligence Approach

D1336255

Springer
London
Berlin
Heidelberg
New York
Barcelona
Hong Kong
Milan
Paris
Singapore
Tokyo

Leandro N. de Castro and Jonathan Timmis

Artificial Immune Systems: A New Computational Intelligence Approach

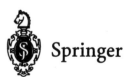 Springer

Leandro N. de Castro, BSc, MSc, PhD
Jonathan Timmis, BSc (hons), PhD

Computing Laboratory, University of Kent at Canterbury, Canterbury, Kent, CT2 7NF, UK

British Library Cataloguing in Publication Data
A catalogue record for this book is available from the British Library

Library of Congress Cataloging-in-Publication Data
de Castro, Leandro N., 1974-
    Artificial immune systems : a new computational intelligence approach / Leandro N. de Castro and Jonathan Timmis.
        p. cm.
    Includes bibliographical references and index.
    ISBN 1-85233-594-7 (alk. paper)
        1. Neural networks (Computer science) 2. Immune system – Computer simulation. 3. Artificial intelligence. I. Timmis, Jonathan, 1970- II. Title.
    QA76.87 .D43 2002
    006.3—dc21

                                                            2002070458

ISBN 1-85233-594-7 Springer-Verlag London Berlin Heidelberg
a member of BertelsmannSpringer Science+Business Media GmbH
http://www.springer.co.uk

Typesetting: Camera ready by authors
Printed and bound at the Athenæum Press Ltd., Gateshead, Tyne and Wear
34/3830-543210 Printed on acid-free paper SPIN 10867470

To my parents: José, Lásara

Leandro Nunes de Castro

To my parents: Jim, Sheila

Jonathan Timmis

Novel paradigms are proposed and accepted not necessarily for being faithful to their sources of inspiration, but for being useful and feasible

Preface

When one reads through the current literature on artificial immune systems (AIS), a common observation is: "the field of AIS is too young to be well defined, and its scope and limitations are still unknown". Indeed, as remarked by I. Stewart while referring to chaos in his best seller *Does God Play Dice?* "few were willing to offer a precise definition. This isn't unusual in a 'hot' research area – it's hard to define something when you feel you still don't fully understand it." Despite this, we feel that in order to help promote and consolidate the emerging area of AIS, an attempt should be made at drawing together what sometimes seems to be very disparate work. In this book we make an effort to bring many ideas from AIS together into a single text that can provide some basics for AIS. It is our hope that this will make the field more accessible to the wider community and also begin the process of *formalizing* AIS through the introduction of an engineering framework.

The majority of the ideas contained in this volume constitute an outcome of Leandro's Ph.D. thesis undertaken at the State University of Campinas – Unicamp, Brazil. Between the two of us, we reviewed, extended, discussed, and improved these ideas in order to achieve the final result that is now this book. The motivation to write this book came from several parts: from the referees of Leandro's viva, from several conversations we had with one another, and from comments of many researchers and research students in the broad area of computational intelligence. Most importantly, we felt that the field lacked a textbook, but we (of course!) do not claim this text is going to answer all questions. Indeed, we see this very much as a first attempt and hopefully not the last one. We hope it will help to mature the field and inspire researchers in AIS and many other areas to gain a better understanding of such a new, rich, and exciting research area.

In order to set the scene for our book, we begin discussing themes such as computing with biological metaphors and computational intelligence. There then follows a discussion on the fundamentals of the biological immune system. It was very difficult to decide how deep we should go into biological terminology, and it is possible that some readers may think that we have gone a bit over the top. However, we feel what we have produced is a compromise of offering a text that makes the biological language simple for computer scientists and engineers, but one that is accurate and provides enough terminology so as to prepare the reader to understand the contents of the book itself and also the related literature on AIS.

From biology, there emerges a proposed framework on how to engineer an AIS. We observed from the literature that there were a number of *common* building blocks, which would make an ideal common framework to design AIS. We then try to exhaustively survey the publications on AIS. Instead of briefly describing every work cited, we identify the major application domains, describe one work of each research school and reference the others. We focus on the immune metaphors employed by the authors and how their approaches suit the framework introduced.

We then again turn back to biology. Chapter 5 is strongly biological and one would probably raise the question "do we actually need all this biology?" It is worth noting that by presenting biology in a broader context, it allows us to understand the wider picture played by the immune system with other organisms. When viewed in relation to other systems, the evolution of species, and cognition, it is easier to explain some of the immune system's behavior and to compare this behavior with the behavior of other systems. Chapter 5 also serves the purpose of reviewing the biological motivation for the development of several computational intelligence tools, such as neural networks and evolutionary algorithms, to be discussed in Chapter 6.

Artificial immune systems are hybrid systems almost by their very nature, and thus, this book could not restrict itself to a discussion of this single theme. It goes far beyond the AIS domain and discusses several other computational intelligence paradigms. Among these, we focus on artificial neural networks and evolutionary algorithms. One of our motivating factors for this is the fact that it is not unusual to hear questions concerning the distinction between an AIS and a genetic algorithm, immune network models and neural networks, and so on. One point to note is that, the flavor of the book might be seen deliberately philosophical in parts. This is an attempt on our end to place emphasis on underlying concepts, knowing that in this rapidly developing area the specifics may change very quickly.

That's what our book is about; computational intelligence focused on the emerging field of artificial immune systems. We hope that it helps to shape the field and that it serves as a guide for you to understand and engineer your own AIS.

Leandro Nunes de Castro & Jonathan Timmis
Canterbury, April 2002

Acknowledgements

Throughout the writing of the book there were several active researchers on immunology, AIS, and computational intelligence who contributed directly or indirectly to the final result presented here. We benefited from comments and suggestions of Myriam Regattieri, Dagmar Machado, Paulo França, Simon Garret, Marco Janssen, Beatriz González, Jungwon Kim, Fernando Gomide, Ricardo Gudwin, Márcio Netto, Felipe França, Modupe Ayara, Dawei Guan, Tom Knight, Christiano Lyra, Ernesto Costa, Patrícia Vargas, and Roberto Michelin: our thanks to you all. Special thanks and appreciation go to Andrew Watkins and Steve Reid for patiently proofreading the book and providing great feedback. Also, many thanks to Prof. Fernando Von Zuben for his invaluable comments on chapters of the book. Finally, many thanks to the unknown reviewers of this book whose feedback was invaluable.

We are also very grateful to the following researchers and institutions for kindly providing us with permission to reproduce part(s) of their work:

1. Dr. Akio Ishiguro
2. Dr. Mihaela Oprea
3. Dr. Steven A. Hofmeyr
4. Elsevier Science
5. McGraw-Hill Publishing Company
6. Publications Scientifiques – Institut Pasteur
7. Springer-Verlag
8. The Endocrine Society
9. The Immunologist Journal – Hogrefe & Huber Publishers
10. The Institute of Electrical and Electronic Engineers – IEEE

Leandro Nunes de Castro
Jonathan Timmis
April, 2002

I would like to especially thank Prof. Fernando Von Zuben from Unicamp who for many years was my M.Sc. and Ph.D. supervisor and who also provided important feedback on some parts of our book. He is now a very good friend and was responsible for inspiring me, thus planting the first seed of this book. I also would like to thank the Computing Laboratory at UKC, Jon Timmis and Prof. Keith Mander for all the research support I received from them, and for inviting me to work in such a nice and friendly environment. Many thanks to all the great friends I made at UKC.

Leandro Nunes de Castro
April 2002

I would like to especially thank Dr. John Hunt who first introduced me to the field of AIS back in the mid 1990s. Many thanks also to Dr. Mark Neal under whom I worked as a Research Associate and under whom I studied for my Ph.D. He convinced me to do a Ph.D. and I have never looked back – you see, Mark, our many chats in the coffee room in Aberystwyth were not in vain. Also, thanks to Prof. Keith Mander, Head of Department of the Computing Laboratory, UKC who gave me a chance to bring Leandro over to the Computing Laboratory to work on this book. To my many colleagues in the Computing Laboratory for their support and backing this last year, in particular Dr. Peter Kenny, Dr. Rogerio de Lemos, and Dr. Colin Johnson: you are great guys to work with! Thanks also to Leandro, who has been a great inspiration to work with over the past year or so and kept me on my toes. Also, many thanks to my close friend Dr. Sarah Cardwell for her friendship and support here at Canterbury, and my other friends who live further away and in so many different ways have been great friends and offered support, in particular: Dr. Andreas Karwath, Alex McManus, Dr. Steve Reid, Dr. Carolyne Timmis and Mathew White. Finally, Zoë Townsley, who over this past year has been so patient with me, and my work – I hope you think it has been worth it.

Jonathan Timmis
April 2002

About the Authors

Leandro Nunes de Castro

Dr. Leandro Nunes de Castro is an Electrical Engineer by the Federal University of Goiás – UFG/Brazil, M.Sc. and Ph.D. by the State University of Campinas – Unicamp/Brazil. He was a Research Associate at the Computing Laboratory at the University of Kent at Canterbury – UKC/England from June 2001 to May 2002, during which period this book was written. His major research field is Artificial Immune Systems, but his research interests and publications also include Artificial Neural Networks, Evolutionary Algorithms, Fuzzy Systems, Artificial Life and Swarm Intelligence. He has been an IEEE member since 1998, an INNS member since 1998, and a member of SBA since 1999. He has been a referee for a number of conferences and journals, including IEEE publications and the Soft Computing Journal. He has also served as a member of the program committee for a number of workshops on artificial immune systems. He is currently a Research Fellow at the Computer and Electrical Engineering School (FEEC) at Unicamp, Brazil, financially supported by CNPq (Profix. n. 540396/01-0).

Jonathan Timmis

Dr. Jonathan Timmis has been a lecturer in Computer Science in the Computing Laboratory, University of Kent at Canterbury (UKC) since June 2000. Prior to that he studied at the University of Wales, Aberystwyth (UWA) where he obtained a first class honors degree in Computer Science and his Ph.D. in Artificial Immune Systems. He spent 2 years working as a Research Associate on immune inspired machine learning at UWA before moving to UKC. His research interests primarily lie in biologically inspired techniques, particularly in the development and use of novel immune inspired algorithms in the data mining, fault tolerance and software engineering domains. He works closely with a number of industrial collaborators, attempting to transfer laboratory ideas to the industrial world. He has given a number of tutorials on Artificial Immune Systems at international conferences, reviews for a number of international journals, served on the program committee for a number of workshops on Artificial Immune Systems and is conference co-chair on the first international conference on Artificial Immune Systems in September 2002. He is a member of the IEEE.

Table of Contents

3. A Framework for Engineering Artificial Immune Systems

4. A Survey of Artificial Immune Systems

5. The Immune System in Context with Other Biological Systems

6. AIS in Context with Other Computational Intelligence Paradigms

8. Conclusions and Future Trends

Chapter 1

Introduction

For metaphors to be good science...You need to say: there's a process going on in both these examples; it's the same process; I can formulate what that process is; and I can do some maths and science with that process. If everything works at that level, your metaphor's got some backbone to it.

– I. Stewart

1.1   The Scope of the Book

What is an artificial immune system? Where have they been used? What are they for? How can I design my own artificial immune system? What is the difference between an artificial immune system and other computational intelligence paradigms? Is the immune system isolated from other bodily systems? Why do artificial immune systems behave the way they do?

These are just a small sample of questions that describe what this book is about. "Artificial Immune Systems: A New Computational Intelligence Approach" is one of the first attempts to introduce, formalize, survey, compare, and assess this novel computational paradigm. The approach adopted in this book is that of the Ockham's Razor (also spelled Occam's Razor). In the 14th century William of Ockham proposed, "it is vain to do with more what can be done with fewer". It is acknowledged that the contents presented in this text are not simple in nature, but taking the Occam's Razor approach an effort has been made to simplify as much as possible with a view to introducing the field at a high and sometimes abstract level and perspective, thus hopefully making it more accessible and understandable.

Artificial immune systems (AIS) are introduced and a framework to engineer them is proposed. The framework is based upon a set of general-purpose algorithms and models to create abstract (or artificial) components of the immune system. These derive from a number of significant works from the literature on AIS and theoretical immunology. The majority of these works were developed with a single application in mind. Here, these ideas have been taken and abstracted out to form basic models and algorithms based on immune components that can be used in a variety of application areas.

From the biological perspective, this book covers topics such as the nervous and endocrine systems, ecosystems, evolutionary biology and cognition, all in addition to the immune system. As one aspect of this book is the description of other biological systems, it is interesting to identify a hierarchy for them; two separate but interrelated levels are illustrated in Figure 1.1.

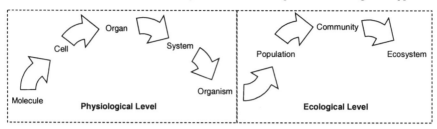

Figure 1.1.   A hierarchical division of biological systems.

The first level, defined as the *physiological level*, is concerned with the study of function in living matter; it attempts to explain the physical and chemical factors that are responsible for the origin, development, and progression of life. The second level, named *ecological level*, deals with the study of the interactions among individual organisms, and organisms and their environment.

This book goes beyond the scope of artificial immune systems and depicts the importance of the immune system as a system that works in collaboration with other bodily systems in order to provide and maintain life. For instance, similarities, differences, and pathways of interactions of the immune, nervous, and endocrine systems are traced. The analysis goes even further: a discourse is presented on how the research on biological and artificial immune systems has been used to trace parallels and has helped to provide new insights into other sciences like ecology. Therefore, the subjects covered will range from the cellular and molecular interactions within the immune system, to the interactions of the immune and other systems, and then some of these implications to the study of other research fields.

An important aspect of this book is the realization that AIS are another computational intelligence paradigm. It is therefore vital that, within this book, AIS are placed in context with other related paradigms. A result of this undertaking is the identification of new avenues to be followed in the development of hybrid systems. In order to consolidate all the information within the book, a number of case studies, mostly real-world applications, are described in detail. This will hopefully assist the reader in bringing together all the ideas presented in this book and show that AIS are applicable not only as an academic research subject, but also as an engineering and industry-based topic. The book is concluded with an overview of its own contents and the emerging field of AIS. Trends for future research are stressed throughout the whole text and are emphasized in the concluding chapter.

In the context of this book, computational intelligence (CI) paradigms are composed of those systems capable of adapting their behavior in order to reach their goals, usually to solve a particular problem, in a range of environments. This definition of computational intelligence is based on the one discussed by Fogel (2000), where the author presents a philosophical discussion of evolutionary computation as a new CI approach. Under this perspective, artificial neural networks (ANN), evolutionary algorithms (EA), fuzzy systems (FS), case-based reasoning (CBR) and classifier systems (CS) are considered to be CI paradigms.

1.2   Why Biology is a Good Metaphor?

For many centuries, observing the natural world has allowed human beings to devise theories about how the many parts of nature behave. Two examples are Newton's laws of physics and Kepler's model of planetary orbits. However, the world need not just be observed and explained but utilized as inspiration for the design and construction of artifacts, based on the simple principle that nature has been doing quite a good job for millions of years. For example, the mechanical designs for new materials, such as Velcro (a plant burr [burdock]) and bulletproof vests (spider silk), were inspired by the natural world (Paton, 1994). Additionally, the development and progress of computer science, engineering, and technology has greatly contributed to the study of the world, particularly the biological systems and sciences.

Recently, computing and engineering have been used to gain a better understanding of biological processes and functions through modeling and simulation of these natural systems. The reciprocal is also true: computing and engineering have been enriched with the introduction of biological ideas to help developing solutions to problems. This can be exemplified by artificial neural networks, evolutionary algorithms, artificial life (ALife), and cellular automata (CA). This inspiration from nature is a major motivation for the development of artificial immune systems.

A new field of research emerged under the name of *bioinformatics* referring to the information technology (e.g., computational methods) applied to the management (acquisition and archiving) and analysis of biological data. It has implications in diverse areas, ranging from computational intelligence and robotics to genome analysis (Attwood & Parry-Smith, 1999). In contrast, the field of *biomedical engineering* was introduced in order to encompass the application of engineering principles to biological and medical problems (Schwan, 1969) and is intimately related to the bioinformatics.

As a result of these bilateral interactions between computing and biology, it is possible to identify three different approaches, namely, *biologically motivated computing*, *computationally motivated biology* and *computing with biological mechanisms*. The first of these is adopted in this book. Biology provides sources of models and inspiration for the development of computational systems (e.g., ANN and EC). In the second approach, computing provides models and inspiration for biology (e.g., ALife and CA). The last approach involves the use of information processing capabilities of biological systems to replace, or at least supplement, the current silicon-based computers (e.g., Quantum and DNA computing).

What then is the distinction then, between a *model* and a *metaphor*? A model is usually aimed at providing a representation or reproducing the functioning (behavior) of one "thing" in terms of "something" else. As an example, consider an equation of motion that mimics the behavior of a set of immune cells when a disease-causing agent invades our organisms. This equation is supposed to reproduce at least approximately the dynamics of our immune cells. Metaphors in contrast, are aimed at creating (often simple) abstract and high level representations of a component or function. A metaphor uses inspiration to construct this basic functionality and is typically used in an area other than the one where the inspiration came from.

A simple example is that of the spider's web. This served as a metaphor for the design of bulletproof vests, but you do not see many spiders carrying guns or shooting at each other! It is worth noting however, that the metaphors should attempt to be as accurate as possible, but typically, deviations from the natural system are inevitable in order to fit into the problem area.

Paton (1992) identified four properties of biological systems important for the development of metaphors: architecture, functionality, mechanism, and organization. The architecture refers to the form or structure of the system; functionality corresponds to its behavior; mechanisms are the working together of the parts, and the organization refers to the ways the activities of the system are expressed in the dynamics of the whole. The next chapter describes the vertebrate immune system covering these aspects and the immune system will be extended to the top most physiologic level in Chapter 5 by putting it in context with other major bodily systems. Finally, extrapolations will be made even further and reach the ecological level with a discussion of how the immune system's behavior relates with the natural selection of species and how it has been used to study ecological systems.

1.3   The Nature of Interdisciplinary Research

As a book dedicated to biologically motivated computing, particularly immune-inspired systems, one question that might already have come into the mind of the reader is related to "how much of biology will I have to know in order to devise or understand artificial immune systems?" There are a few issues involved in answering this question. The previous section suggested that maintaining the accuracy of the metaphor is important, and thus, minimum background knowledge on immunology is required. This is one reason why a whole chapter on the fundamentals of the immune system is provided.

Usually, in texts about other biologically motivated computing paradigms, such as artificial neural networks and evolutionary algorithms, very little is said about the biological motivation, often no more than a single section. By comparison, Chapter 2 might be going far over the top on biology. The argument is simple. This is the first textbook in the field, and it makes perfect sense to contain within one volume the basics of immunology for the reader, to save them wading through several papers or specific textbooks on immunology. The approach of this book is to try and simplify the required information. In addition, the reader is guided to some of the relevant literature on immunology and artificial immune systems through further reading.

Due to the young age of the field of AIS, novel algorithms are constantly being proposed. This is in contrast to a great deal of the research on ANN and EA where most researchers are concerned with improving the performance or modifying the behavior of already existing algorithms. It is likely that there will come a time when the research on AIS reaches the same stage. This is another reason why a basic description of the immune system is necessary.

When considering how much into biology one should go, the reader should take into account his/her own goals. If it is the intent to devise new metaphors or develop new models of immune components, mechanisms, and functioning, then there is a wide range of immunological background that this single text does not and could not possibly cover, even if it were entirely dedicated to the science of immunology. Alternatively, if the goal is to try to improve already existing algorithms, then a more subtle biological background is required.

It is important to stress that novel fields of research, like bioinformatics, biological engineering, and now biologically motivated computing, have emerged from the bilateral interaction of biology, engineering, and computer science (and others). This synergy has already demonstrated its usefulness, and we are certainly very far from reaching a minor percentage of its true potentiality.

1.4   Structure of the Book

In Chapter 2, a high-level, information-processing perspective of the fundamentals of the vertebrate immune system is presented. The focus is on the main cells, molecules and organs that compose the system, together with their structures and primary roles. Among the many theories used to explain how the immune system works, the focus is on those that are currently being modeled and explored in the development of AIS.

From an artificial immune system perspective, Chapter 3 is the core of the book. Here, the reader is instructed how to use/adapt the immune system as a metaphor is appropriate for the development of computational problem solving techniques. A definition of an artificial immune system is presented. A framework for engineering AIS is then proposed. The framework is one of the central focuses of this book. This framework is composed of a formalism to create abstract models of immune cells and molecules, and to quantify their interactions, and a set of algorithms claimed to be general-purpose building blocks for the design of AIS. The framework is concluded with some AIS design guidelines.

Chapter 4 reviews a large number of works from the literature that fit into the definition proposed in Chapter 3 for AIS. The major schools and application domains are identified, together with their main contributors. One work from each application domain (or author) is reviewed and the reader is guided to their related references. The focus is on the metaphors employed and how the AIS fit into the framework proposed. The papers containing hybrids of AIS with other computational intelligence paradigms for the sake of improvement of one of the methodologies are reviewed in Chapter 6. It should be noted that by the time you read this book this chapter will be out of date. However, it is intended to be a comprehensive survey up to January 2002.

In Chapter 5 attention is turned back to biology. First, some fundamentals of the nervous and endocrine systems are presented. This is to provide the basis for the study of a new science named *psychoneuroimmunology* and a discussion of the similarities and differences among the nervous, immune, and endocrine systems. One reason for introducing all these subjects is that some of the pioneering works on AIS research started with a trade-off among these biological systems. The chapter then follows with the basics of evolutionary biology, ecosystems and cognition.

These topics are tackled because they lead to theoretical and philosophical explanations of the behavior of the immune system and thus some artificial immune systems. Also, many of the concepts discussed in this chapter under a biological perspective are used in the development of the computational paradigms reviewed in Chapter 6.

Chapter 6 returns the context of the book to computing. It starts with the review of the fundamentals of neural networks, and evolutionary algorithms. After this review, a discourse of the main differences between AIS, neural networks and evolutionary algorithms is given. The text follows with a description of hybrids of these methodologies with AIS. Other approaches such as case-based reasoning, DNA computing, fuzzy systems, and classifier systems are also put in context with AIS. The chapter is concluded with future trends on the development of hybrids between the many computational intelligence paradigms reviewed and AIS.

Based upon the framework for engineering AIS, Chapter 7 presents four case studies in detail. The first case is an autonomous navigation task for a robotic system. Second, an artificial immune system for network intrusion detection is reviewed. Then, a job-shop scheduling application is studied and, finally, an AIS for data analysis and optimization is described. The goal is to illustrate in full the process of engineering an AIS, and to provide the reader with a knowledge of how to design his/her own AIS using the framework introduced.

Chapter 8 concludes the book by discussing the framework, the use of biological metaphors, and the new and future trends of AIS. The three appendices aim to present a glossary of the biological terminology required to properly understand the subjects studied, outline pseudocode for the basic immune algorithms, list-related journals and magazines on immunology and computational intelligence, and provide personal and organizational URL addresses in which to search for information about AIS.

1.5   Suitability of the Book and how to use it

It is hoped that this book serves many different fields of research and activities, such as biologically motivated computing, bioinformatics, computational intelligence, computer science and industrial parties. First, the book is an introductory level text aimed at providing the reader suitable background on relevant immunology. This is essential for the development and comprehension of artificial immune systems. Secondly, the reader is provided with a framework for guidance on how to engineer new AIS of his/her own. This structure has the benefit of appealing to both the "newcomer" to biologically inspired computation, particularly immune inspired computation, and mature researchers. Thirdly, the reader is provided with an up-to-date review of the current research that is being undertaken in AIS. This is designed to make the reader aware of the wider picture of AIS and its use as both an academic discipline and a practical paradigm.

If the reader is basically interested in the fundamentals of AIS and where they have been applied, Chapters 2, 3, 4 and 7, are the most relevant ones. Nevertheless, Chapters 4 and 7 require some background on other computational intelligence paradigms such as neural networks, evolutionary algorithms, fuzzy systems, and classifier systems. For those who do not possess this background knowledge, an introductory theory for these and other paradigms is provided in Chapter 6. In addition, Chapter 6 discusses several soft-computing hybrids with AIS. Chapter 5 is not particularly essential for the design of AIS, but it puts the immune system into the broader context of other biological systems. This leads to a better understanding of the behavior of AIS and opens new avenues for the development of novel computational and hybrid methodologies.

Each chapter contains its own list of references and suggestions for further reading. In both cases, the references constitute those works consulted by the authors during their research and the writing of this volume. With the exception of Chapter 4, no attempt has been made to provide an exhaustive list of references for the reader, but rather a set of suitable sources of information on the subjects studied in this book is offered. There is also a supporting website for the book, which can be found at http://www.cs.ukc.ac.uk/aisbook/

References

Attwood, T. K. & Parry-Smith, D. J. (1999), *Introduction to Bioinformatics*, Prentice Hall.

Fogel, D. B. (2000), *Evolutionary Computation: Toward a New Philosophy of Machine Intelligence*, 2nd ed., IEEE Press.

Paton, R. (ed.) (1994), *Computing with Biological Metaphors*, Chapman & Hall.

Paton, R. (1992), "Towards a Metaphorical Biology", *Biology and Philosophy*, 7, pp. 279-294.

Schwan, H. P. (1969), *Biological Engineering*, McGraw-Hill.

Chapter 2

Fundamentals of the Immune System

By defining and defending the self, the immune system makes life possible; malfunction causes illness and death

– G. J. V. Nossal

2.1 Introduction

In Roman times people who were "free of burden", be that from taxes imposed by Caesar, a law, or a disease, were said to be *immunis*, the Latin word from which *immunology* is derived. Immunology can be defined as the study of the defense mechanisms that confer resistance against diseases. The system whose main function is to protect our bodies against the constant attack of external *microorganisms* is called the *immune system*. The immune system specifically recognizes and selectively eliminates foreign invaders by a process known as the *immune response*.

Individuals who do not succumb to a disease when infected are said to be *immune*, and the status of a specific resistance to a certain disease is called *immunity*. As the immune system plays a major role for the survival of an animal, it has to act efficiently and effectively. There are a large number of distinct components and mechanisms acting on the immune system. Some of these elements are optimized to defend against a specific invader, while others are directed against a great variety of *infecting agents*. The circulation of immune cells, as well as their traffic through the organism, is essential to *immunosurveillance* and to an efficient immune response. In addition, there is a great redundancy within the immune system, to allow for many distinct defense mechanisms to be activated against a single agent.

From a biological and computational perspective, the presence of *adaptive* and *memory* mechanisms in the immune system is of great importance. The immune system possesses the capability of extracting information from the infectious agents (environment) and making it available for future use in cases of re-infection by the same or a similar agent.

This chapter is organized as follows. Section 2.2 begins with a brief history of immunology. In Sections 2.3 and 2.4 the fundamentals of the immune system and a general overview of its main defense mechanisms, including the primary and secondary immune responses, are reviewed. Section 2.5 describes the physiology of the immune system. Sections 2.6 and 2.7 introduce the innate and adaptive immune systems, respectively. Section 2.8 discusses the B-cell and T-cell receptors in more detail, stressing their mechanisms of formation. Section 2.9, discusses theories on how the immune system learns and maintains a memory of past encounters. Self/nonself discrimination in the immune system is reviewed in Section 2.10, followed by the final Section, 2.11, on the immune network theory.

2.2   Brief History and Perspectives on Immunology

2.2.1. The Early Years

Immunology is a relatively new science. Its origins have been attributed to Edward Jenner who, in 1796, discovered that by introducing small amounts of *vaccinia*, or *cowpox*, in an animal would induce protection against the often lethal disease *smallpox*; this process was named *vaccination*. Vaccination is an expression that is still used to describe the inoculation of healthy individuals with weakened samples of the agents responsible for causing the disease. This process is aimed at promoting protection against future infection of that disease.

When Jenner discovered the process of vaccination, very little was known about the functioning of the immune system. In the 19th century, Robert Koch proved that pathogenic microorganisms caused infectious diseases; each of which is responsible for a specific *infection* or *pathology*. It is now considered that there are four categories of disease causing microorganisms, or *pathogens,* these are: *viruses, bacteria, fungi,* and *parasites*.

The discoveries of Koch and other researchers from the 19th century contributed to the development of the science of immunology, which in time allowed for the vaccination against other forms of diseases. In the 1880s, Louis Pasteur successfully designed a vaccine against *chickenpox* and developed what was called an *antirage*. This was the first successful *inoculation* of a child bitten by a mad dog.

Pasteur, though well versed in the development of vaccines, had little knowledge about the mechanisms involved in the process of *immunization* (that is, the use of these vaccines in protecting from infection). He suggested that elements in the vaccinia were capable of removing nutrients essential to the body and, thus, avoiding the growth and proliferation of the disease-causing agents. Around ten years later, in 1890, Emil von Behring and Shibasaburo Kitasato demonstrated that protection induced by vaccination was not due to the removal of nutrients, but was associated with the appearance of protecting elements in the blood serum of inoculated individuals. They discovered that people who had been inoculated against diseases contained certain agents that could in some way bind to other infectious agents. These agents were named *antibodies*. Emil von Behring received, in 1901, the first Nobel Prize in Medicine for his work on antibody production.

The first major controversy in immunology appeared when Elie Metchnikoff demonstrated in 1882, primarily in invertebrates and later in mammals, that some cells were capable of "eating" microorganisms. These cells were named *phagocytes*, and he proposed they were the main operative defense mechanisms against the invading microorganisms. He suggested that antibodies were of little importance within the immune system. The conflict was resolved in 1904 when Almroth Wright and Joseph Denys demonstrated that antibodies were capable of binding with bacteria and promoting their destruction by phagocytes.

Still in the 1890s, Paul Ehrlich formulated a theory named *side-chain theory*. The main premise of this theory was that the surfaces of white blood cells, such as

B-cells, are covered with several side-chains, or *receptors*. He also developed a technique by which it was possible to estimate the amount of antibodies contained in the blood. The receptors on the surfaces of B-cells form chemical links with the *antigens* encountered. In a broad sense, any molecule that can be recognized by the immune system is referred to as *antigen*. Given any antigen, at least one of these receptors would be able to recognize and bind with the antigen. It was shown that an explosive increase in the production of antibodies is observed after exposure and binding with a given antigen.

In order to produce the required antibodies to fight the infection from antigens, a theory was proposed, called the *providential* (or *germinal*) theory. This theory stated that antibodies might be constructed from the collection of genes, or *genome*, of the animal. Therefore, it was suggested that the contact of a receptor on a B-cell with a given antigen would be responsible for *selecting* and *stimulating* the B-cell. This would give rise to a large production of these receptors, which would then be secreted to the blood stream as antibodies. These selection and stimulation events allowed for the characterization of Ehrlich's theory as *selectivist*, where antigens were responsible for selecting and stimulating a B-cell. This theory was intriguing, as it implied the idea that it was possible to generate an almost limitless amount of antibodies from a finite genome. The theory also suggested that the antigens were themselves responsible for selecting an already existing set of cells through their receptors. The Nobel Prize of 1908 was shared by Ehrlich and Metchnikoff.

In the period between 1910 and 1930, experiments performed by people such as Obermayer, Pick, Jules Bordet and Karl Landsteiner with *artificial haptens* (antigens that do not exist in nature, i.e., artificially synthesized), led to the abandonment, for more than half a century, of Ehrlich's selectivist theory. Jules Bordet received the 1919 Nobel Prize for the discovery of a set of proteins that act together in the attack of extra cellular pathogenic agents. This set of proteins was termed the *complement system* or simply the *complement*. In 1930, Karl Landsteiner received the Nobel Prize for the identification of the different blood types, resulting in the success of the blood transfer procedures.

Between 1914 and 1955 it was thought that no *selective* theory about the formation of antibodies would ever be correct. The theoretical proposals about such formations were mainly considered as sub-cellular. This means that research focus was on the creation of the antibody molecules produced by cells, with the conclusion that the antigen would bring to the cell information concerning the complementary structure of the antibody molecule. This theory is called *template instruction theory*. Pioneering work was performed by Anton Breinl and Felix Haurowitz, and more recently developed and defended by the Nobel Prize winner Linus Pauling. Pauling postulated that all antibodies possess the same *amino acid* sequences, but that their tri-dimensional configuration would be determined during the synthesis in direct contact with the antigen, which would serve as a *template*.

From this brief tour of early immunology it can be seen that there were conflicts of opinion. This was particularly apparent in the discussion about what defined the structure of the antibody. On the one hand, the germinal or selective theories suggested that the genome was responsible for the definition of the antibody structure; on the other, the instructionist or template theory suggested that the antigens played a part in antibody formation.

2.2.2. Recent Perspectives

Niels K. Jerne revived the selective theories of antibody formation in the early 1950s. Jerne assumed that a diverse population of *natural antibodies* would appear during development, even in the absence of antigen interaction. The antigen would be matched through the selection of circulating antibodies containing structures complementary to this antigen. The quality of an immune response to a given antigen would depend upon the concentration of the circulating antibody of a specific type and could be enhanced by the previous exposition to the antigen.

It remained for Burnet (and also to Talmage) to assert that each cell produces and creates on its surface a single type of antibody molecule. The *selective event* is the stimulus given by the antigen, where those cells that produce antibodies complementary to it will proliferate (*clonal expansion*) and secrete antibodies. *Clonal selection* (or *clonal expansion*) *theory* (Section 2.9), formalized in Burnet (1959), assumed that random processes generated antibody diversity. This would take place during neo-natal life, such that, immediately after birth, the animal would have a fixed repertoire of antibodies. In addition, he postulated the death of any cell possessing antibodies capable of recognizing *self-antigens*, named *self-reactive cells*, during this period of diversity generation. Peter Medawar confirmed experimentally the clonal selection theory proposed by Burnet. The studies on how the body reacts to the invading agents and how the organism becomes *tolerant* (does not respond) to its own cells and tissues resulted in another Nobel Prize in immunology, this time for Medawar and Burnet.

In 1971, Jerne argued that the elimination of self-reactive cells would constitute a powerful *negative selection* mechanism. This would favor the cellular diversity in cells that could potentially recognize antigens similar to the self. Considerations on how the self-antigens, particularly those of the antibody molecules, named *idiotopes*, could affect the diversity generation and the regulation of the immune responses, lead to the Jerne's proposal of the *immune network theory*. For this work, Jerne was awarded the Nobel Prize in 1984.

More recently, Susumo Tonegawa (1983) formalized his studies concerning the structure and diversity of the antibody molecules. He proposed that within the genome of a germinal cell, a newly created cell, is contained (in multiple gene segments scattered along a chromosome) the genetic information to code for an antibody molecule. This work resulted in another Nobel Prize for immunology in 1987.

Table 2.1 summarizes the main concepts, periods and their respective researchers up to the 1990s.

Table 2.1. Periods of the history of Immunology (reproduced with permission from [Jerne, 1974]. © *Institut Pasteur, 1974*).

Tendencies	Period	Pioneers	Concepts
Application	1796-1870	E. Jenner R. Koch	Immunization Pathology
	1870-1890	L. Pasteur E. Metchnikoff	Immunization Phagocytosis
Description	1890-1910	E. von Behring & S. Kitasato P. Ehrlich	Antibodies Cell receptors
	1910-1930	J. Bordet K. Landsteiner	Specificity/Complement Haptens/Blood types
Mechanisms (System)	1930-1950	A. Breinl & F. Haurowitz L. Pauling	Antibody synthesis Instructionism
	1950-1980	M. Burnet & Talmage N. Jerne	Clonal selection Network and cell co-operation
Molecular	1980-1990	S. Tonegawa	Structure and diversity of receptors

According to Zinkernagel (2000), the progress made in cell biology, genetics, molecular biology, and developmental biology will help scientists to better understand general rules and exceptions of immunity. These insights might lead to the improvement of immunity against infections and tumors. Among the many challenges for the immunology to the 21st century, Abbas and Janeway (2000) stress the increase in the understanding of the mechanisms that control the *adaptive immune response*. This would assist in the transformation of an immune response from an aggressive to a benign state. This could also help to control undesired immune functions, such as the response to allergens, self-antigens (autoimmune diseases), and grafted tissues. In addition, an increase in the efficiency and efficacy of an immune response to certain viruses such as HIV, tuberculosis, and some tumors, could possibly be reached through the control of the adaptive immune response.

2.3 Fundamentals and Main Components

The immune system is a natural, rapid and effective defense mechanism for a given host against infections. It consists of a two-tier line of defense, these are known as the *innate immune system* and the *adaptive immune system*. Both systems depend upon the activity of *white blood cells*, the *leukocytes*, where the innate immunity is mediated mainly by *granulocytes* and *macrophages*, and the adaptive immunity is mediated by *lymphocytes*, as summarized in Figure 2.1.

The cells of the *innate immune system* are immediately available to combat against a wide variety of bacteria, without requiring previous exposure to them. This reaction will occur in the same way in all normal individuals.

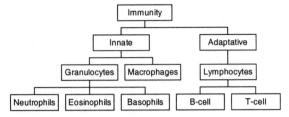

Figure 2.1.   Immune lines of defense and their respective main mediators.

The phagocytes are composed of *macrophages* and *neutrophils*, which possess the capability of ingesting and digesting several microorganisms and antigenic particles. Some phagocytes, like the macrophage, also have the ability to present antigens to other cells, being termed *antigen-presenting cells* (APC). The granulocytes, or *polymorfonuclear leukocytes*, constitute a special group of white blood cells with multiglobule nuclei containing cytoplasmatic *granules* filled with chemical elements (*enzymes*), as illustrated in Figure 2.2. The *neutrophils* are the most abundant cellular elements and are the most important mediators of innate immunity. The importance of the *eosinophils* is their role in the defense against infections by parasites. However, the main function of the *basophils* is still not well understood (Janeway *et al.*, 1999).

The antibody production in response to a determined infectious agent is called a *specific immune response*, also known as an *adaptive immune response*. Within the adaptive immune system, antibodies are produced only in response to specific infections. The presence of antibodies in an individual reflects the infections to which that individual has already been exposed. Cells of the adaptive system are capable of developing an immune memory, i.e., they are capable of recognizing the same antigenic stimulus when it is presented to the organism again. This capability avoids the re-establishment of the disease within the organism. Thus, the adaptive immune response allows the immune system to improve itself with each encounter of a given antigen.

The immune system is made up of a number of components, one of these being lymphocytes. Lymphocytes mediate the adaptive immune response and are responsible for the *recognition* and *elimination* of the pathogenic agents. These agents in turn proportion immune memory that occurs after the exposition to a disease, or vaccination. Lymphocytes usually become active when there is some kind of interaction with an antigenic stimulus leading to the activation and proliferation of the lymphocytes. There are two main types of lymphocytes: *B lymphocyte* (or *B-cell*) and *T lymphocyte* (or *T-cell*). The B- and T-cells express in their surfaces antigenic receptors highly specific to a given antigenic determinant (Section 2.8).

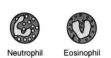

Neutrophil   Eosinophil   Basophil

Figure 2.2.   Presence of granules (small bubbles) filling the polymorfonuclear leukocytes.

   While the adaptive immune response results in immunity against re-infection to the same infectious agent, the innate immune response remains constant along the lifetime of an individual, independent of the antigenic exposure. Altogether, the innate and adaptive immune systems contribute to an extremely effective defense mechanism. This guarantees that although we spend our lives surrounded by potentially pathogenic infections, we rarely develop a disease. These two systems are of great importance and will therefore be discussed in greater detail in Sections 2.6 and 2.7, respectively.

2.4   Basic Immune Recognition and Activation Mechanisms

The immune system consists of a complex set of cells and molecules that protect our bodies against infection. Our bodies are under constant attack by antigens (Ag) that can stimulate the adaptive immune system. Antigens might be foreign, i.e., surface molecules present on pathogens, or self-antigens, which are composed of portions of cells or molecules of our own body.

   Figure 2.3 illustrates a simplified view of the main immune recognition and activation mechanisms. Part (I) of the diagram shows how specialized antigen presenting cells (APCs), such as macrophages, circulate throughout the body ingesting and digesting antigens. These antigens are fragmented into *antigenic peptides* (Nossal, 1993). Part of these peptides bind to molecules of the *major histocompatibility complex* (MHC) which are in turn presented in the APC cell surface as an MHC/peptide complex (II). The T-cells carry surface receptors that allow them to recognize different MHC/peptide complexes (III). Once activated by the MHC/peptide recognition, the T-cells become activated, divide and secrete *lymphokines*, or chemical signals, that stimulate other components of the immune system to enter into action (IV).

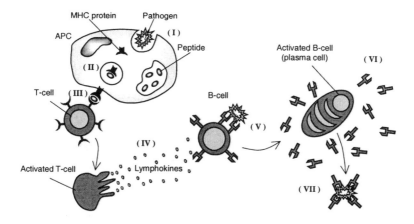

Figure 2.3.   Simplified view of the immune recognition and activation mechanisms.

In contrast, the B-cells have receptors with the ability to recognize parts of the antigens free in solution without the assistance of MHC molecules (V). The surface receptors on these B-cells respond to a specific antigen. When a signal is received by these B-cell receptors, the B-cell is activated and will proliferate and differentiate into *plasma cells* that secrete antibody molecules in high volumes (VI). These released antibodies (which are soluble forms of the B-cell receptors) are used to neutralize the pathogen (VII), leading to their destruction mainly by the enzymes of the complement system (Section 2.6). Some of these activated B- and T-cells will differentiate into *memory cells*. These will remain circulating through the organism for long periods of time, thus guaranteeing future protection against the same (or a similar) antigen that elicited the immune response.

2.5   Physiology of the Immune System

There are many organs distributed throughout the body that make up the immune system. These organs, called *lymphoid organs*, are responsible in part for the production, growth, and development of lymphocytes, mainly B- and T-cells. In the lymphoid organs, the lymphocytes interact with several types of cells, either when they are being produced, or during the start of an adaptive immune response. The lymphoid organs can be divided into *primary* (or *central*), which are responsible for the production and maturation of lymphocytes, and *secondary* (or *peripheral*) where the lymphocytes interact with the antigenic stimuli, thus initiating adaptive immune responses. Figure 2.4 shows the lymphoid organs located in the body.

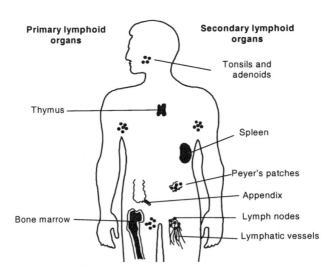

Figure 2.4.   Anatomy of the immune system (lymphoid organs).

The location and main roles of the lymphoid organs are:

1. Primary lymphoid organs:

- *Bone marrow*: soft tissue located inside the most elongated bones. It is the major site of *haematopoiesis* (production of blood cell types, including *red blood cells*, monocytes, granulocytes, lymphocytes, and *platelets*). It provides the environment for antigen-independent differentiation of B-cells and antigen processing.
- *Thymus*: located behind the sternum, above and in front of the heart. It provides the environment for antigen-independent differentiation of T-cells and produces hormonal factors important for T-cell maturation. The thymus has an interactive role with the *endocrine system* as *thymectomy* (thymus extraction) leads to a reduction in pituitary hormone level as well as atrophy of some *glands* (see Chapter 5 for an introduction to the interactions of the immune, endocrine, and nervous systems).

2. Secondary lymphoid organs:

- *Tonsils and adenoids*: the tonsils are embedded in the lateral walls of the opening between the mouth and the pharynx, while the adenoids are located at the back of the nose in the upper part of the throat. These large collections of lymphoid cells are primarily associated with the protection of the respiratory system.
- *Lymph nodes*: small solid structures found at varying points along the lymphatic system. They act as convergence sites of a large number of vessels that collect the extra-cellular fluid from tissues, carrying it back to the blood. This cellular fluid is continuously produced by filtering the blood and is named *lymph*. The lymph nodes are also the sites where the adaptive immune response occurs.
- *Appendix and Peyer's patches*: located in the walls of the small intestine. They are specialized lymph nodes containing immune cells to protect the digestive system.
- *Spleen*: is a large, encapsulated, bean shaped organ with a spongy interior and is situated on the left side of the body below the diaphragm. It is the only lymphoid organ that crosses the blood stream. The spleen therefore constitutes the site where the lymphocytes fight against the microorganisms that invade the blood stream. The spleen contains a *red pulp* that is responsible for removing old blood cells, and a *white pulp* of lymphoid cells that respond to the antigens carried by the blood.
- *Lymphatic vessels*: network of channels spread throughout the body. They transport the lymph to the blood and lymphoid organs. The lymph is transported from the tissues to the lymph nodes through the *afferent lymphatic vessels*. It enters a node through a series of cavities, percolates through the tissues of the lymph node, and exits through the *efferent lymphatic vessels*.

The immune system can be considered to have a layered architecture, with regulation and defense mechanisms spread in several levels (Figure 2.5).

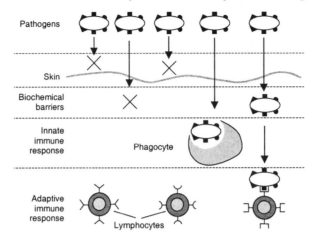

Figure 2.5. Multilayer architecture of the immune system.

The protection layers can be divided as follows (Janeway *et al.*, 1999; Rensberger, 1996; Hofmeyr, 2000):

- *Physical barriers*: our skin serves as a shield to protect against invaders, either malefic or not. The respiratory system also helps to keep potential infections at bay. These defense mechanisms include the trapping of irritants in nasal hairs and mucus, carrying mucus upward and outward on cilia, coughing and sneezing. The skin and the mucous membranes lining the respiratory and digestive tracts also contain macrophages and antibodies.
- *Biochemical barriers*: fluids such as saliva, sweat and tears contain destructive enzymes. Stomach acids will kill most microorganisms ingested in food and drinks. The pH levels and temperature of the body present unfavorable living and breeding conditions for some invaders.
- *Innate and adaptive immune systems*: constitute the two main lines of defense of the immune system and thus will be discussed separately in Sections 2.6 and 2.7, respectively.

2.6   Innate Immune System

The innate immune system is the first line of defense against several types of microorganisms and is considered essential to the control of common bacterial infections. The innate immune system is made up of phagocytic cells, like the macrophages and neutrophils, soluble factors like the complement system, and a limited number of enzymes. Some authors, like Scroferneker and Pohlmann (1998), classify the physical barriers as part of the innate immune system; however, they will be viewed separately in this book.

The cells of the innate immune system perform a crucial role in the process of initiating and controlling the adaptive immune response. A number of days may pass before the infection is attacked by the components of the adaptive immune system. Therefore in the interim period, the innate immune system is responsible for controlling the infection.

The macrophages and neutrophils have surface receptors that evolved to recognize and bind to common molecular patterns found only in microorganisms. The bacterial molecules that bind to these receptors stimulate the cells to engulf the bacteria and also induce the secretion of active molecules such as *cytokines*. Cytokines are proteins secreted by cells that affect the behavior of other cells, and lymphokines are cytokines secreted by lymphocytes. These surface receptors are constructed and coded in a site termed *germinal center* and are known as *pattern recognition receptors* (PRR). The PRR have the ability to recognize molecular patterns associated with pathogenic microbes, named *pathogen associated molecular patterns* (PAMP). PAMPs are only produced by the invading microbes and never by the host organism. Therefore, their recognition by a PRR signals the presence of a pathogen.

This way, the structures recognized by the innate immune system have to be absolutely distinct from the self-antigens in order to avoid damage to the cells and tissues of the host. The consequence of this mechanism is that the innate immune system plays a role in the process of distinguishing between the *self* and the *nonself*. When a PAMP is recognized, it activates effector mechanisms of the innate immune system, including the phagocytosis, the synthesis induction of anti-microbial peptides, and the synthesis induction of nitric oxide in the macrophages. Additionally, the PAMPs induce the construction of an endogenous set of signals under the form of *effector*, *inflammatory cytokines*, and *chemokines*. These are responsible for the recruiting of lymphocytes to the sites of infection and for the regulation of the activation of the appropriate effector mechanisms. The control of effector T-cell differentiation of a certain type is one such example.

An important aspect of the interaction between the innate and the adaptive immunity is that the recognition of a PAMP by a PRR induces the expression of *co-stimulatory molecules* in antigen presenting cells. This promotes an adaptive immune response against the pathogenic agent whose PAMP has been recognized. The antigenic recognition by a B-cell in the absence of this co-stimulatory signal, for example, might result in the cell death, or *anergy*. This will be discussed in detail in Section 2.10.

2.6.1. The Complement System

The *complement system* is composed of several plasma proteins that interact in a sequential and regulated way to eliminate foreign cells and microbial infections. It can promote the lesion of certain membranes and perform other biological functions such as participating in the *inflammatory responses*. An inflammatory response is characterized by the increase in the local blood flow and permeability between the blood and tissues. These changes mean that a large number of immune cells have been recruited to the site of infection.

The main functions of the complement system are:

- *Chemotaxis*: attraction of phagocytes to the sites of infection;

- *Opsonization*: the coating of an organism with proteins so as to make it palatable to phagocytes;
- *Anaphylaxis*: increase in the blood flow to the infection sites and increase of vessel permeability;
- *Lysis*: damage in the plasma membrane of the cells, some bacteria and viruses among others.

The elements that are part of the complement activation cascade (or *complement cascade*) are inactive in the blood stream and other biological fluids. In the *classical pathway of complement activation,* an antibody is bound to an antigen. This requires the interaction of the adaptive immune system, through the presence of antibodies. However, the *alternative pathway of complement activation* is due to microorganisms, *toxins* and *lipopolysaccharides* contained within a small number of bacteria. Figure 2.6 illustrates the complement cascade activated via the classical pathway of activation.

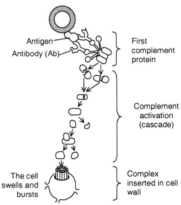

Figure 2.6. Complement activation (cascade reaction).

2.6.2. Cytokines and Natural Killer Cells

During an immune response, signals are sent among cells. Cytokine is the general term given to the molecules involved in this cell signaling process. Lymphokines or *interleukines* (IL) are cytokines secreted by lymphocytes. The primary function of the cytokines is to induce an inflammatory response. Another effect of the cytokines is to increase the body temperature; this is associated with a *fever*. It is believed that the fever, to a certain degree, is beneficial because the activity of some pathogens is reduced with the temperature increase, while the adaptive immune response increases in intensity (Hofmeyr, 2000).

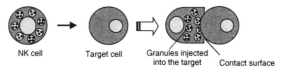

Figure 2.7. Action of a natural killer cell (NK cell).

Cytokines also reinforce the innate immune response by allowing the liver to produce substances known as *acute phase proteins* (APP). These APP bind to the bacteria, activating the macrophages or the complement system. There are four main groups of cytokines: the *interferons* (IFN), the *interleukines* (IL), the *colony stimulator factors* (CSF), and the *tumor necrosis factor* (TNF). The interferons are particularly important as they limit the expansion of viral infections. They are also used for activation of other cells, such as the *natural killer (NK) cells*.

The NK cells are a lethal type of lymphocyte and possess granules filled with chemical elements capable of damaging their target cells. They are designated as natural killer cells as they do not have to be stimulated via APC to start acting. Primarily, they attack tumor cells and help to protect against a variety of viruses. These cells also contribute to the regulation of the immune response, secreting various types of lymphokines. Figure 2.7 illustrates the action of a natural killer cell.

2.7 Adaptive Immune System

All living beings have the ability to present a resistance to pathogens. However, the nature of this resistance differs according to the type of organism. Traditionally, research in immunology has studied almost exclusively the *vertebrate* (animals containing bones) defense reactions and, in particular, the immune system of mammals, exemplified by mice and humans. Vertebrates have developed a defense system whose main characteristic is one of being preventive, i.e., the vertebrate immune system can prevent infection against many kinds of antigens that can be encountered, both natural and artificially synthesized.

Lymphocytes are the most important cells of the adaptive immune system. They are present only in vertebrates who have evolved a system to proportionate a more efficient and versatile defense mechanism against future infections. This is when compared to those mechanisms of the innate immune system. However, the cells of the innate immune system have a crucial role in the initiating and regulating of the adaptive immune response.

Each *naïve lymphocyte* (i.e., one that has not been involved in an immune response) that enters the blood stream carries antigen receptors of single specificity. The specificity of these receptors is determined by a special mechanism of gene rearrangement that acts during the lymphocyte development in the bone marrow and thymus. It can generate millions of different variants of the encoding genes. So, though an individual lymphocyte carries a single specificity receptor: the specificity of every lymphocyte is different. There are millions of lymphocytes circulating throughout our bodies and therefore they present millions of different specificities.

McFarlane Burnet formalized, in 1959, the selective theory finally accepted as the most plausible explanation for the behavior of an adaptive immune response. This explained why antibodies can be induced in response to virtually any antigen, and are produced in each individual only against those antigens to which it was exposed. The author postulated the existence of many cells that could potentially produce different antibodies. Each of these cells had the capability of synthesizing an antibody of distinct specificity and exhibits, on its surface, this antibody type that was bound to the membrane and acted as an antigen receptor. After binding with the antigen, the cell is activated to proliferate and produce a large *clone*. A clone can be understood as a cell or set of cells that are the progeny of a single parent cell; and the clone size refers to the number of offspring generated by the parent cell. These cells would now secrete antibodies of the same specificity to its cell receptor. This principle was named *clonal selection theory* (or *clonal expansion theory*) and constitutes the core of the adaptive immune response. Its implications to the immune learning and memory are significant and are therefore studied separately in Section 2.9.

Based upon this clonal selection theory, the lymphocytes can therefore be considered to undergo a process similar to *natural selection* (Darwin, 1859) within an individual organism. Only those lymphocytes that meet an antigen that can interact with its receptor are activated to proliferate and differentiate into effector cells. In Chapter 5, we will discuss the *natural selection theory* that inspired the development of *evolutionary computation*, relating the evolution of immune cells with the evolution of species. This aspect is particularly important to the characterization of some artificial immune systems.

2.8   Pattern Recognition

From the viewpoint of *pattern recognition* in the immune system, the most important characteristics of B- and T-cells is that they carry *surface receptor molecules* capable of recognizing antigens. B-cell and T-cell receptors recognize antigens with distinct characteristics. The B-cell receptor (BCR) interacts with antigenic molecules free in solution, while the T-cell receptor (TCR) recognizes antigens processed and bound to a surface molecule called *major histocompatibility complex* (MHC) (see Figure 2.3). Notice that these cells also present receptors for soluble factors, such as lymphokines and in some cases hormones, which will not be considered in this chapter (see Section 5.3, Figure 5.6, for an illustration).

The antigen B-cell receptors are bound to the cell membrane and will be secreted in the form of antibodies when the cell becomes activated. The main role of the B-cell is the production and secretion of antibodies in response to pathogenic agents. Each B-cell produces a single type of antibody, a property named *monospecificity*. These antibodies are capable of recognizing and binding to a determined protein. The secretion and binding of antibodies constitute a form of signaling other cells so that they can ingest, process, and/or remove the bound substance.

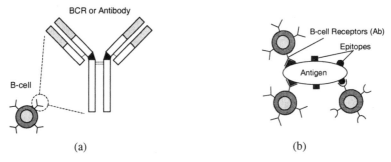

(a)   (b)

Figure 2.8. B-cell. (a) B-cell detaching the antibody molecule on its surface. (b) The portion of the antigen that is recognized by an antibody is called epitope. While antibodies are monospecific, antigens might present several different types of epitopes.

Figure 2.8(a) illustrates the B-cell detaching the antibody molecule on its surface. The immune recognition occurs at the molecular level and is based on the *complementarity* between the binding region of the receptor and a portion of the antigen called *epitope*. Whilst antibodies present a single type of receptor, antigens might present several epitopes. This means that different antibodies can recognize a single antigen, as illustrated in Figure 2.8(b).

While B-cells present antibody molecules on their surface, and maturate within the bone marrow, the maturation process of T-cells occurs in the thymus. T-cell functions include the regulation of other cells and the direct attack of the cells that cause an infection of the host organism. T-cells can be divided into two major subgroups: *helper T-cells* (T_H) and *killer* (or *cytotoxic*) *T-cells* (T_K). T-cell antigenic receptors (TCR) are structurally different when compared to B-cell receptors, as illustrated in Figure 2.9(a). The TCR recognizes antigens processed and presented in other cells by a surface molecule called major histocompatibility complex, or MHC. Figure 2.9(b) illustrates the T-cell receptor and the binding with the MHC/peptide complex.

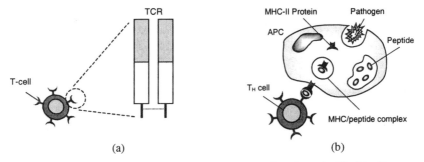

(a)   (b)

Figure 2.9. T-cell. (a) T-cell detaching the TCR on the cell surface. (b) The T-cell receptor binds with the complex formed by a self-MHC molecule and an antigenic peptide.

There are two major classes of MHC molecules (Germain, 1994, 1995), named MHC class I (MHC-I) and MHC class II (MHC-II). The class I molecules can be found in all cells, while the class II molecules are found in the antigen presenting cells (APC), which include B-cells, macrophages, and *dendritic cells* (Banchereau & Steinman, 1998). The killer T-cells recognize antigens bound to MHC-I molecules, allowing the detection of virus infected cells. The helper T-cells interact with antigens bound to MHC-II molecules. APCs capture antigenic protein from the surrounding area and process it by ingesting and digesting the antigen. This causes a fragmentation of the antigen into small particles named *peptides*. Some of these peptides bind to the MHC-II molecule and the MHC/peptide complex is transported to the cell (APC) surface, where they can interact with a T_H cell. This process is illustrated in Figure 2.9(b).

Both MHC classes bind to peptides and present them to T-cells. Class I is specialized in the presentation of proteins synthesized within the APC (intracellular pathogens), such as viral proteins produced by an infected cell. In contrast, class II is specialized in the presentation of fragments of molecules rescued from the environment. Both systems present peptides of *self-molecules* and also of foreign, *nonself* molecules. The T-cells then also play a role in the discrimination between what is *self* and what is *nonself*, a matter to be discussed in Section 2.10.

2.8.1. The B-Cell Receptor (BCR)

The antibody molecule is said to be bi-functional as it is able to bind with an antigen or to perform a biological (effector) activity. The basic make-up of an antibody, or immunoglobulin (Ig), molecule is four *polypeptide chains*: two identical light (L) and two identical heavy (H) chains (Tonegawa, 1983). This is illustrated in Figure 2.10.

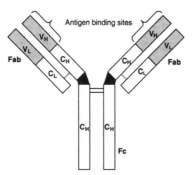

Figure 2.10.   Antibody molecule. The variable region (V-region) is responsible for the antigenic recognition and binding, and the constant region (C-region) is responsible for a variety of effector functions, such as complement fixation. The molecule is symmetric presenting two identical sites to bind with the antigen (Fab) and a site (Fc) that binds with cell receptors on effector cells, or interact with the complement proteins. Indexes H and L refer to the heavy and light chains, respectively.

Extensive analyses of the immunoglobulin polypeptide chains revealed that they are composed of an amino-terminal region that is highly variable (*variable region*) and a carboxiterminal region that can assume one of a few types (*constant region*). The variable region, or V-region, is responsible for the antigenic recognition and contains particular variable sub-regions whose composition might be a consequence of the contact with an antigen (Section 2.9). These sub-regions are usually named *complementary determining regions*. The constant region, or C-region, is responsible for a variety of effector functions, such as complement fixation and ligation to other cell receptors of the immune system.

It has been discovered that a polypeptide chain of an antibody molecule is coded in multiple gene segments scattered along a chromosome of the genome. These gene segments are brought together to form a complete molecule of an antibody, which is active in the B-cell. Additionally, somatic mutations with high rates (*somatic hypermutation*) can be introduced in a gene of the antibody molecule. The genetic recombination together with the somatic hypermutation contributes to the increase of the diversity of the genetic information coded in the genome.

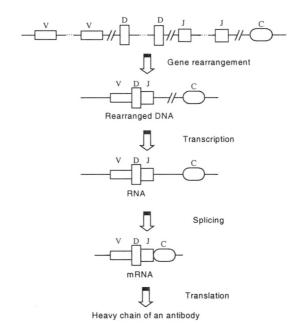

Figure 2.11.   The gene rearrangement process that results in the production of the heavy chain of an antibody molecule: the gene fragments (exactly one from each library) are concatenated in an orderly fashion. Each chain receives in its extremity a constant (C) fragment. A *transcription* process joins C to V(D)J and the RNA *splicing* brings together the joined sequences of the V-region to the sequences that code the C-region. This results in the heavy chain of an antibody molecule (reproduced with permission from [Oprea, 1999]. © *Mihaela Oprea, 1999*).

It is known that processes of DNA rearrangement combine genetic information in order to code for the antibody molecules. This means that genes contained in several gene libraries are concatenated to form the heavy and light chains of the antibody molecules. In the light chain, for example, two separate gene segments code the V-region. The first segment is named V (for variable) and the second J (for junction). The junction of a V segment with a J segment originates a continuous DNA segment that codes for the whole V-region of the light chain. In contrast, three gene segments code the V-region of the heavy chain. Beyond the V and J segments, a third segment named D (for diversity) is found between the segments V and J of the heavy chain. Figure 2.11 illustrates the synthesis process of the heavy chain of an antibody molecule.

The presence of both combinatorial recombination and somatic mutation as mechanisms for the diversification of antibody genes is intriguing (Tonegawa, 1983). The question, "why have two systems evolved to accomplish the same task?" could be asked. Both mechanisms are under strict control during the development of B-cells. The recombination of the immunoglobulin gene segments is performed first and is completed by the time the cells are first exposed to antigens. This creates a population of cells that vary widely in their specificity. The mutational mechanism is then activated during the proliferation of the selected B-cells. By altering individual nucleotide bases, the mutations followed by selection fine-tune the immune response, creating antibody molecules that better match the selective antigen. In Section 2.9, the somatic hypermutation and *receptor editing* (or V(D)J recombination) mechanisms that are responsible for altering the structure of lymphocyte receptors during an immune response will be discussed.

Therefore, it can then be concluded that in a first stage receptor diversity is due to the generation of lymphocytes through random recombination of gene fragments contained in several libraries. The B-cells rearrange the available elements in the gene libraries to produce a vast array of cells expressing distinct antigenic receptors. In a second stage, the process of somatic hypermutation is used to increase the Ag-Ab (antigen-antibody) *affinity*, thus increasing the immune diversity and capacity of response. The *affinity* can be understood as the strength of binding between two binding sites, such as a cell receptor and an epitope. The combined action of these two mechanisms of generation and diversification of antibodies makes the immune system capable of synthesizing an almost infinite number of cell receptors from a finite genome.

Humoral Immune Response

The *humoral immune response*, also known as *antibody mediated immune response*, is the response that can be transferred in cellular fluids and is characterized by the presence of soluble substances. These substances primarily take the form of antibodies produced by B-cells, which in turn lead to the destruction of the extracellular microorganisms and avoid the dissemination of the intracellular infections. The proteins of the complement system can also be considered as part of the humoral immune response.

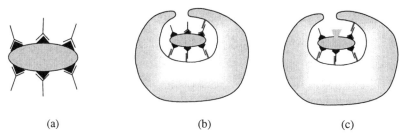

        (a)   (b)   (c)

Figure 2.12.   Antibody roles during a humoral immune response. (a) Neutralization. Antibodies attach to the pathogen inhibiting its toxic effects. (b) Opsonization. A phagocytic cell more easily recognizes a pathogen covered with antibodies. (c) Complement activation leading to the cell burst. The pathogen is recognized by the phagocyte that promotes its destruction.

There are basically three ways through which the antibodies contribute to immunity (Janeway *et al.*, 1999), as illustrated in Figure 2.12:

- *Neutralization*: the antibodies that bind to the pathogen inhibit its toxic effects, providing that this pathogenic agent binds with the specific molecules in the target cell;
- *Opsonization*: the antibodies cover the pathogens such that other accessory cells (phagocytes) recognize the Fc portions of antibody groups and ingest and digest the pathogen; and
- *Complement activation*: the antibody binding to a pathogen surface might activate the proteins of the complement system, promoting the opsonization and cleavage of some bacteria.

2.8.2. The T-Cell Receptor (TCR)

There are four polypeptide chains that can be used to form two types of TCR, each of which contains two of these four chains. Two polypeptide chains are bound one to the other through a disulfide bridge to form a TCR, in a structure similar to a Fab fragment of an antibody molecule, as illustrated in Figure 2.13. The diversity of the V-region of a TCR is generated similarly to the diversity of the antibody molecules, but with a few distinct characteristics.

The four polypeptide chains that can be used to form a TCR are coded into four distinct gene libraries (α, β, γ, and δ) that are similar to the gene segments that code for the light and heavy chains of an antibody molecule. All four libraries contain the V, J, and C gene segments, whilst libraries β and δ also contain D segments.

Another difference from the immunoglobulin gene libraries is that each gene library of a TCR presents two C-region genes. In the libraries α/δ, these two C-region genes are functionally and structurally different, such that one codes the C-region α (Cα) and the other codes the C-region δ (Cδ). All T_H and T_K cells rearrange and express α and β genes, whilst a small subpopulation uses γ and δ genes.

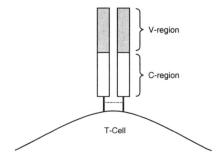

Figure 2.13.   The TCR is composed of two out of four polypeptide chains (α, β, γ, and δ), such that each chain contains a portion similar to the constant and variable domains of an antibody molecule.

As previously stated, the BCR has two identical binding sites (Figure 2.8) and the ability to be secreted. However, the TCR is different from the BCR in that the former presents a single binding site and is always a surface molecule (Figure 2.9). Like the B-cell case, the T-cell activation requires more than the binding between the TCR and the MHC/peptide complex; co-stimulatory signals are required. The co-stimulation is also important to determine if the binding is going to result in cell activation or is going to induce *tolerance* (Section 2.10).

Cellular Immune Response

The *cellular immune response*, also known as *cell mediated immune response*, describes any adaptive immune response in which specific cell types, such as T-cells and macrophages, are the most important mediators. It embodies all adaptive immune responses that cannot be transferred to a naive receptor through serum antibodies.

Through the study of the function and interrelations of T-cells, it has been possible to determine most of the mechanisms involved in the body's responses to aggressive agents, such as tumors, grafted tissues, viral infections, and hypersensitivity. A cellular immune response might be divided as follows:

- *Antigenic recognition*: occurs through the recognition of an MHC/peptide complex by a TCR;
- *Cell activation and proliferation*: the response of a T-cell to the antigenic recognition consists of a series of cellular events called T-cell activation. When stimulated, the TCR generates intracellular signals that increase transitorily the transcription of certain genes normally at rest in non-stimulated cells. As a consequence, there is an increase in the production of effector and mitotic proteins of the T-cells. The response of T-cell to the antigenic stimulus extends for short periods of time and is rapidly turned off when the antigen is eliminated; and
- *Effector phase*: the activated T-cell has the capability of secreting chemicals, or lymphokines. These stimulate the T-cell's own growth and mobilize other

immune components with the purpose of eliminating the antigen. Additionally, the T_K cell can also kill other cells on contact, as done by the NK cell.

2.9   The Clonal Selection Principle

As each lymphocyte presents a distinct receptor specificity, the number of lymphocytes that might bind to a *ligand* is restricted. In order to produce enough specific effector cells to fight against an infection, an activated lymphocyte has to first proliferate and then differentiate into these effector cells. This process, called *clonal expansion,* occurs inside the lymph nodes in a microenvironment named the *germinal center* (GC) and is characteristic in all adaptive immune responses (Weissman & Cooper, 1993; Tarlinton, 1998).

The *clonal selection principle* (or *clonal expansion principle*) is the theory used to describe the basic properties of an adaptive immune response to an antigenic stimulus. It establishes the idea that only those cells capable of recognizing an antigenic stimulus will proliferate and differentiate into effector cells, thus being selected against those that do not. Clonal selection operates on both T-cells and B-cells. The main difference between B- and T-cell clonal expansion is that B-cells suffer somatic mutation during reproduction and B-effector cells are active antibody secreting cells. In contrast, T-cells do not suffer mutation during reproduction, and T-effector cells are mainly active lymphokine secretors or T_K cells. The presence of mutational and selectional events in the B-cell clonal expansion process allow these lymphocytes to increase their repertoire diversity and also to become increasingly better in their capability of recognizing the selective antigens. Due mainly to the genetic variation, selection, and adaptation capabilities of B-cells, discussion will be focused on the clonal selection of the B-cells, whereas T-cell clonal expansion will be restricted to the discussion presented in the cellular immune response section above.

When an animal is exposed to an antigen the B-cells respond by producing antibodies. Each B-cell secretes only one kind of antibody, which is relatively specific for the antigen. Figure 2.14 presents a simplified description of the clonal selection principle. Antigenic receptors on a B-cell bind with an antigen (I) and coupled with a *second signal* (or *co-stimulatory signal*) from accessory cells, such as T_H cells, allow an antigen to stimulate a B-cell. This stimulation of the B-cell causes it to proliferate (divide) (II) and mature into terminal (non-dividing) antibody secreting cells, called *plasma cells* (III). While plasma cells are the most active antibody secretors, the rapidly dividing B-cells also secrete antibodies, albeit at a lower rate. The B-cells, in addition to proliferating and differentiating into plasma cells, can differentiate into long-lived *B-memory cells* (IV). Memory cells circulate through the blood, lymph, and tissues and probably do not manufacture antibodies. However, when exposed to a second antigenic stimulus they rapidly commence differentiating into plasma cells capable of producing high affinity antibodies. These are *pre-selected* for the specific antigen that had stimulated the *primary response*. The theory also proposes that potential self-reactive developing lymphocytes are removed from the repertoire previously to its maturation (Section 2.10).

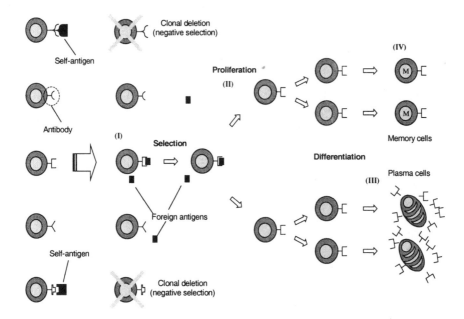

Figure 2.14.   The clonal selection principle. During the generation of the lymphocyte repertoire, some cells carry receptors that bind to self-antigens, thus being eliminated in an early phase of the development, i.e. before they are able to perform an immune response. This process leads to the self-tolerance. When the antigen interacts with the receptor in a mature lymphocyte, the cell is activated and commences proliferating. A clone will arise and differentiate into effector and memory cells.

In summary, the main properties of the clonal selection theory are:

- *Negative selection*: elimination of newly differentiated lymphocytes reactive with antigenic patterns carried by self components, named *self-antigens* (Section 2.10);
- *Clonal expansion*: proliferation and differentiation on contact of mature lymphocytes with foreign antigens in the body;
- *Monospecificity*: phenotypic restriction of one pattern to one differentiated cell and retention of that pattern by clonal descendants;
- *Somatic hypermutation*: generation of new random genetic changes, subsequently expressed as diverse antibody patterns, by a form of accelerated somatic mutation; and
- *Autoimmunity*: the concept of a *forbidden clone* resistant to early elimination by self-antigens as the basis of *autoimmune diseases*.

2.9.1. Immune Learning and Memory

In order for the immune system to be protective over periods of time, antigen recognition is not enough. The immune system must also have sufficient resources to mount an effective response against pathogens encountered at a later stage. As in typical *predator-prey* situations (Taylor, 1984), the size of the lymphocyte sub-population (clone) specific for the pathogen with relation to the size of the pathogen population is crucial to determining the outcome of infection (Section 5.6). *Learning* in the immune system involves raising the population size and the affinity of those lymphocytes that have proven themselves to be valuable during the antigen recognition phase. Thus, the immune repertoire is biased from a random base to a repertoire that more clearly reflects the actual antigenic environment.

As the total number of lymphocytes in the immune system is regulated, increases in the sizes of some clones mean that other clones may have to decrease in size. However, the total number of lymphocytes is not kept absolutely constant. If the immune system learns only by increasing the population sizes of specific lymphocytes, it must either "forget" previously learned antigens, increase in size, or constantly decrease the portion of its repertoire that is generated at random and that is responsible for responding to novel antigens (Perelson & Weisbuch, 1997).

In the normal course of the evolution of the immune system, an organism would be expected to encounter a given antigen repeatedly during its lifetime. The initial exposure to an antigen that stimulates an adaptive immune response (an *immunogen*) is handled by a small number of B-cells, each producing antibodies of different affinity. Storing some high affinity antibody producing cells from the first infection, so as to form a large initial specific B-cell sub-population (clone) for subsequent encounters, considerably enhances the effectiveness of the immune response to secondary encounters. These are referred to as *memory cells*. Rather than 'starting from scratch' every time, such a strategy ensures that both the speed and accuracy of the immune response becomes successively stronger after each infection. This scheme is intrinsic of a *reinforcement learning strategy* (Section 6.2), where the system is continuously learning from direct interaction with the environment. In the next section, mechanisms by which B-cells become increasingly more specialized in the antigenic recognition will be introduced. Meanwhile, we will continue discussing the outcomes of these mechanisms.

To illustrate an immune response (memory), consider that an antigen Ag_1 is introduced in an animal at time 0 (Figure 2.15). A few specific antibodies to Ag_1 will be available at the serum, and after a *lag* phase, the antibodies against Ag_1 will start increasing in concentration and affinity up to a certain level, and when the infection is eliminated, its concentration begins to decline. This first phase is known as the *primary response*. When another antigen Ag_2 (different from Ag_1) is introduced, the same pattern of response is presented, but for a kind of antibody with different specificity from the one who recognized Ag_1. This demonstrates the specificity of the adaptive immune response. On the other hand, one important characteristic of the immune memory is that it is associative. B-cells adapted to a certain type of antigen Ag_1 can present a faster and more efficient *secondary response* not only to Ag_1, but also to any structurally related antigen, e.g., Ag_1'.

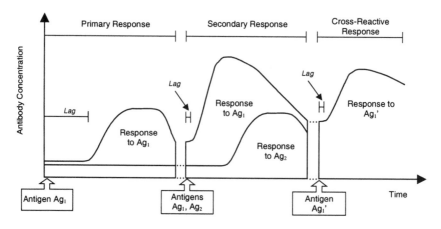

Figure 2.15. Primary, secondary and cross-reactive immune responses. After an antigen Ag_1 is seen once (primary response), subsequent encounters with the same antigen (secondary response), or a similar one Ag_1' (cross-reaction), will promote a faster and more effective response not only to Ag_1, but also to Ag_1'. Primary responses to antigens Ag_1 and Ag_2 are qualitatively equivalent.

The phenomenon of presenting a more efficient secondary response to an antigen structurally related to a previously seen antigen is called *immunological cross-reaction*, or *cross-reactive response*. This is also a sort of *associative memory*, such as the one contained in the processes of vaccination. The immunological cross-reaction is equivalent to the *generalization capability*, or simply *generalization*, discussed in other computational intelligence fields, like *neural networks* (Section 6.2). Figure 2.15 illustrates the primary, secondary, and cross-reactive immune responses.

By comparison with the primary response, the secondary response is characterized by a shorter lag phase, a higher rate of antibody production, and longer persistence of antibody synthesis. Moreover, a dose of antigen substantially lower than that required to initiate a primary response can cause a secondary response.

As a summary, immune learning and memory are acquired through:

Learning:
- Repeated exposure to an antigenic stimulus;
- Increase in size of specific B-cell sub-populations (clones); and
- Affinity maturation of the antigenic receptor (antibody).

Memory:
- Presence of long living lymphocytes that persist in a resting state until a second encounter with the antigen;
- Repeated exposure to an antigen even in the absence of infection, or low-grade chronic infection; and
- Cross-reactivity.

Like the clonal selection principle, the *immune network theory* (or *idiotypic network theory*), to be discussed in Section 2.11, presents a conceptually different approach to explain phenomena such as immune learning and memory.

2.9.2. Affinity Maturation

In a T-cell dependent immune response, the repertoire of antigen-activated B-cells is diversified basically by two mechanisms: *hypermutation* and *receptor editing*. Only high-affinity variants are selected into the pool of memory cells. This maturation process together with the clonal expansion takes place in the germinal centers (Tarlinton, 1998).

Antibodies present in a secondary response have, on average, a higher affinity than those of the early primary response. This phenomenon, which is restricted to T-cell dependent responses, is referred to as the *maturation of the immune response*. This maturation requires that the antigen-binding sites of the antibody molecules in the matured response be structurally different from those present in the primary response. Three different kinds of mutational events have been observed in the antibody V-region (Allen *et al.*, 1987):

- Point mutations;
- Short deletions; and
- Non-reciprocal exchange of sequence following gene conversion (repertoire shift).

During the clonal expansion, random changes are introduced into the variable region (V-region) genes, and occasionally one such change will lead to an increase in the affinity of the antibody. These higher-affinity variants are then selected to enter the pool of memory cells. The repertoire is not only diversified through a hypermutation process but mechanisms exist such that rare B-cells with high affinity mutant receptors can be selected to dominate the response. Due to the random nature of the somatic mutation process, a large proportion of mutating genes become non-functional or possibly develop harmful anti-self specificities. Those cells with low affinity receptors, or the self-reactive cells, must be efficiently eliminated (or become anergic). This is necessary so that they do not significantly contribute to the pool of memory cells.

Some B-cells can contain damaged and, therefore, disabled antigen-binding sites. The way in which these B-cells are eliminated is not fully understood. *Apoptosis* in the germinal centers is likely. Apoptosis is a process of programmed cell death, which is encoded in every cell where a cascade of intracellular events results in the DNA condensation, fragmentation, death and phagocytosis of the cell residuals (McConkey *et al.*, 1990; Cohen, 1993).

Through the study of the development of antibody repertoire expressed on B-cells in the germinal center, it has been clearly demonstrated that somatic mutation followed by selection plays a key role in the maturation of the immune response. Two processes are of vital importance for the maturation – hypermutation of the variable region and selection of higher-affinity variants.

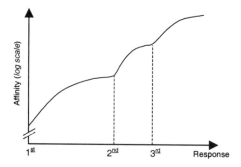

Figure 2.16.   Qualitative illustration of the affinity maturation process during successive adaptive immune responses.

The increase in antibody affinity from the primary to the secondary response, shows that maturation of the immune response is a continuous process, as illustrated in Figure 2.16. Therefore, there are four essential features of the adaptive immune responses:

- *Sufficient diversity* to deal with a universe of antigens;
- *Discrimination of self from nonself*;
- *Adaptability* of the antibodies to the selective antigens; and
- Long lasting *immunological memory*.

In the original clonal selection theory, formalized by Burnet (1959), it was suggested that memory would be provided by expanding the size of an antigen-specific clone, with random mutation being allowed to enhance affinity. Furthermore, self-reactive cells would be clonally deleted during development. Recent results suggest that the immune system practices molecular selection of receptors in addition to clonal selection of lymphocytes (Nussenzweig, 1998). Instead of the expected clonal deletion of all self-reactive cells, occasionally B lymphocytes were found that had undergone *receptor editing*: these B-cells had deleted their self-reactive receptors and developed entirely new receptors by V(D)J recombination.

Although editing and receptor selection were not part of Burnet's model, the clonal selection theory could certainly accommodate receptor editing if receptor selection occurred before cellular selection. Any high affinity clone developed by somatic hypermutation or editing would be expected to be preferentially expanded, but a few low affinity cells are also allowed to enter the repertoire, thus maintaining the population diversity.

George and Gray (1999) argued that there should be an additional diversity-introducing mechanism during the process of affinity maturation. They suggested that receptor editing offers the ability to escape from *local optima* on an *affinity landscape* (Section 3.6). Figure 2.17 illustrates this idea by considering all possible antigen-binding sites depicted in the *x*-axis, with the most similar ones adjacent to each other. The Ag-Ab affinity is shown on the *y*-axis.

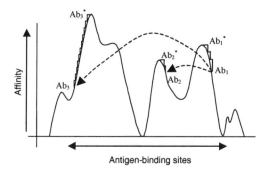

Figure 2.17.   Schematic representation of the shape-space for an affinity landscape. Somatic mutations followed by selection allow the finding of local optima,
while receptor editing introduces diversity, leading to possible new candidate
receptors located in regions of the shape-space that can lead to the determination of the global optimum.

In Figure 2.17, assume that a particular antibody (Ab_1) is selected during a
primary response, then point mutations followed by selection allow the immune
system to explore local areas around Ab_1 by making small steps towards an antibody with higher affinity, leading to a local optimum (Ab_1^*). As mutations with
lower affinity are lost, the antibodies cannot go down the hill. Receptor editing allows an antibody to take large steps through the landscape, landing in a locale
where the affinity might be lower (Ab_2). However, occasionally the leap will lead to
an antibody on the side of a hill where the climbing region is more promising (Ab_3),
reaching the global optimum. From this locale, point mutations followed by selection can drive the antibody to the top of the hill (Ab_3^*).

In conclusion, point mutations are good for exploring local regions, while editing may rescue immune responses stuck on unsatisfactory local optima. Thus, receptor editing and point mutations play complementary roles in the affinity maturation process. In addition to somatic hypermutation and receptor editing, a fraction of
newcomer cells from the bone marrow is added to the lymphocyte pool in order to
maintain the diversity of the population.

Regulation of the Hypermutation Mechanism

During the cell differentiation process, a hypermutation mechanism operates with a
rate close to 1×10^{-3} per base pair (bp) of the variable regions, per generation. Since
the combined length of these variable regions is around 700bp, on average one mutation per cell division will be introduced (Allen *et al.*, 1987; Berek & Ziegner,
1993). This average mutation per cell division has the outcome that all clones of a
single cell might be similar but never identical to their parent cell. This way, diversity is maintained in the immune repertoire.

A rapid accumulation of mutations is necessary for a fast maturation of the
immune response. However, the majority of the changes will lead to a collection of

poorer or non-functional antibodies. If a cell that has just picked up a useful mutation continues to be mutated at the same rate during the next immune response, then the accumulation of deleterious changes may cause the loss of the advantageous mutation. Thus, a short burst of somatic hypermutation, followed by a pause to allow for selection and clonal expansion, may form the basis of the maturation process. The selection mechanism may provide a means by which the regulation of the hypermutation process is made dependent upon receptor affinity. Cells with low affinity receptors may be further mutated and, if they do not improve their affinities, die through apoptosis. However, in cells that contain high-affinity antibody receptors, hypermutation may be inactivated (Kepler & Perelson, 1993a,b).

2.10 Self/Nonself Discrimination

For each of the two main types of cellular components in the lymphoid system (B- and T-cells) we can consider three classes of repertoires:

- *Potential repertoire*: determined by the number, structure, and mechanisms of expression of germ-line collections of genes encoding antibodies or T-cell receptors, plus the possible somatic variants derived from these (i.e., errors introduced during gene segment joining). It corresponds to the total repertoire that can be generated;
- *Available* (or *expressed*) *repertoire*: defined as the set of diverse molecules that are used as lymphocyte receptors, that is, what can be (but is not at present being) used;
- *Actual repertoire*: that set of antibodies and receptors produced by effector lymphocytes activated in the internal environment which actually participate in the interactions defining the autonomous activity in any given state.

The immune system in its ability to recognize antigens is *complete*. The antibody molecules and T-cell receptors produced by the lymphocytes of an animal can recognize any molecule, either self or nonself, even those artificially synthesized. Antibody molecules have immunogenic *idiotopes*, i.e., they present epitopes that can be recognized by the antigen binding sites on other antibodies. It follows from the completeness axiom that all idiotopes will be recognized by at least one antibody molecule. This argument leads to the concept of *idiotypic networks*, which will be discussed later. The main factors that result in the repertoire completeness are its *diversity* (obtained by mutation, editing, and gene rearrangement) its *cross-reactivity* and its *multispecificity* (Inman, 1978). Cross-reactivity and multispecificity are considered the main reasons why a lymphocyte repertoire smaller than the possible antigen set to be recognized can succeed in its task of recognizing and binding to every antigen. The difference between cross-reactivity and multispecificity is that the former indicates the recognition of related antigenic patterns (*epitopes*) while the latter refers to the recognition of very different chemical structures, providing a minimal amount of complementary interactions occur.

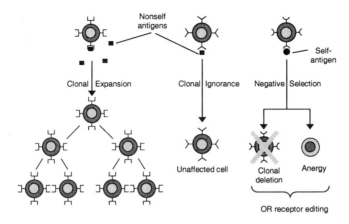

Figure 2.18. Main types of interaction between a lymphocyte and an antigen.

The completeness axiom represents a fundamental paradox, because it states that all molecular shapes can be recognized including our own, which are also seen as antigens, or *self-antigens*. For the immune system to function properly, it needs to be able to distinguish between the molecules of our own cells (self) and foreign molecules (nonself), which are a priori indistinguishable. If the immune system is not capable of performing this distinction, then an immune response will be triggered against the self-antigens, causing autoimmune diseases. Not responding against a self-antigen is a phenomenon called *self-tolerance*, or simply *tolerance* (Kruisbeek, 1995; Schwartz & Banchereau, 1996). Understanding how this is accomplished by the immune system is called the *self/nonself discrimination problem*.

Beyond the large stochastic element in the construction of lymphocyte receptors, an encounter between a lymphocyte receptor and an antigen does not inevitably result in activation of the lymphocyte. Such an encounter may actually causes its death or inactivation (*anergy*). Therefore, there is a form of *negative selection* that prevents self-specific lymphocytes from becoming auto-aggressive. In contrast, a smaller percentage of cells undergo *positive selection* and mature into *immunocompetent* cells to constitute the individuals' available repertoire.

Some of the main results of the encounter between a lymphocyte receptor and an antigen are illustrated in Figure 2.18, and can be listed together with their principal causes:

- *Clonal Expansion* (Section 2.9): recognition of nonself antigens in the presence of co-stimulatory signals;
- *Positive Selection*: recognition of a self-MHC by an immature T-cell, or recognition of a nonself antigen by a mature B-cell;
- *Negative Selection*: recognition of self-antigens in the central lymphoid organs, or peripheral recognition of self-antigens in the absence of co-stimulatory signals; and

- *Clonal Ignorance*: all circumstances in which a cell with potential antigen re-activity fails to react to the antigen, e.g., if the antigen concentration is very low or if the affinity of the receptor for the antigen in question is low.

2.10.1. Positive Selection

The *positive selection* of lymphocytes (T- and B-cells) serves the purpose of avoiding the accumulation of useless lymphocytes with either no receptor at all or with receptors that are unproductive for the organism. As an outcome, the cells that survive positive selection are rescued from cell death and become more efficient in the antigenic recognition process.

Positive Selection of T-cells

All T-cells must recognize antigens associated with self-MHC molecules named self-MHC/peptide complexes, or simply MHC/peptide complexes. Thus, it is primarily necessary to select those immature T-cells, named *thymocytes*, whose receptors are capable of recognizing and binding with self-MHC molecules. One can say that positive T-cell selection allows the immune system to recognize the self.

The process of positive selection assures that the mature T-cells that leave the thymus circulate throughout the body are as a rule only activated by foreign antigens presented by self-MHC molecules. Thus, mature T-cells act in a self-MHC restricted adaptive immune response. This process occurs in the thymus (thus it is called central positive selection, or thymic positive selection) and involves recognition events that lack affinity, avidity, or efficacy needed to cause a clonal expansion.

Among the main consequences of the central T-cell positive selection, one can stress:

- T-cells are selected to develop into functionally mature (immunocompetent) cells;
- Termination of the TCR gene rearrangement process; and
- Increase in the cell life span.

Positive Selection of B-Cells

Rescue of immature T- and B-cells appears similar in that, in each case, the receptor consists of the initially produced chain of the antigen receptor; this is expressed by mature cells plus other developmentally regulated proteins. These receptors are coupled to signal-transducing molecules and possibly exert their function by binding to ligands. The generated signals result in rescue from cell death and maturation that are associated with suppression of rearrangement of immunoglobulin light chain.

Positive selection of mature B-cells also involves the rescue from cell death. As a result of antigen binding and T-cell help (co-stimulation), proliferating B-cells undergo extensive somatic hypermutations of their antibody V-regions. Many mutants are generated that no longer bind the antigen and die through apoptosis. Those few cells with mutated antibodies that bind most efficiently to antigen are rescued from cell death. As a result, some of the rescued cells become long-living memory B-cells.

When compared with the T-cells, positive selection of mature B-cells looks very much like positive thymic selection of immature T-cells. In the T-cell case, thymocytes are rescued from cell death due to recognition of a self-MHC molecule, whilst in the B-cell case, mature B-cells are rescued from cell death due to recognition of a nonself molecule in the presence of co-stimulatory signals.

2.10.2.   Negative Selection

The concept of a *negative* or *down-regulatory signal* following certain lymphocyte-antigen interactions, permits the control of those lymphocytes bearing anti-self receptors. Negative selection of a lymphocyte describes the process whereby a lymphocyte-antigen interaction results in the death (or anergy) of that lymphocyte. The T- or B-cell is simply purged from the repertoire. Geography plays a role in negative selection: the primary lymphoid organs are designed to largely exclude foreign antigens and to preserve the self-antigens, whereas the secondary lymphoid organs are designed to filter out and concentrate foreign material and to promote co-stimulatory intercellular immune reactions.

Negative Selection of T-Cells

The negative selection of T-cells can occur within the thymus or on the periphery. Negative thymic selection is based on the following considerations. The thymus is comprised of a myriad of class I and class II MHC-bearing APCs, including macrophages, dendritic cells, and specialized epithelial cells. As the thymus is protected by a blood-thymic barrier, these APCs primarily present self-peptide/MHC complexes to the emerging T-cell repertoire. Negative thymic selection stems from interactions of immature T-cells with the self-peptides presented by the self-MHC molecules on thymic APC. This results in an activation dependent cell's death to purge potentially auto reactive T-cells from the repertoire. T-cells bearing "useless" TCRs that do not exhibit significant interactions with any self-MHC ligands are lost from the repertoire through positive selection, as discussed previously. The time and extension of this process of deletion depends upon the affinity of the binding between the TCR and the self-antigen. T-cells that bind with higher affinities to self-antigens are more effectively purged from the repertoire than those that bind with lower affinities.

Negative thymic selection however, is not perfect, and some self-reactive T-cells escape into the periphery as fully immunocompetent cells. These can pose the threat of an autoimmune disease taking hold of the host. The inductive signal for T-cell activation requires more than the binding of a TCR with an MHC/peptide complex. For the T-cells on the periphery, several adjunct processes such as the binding of a variety of cell adhesion molecules are necessary for T-cell activation. In the absence of co-stimulatory activity, the union of TCR and an MHC/peptide complex may deliver a down-regulatory signal to the T-cell. The innate immunity is responsible for delivering a great amount of co-stimulatory signals for the adaptive immunity, as briefly discussed in Section 2.6.

Negative Selection of B-Cells

T-cell tolerance alone would be insufficient protection against autoimmunity. Immature B-cells within the bone marrow are especially sensitive to tolerance induction.

Mature B-cells can also be rendered tolerant if they encounter antigen in the absence of both T-cell help and co-stimulatory influences. As with the T-cells, self-reactive B-cells can also escape the central B-cell negative selection. In this case, B-cell activation or tolerance will be the result of the number, strength, and time at which the co-stimulatory signals will arise. A fast and sudden ligation (characteristic of foreign antigens) of the receptor with the antigen will generally induce a clonal response. At the same time, a constant and relatively weak stimulation (typical of self-antigens) leads to tolerance, characterized by the inhibition of the clonal response and further cellular apoptosis. Cases where the antigenic doses are very high might also induce tolerance (Tizard, 1995), as illustrated in Figure 2.19. These peripheral tolerance mechanisms operate on both B- and T-cells.

Table 2.2 summarizes the processes of positive and negative selection, stressing the main variables and mechanisms involved, together with their outcomes.

Table 2.2.   Main variables and mechanisms involved in the negative and positive selection processes, together with their outcomes.

		Positive Selection	**Negative Selection**
Variables	**T-cell**	Level of antigen expression; degree of antigenic affinity	Site and level of antigen expression and affinity; co-stimulation
	B-cell	Level of antigenic affinity; co-stimulation	Site, nature, and level of antigen expression and affinity; co-stimulation
Mechanisms	**T-cell**	Rescue from cell death	Thymic and peripheral clonal deletion; peripheral anergy; clonal ignorance
	B-cell	Rescue from cell death	Bone marrow and peripheral clonal deletion; peripheral anergy; receptor editing
Outcomes	**T-cell**	Become mature, immunocompetent cells; increase in cell life span; termination of TCR gene rearrangement	Cell deletion (apoptosis) or inactivation
	B-cell	Clonal expansion; increase in cell life span; termination of Ig gene rearrangement	Cell deletion (apoptosis) or inactivation; V(D)J recombination

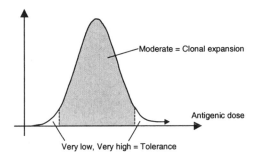

Figure 2.19. High and low zone antigenic doses induce tolerance, whilst moderate doses result in an immune response.

2.11 Immune Network Theory

The clonal selection theory, discussed in Section 2.9, regards the immune system as a set of discrete cells and molecules originally at rest and triggered only by a foreign antigenic stimulation. This section will introduce a conceptually different theory of how the components of the immune systems interact with each other and with the environment (antigens). This theory, named the *immune network theory* (or *idiotypic network theory*), was formally proposed by N. K. Jerne in 1974 (Jerne, 1974) and presents a novel perspective to approach important emergent properties such as learning and memory, self-tolerance, and size and diversity of immune repertoires. An abundance of literature is available on topics such as:

- The biological and experimental reasons supporting this perspective of the immune system structured as a network of interacting elements; and
- The theoretical justification of mathematical models and their respective results.

Some of these mathematical models of the immune network will be studied in Section 3.6. The discussion here will focus on the high-level philosophical behavior of immune networks, as formally introduced by Jerne. This theory is rooted in the demonstration that animals can be stimulated to make antibodies capable of recognizing parts of antibody molecules produced by other animals of the same species or strain. According to Jerne (1974), this made reasonable the assumption that, within the immune system of one given individual, any antibody molecule could be recognized by a set of other antibody molecules.

By the time the network hypothesis was proposed, most immunologists were concerned with the study of the signaling responsible to initiate and interrupt immune responses, the effector mechanisms that may become operative as a result of this interaction, and how antibodies are synthesized (Section 2.2). Keeping in mind the importance of determining and understanding these mechanisms, Jerne introduced the immune network as a novel and fundamental idea to explain phenomena like repertoire selection, tolerance, self/nonself discrimination, and memory (Varela

& Coutinho, 1991). It was suggested that the immune system is composed of a regulated network of molecules and cells that recognize one another even in the absence of antigens. By assuming this pattern of interactions among the components of the immune system, the network hypothesis was in conflict with the recently established clonal selection pattern of immune responses. In fact, several authors assume the immune network paradigm to be absurd (e.g., Langman & Cohn, 1986). However, it is not the concern here to discuss the validity of the immune network theory. Instead, it is the intent to present its general ideas that have been very useful in the development of novel computational tools for the solution of problems in different domains.

To describe the immune network, Jerne suggested the following notation. The portion of an antibody molecule responsible for recognizing (complementarily) an epitope was named *paratope*. An *idiotype* was defined as the set of epitopes displayed by the variable regions of a set of antibody molecules, and an *idiotope* was each single idiotypic epitope. The patterns of idiotopes are determined by the same variable regions of antibody polypeptide chains that also determine the paratopes. Thus, the idiotopes are located in and around the antigen binding site (Hood *et al.*, 1984), and each Fab arm of an antibody molecule displays one paratope and a small set of idiotopes (Jerne, 1974).

The *immune system* was formally defined as an enormous and complex network of paratopes that recognize sets of idiotopes and of idiotopes that are recognized by sets of paratopes. Thus, each element could recognize as well as be recognized. This property lead to the establishment of a network, and as antibody molecules occur both free and as receptor molecules on B-cells, this network intertwines cells and molecules. After a given antibody recognizes an epitope or an idiotope, it can respond either positively or negatively to this recognition signal. A positive response would result into cell activation, cell proliferation, and antibody secretion, while a negative response would lead to tolerance and suppression. Figure 2.20(a) illustrates the paratope and idiotope of an antibody molecule, and Figure 2.20(b) depicts the negative and positive responses of the network theory.

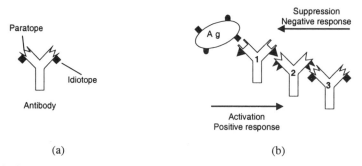

(a)   (b)

Figure 2.20.   Basic concepts of the immune network theory. (a) Antibody molecule illustrating its paratope and idiotope. In reality, the idiotopes might be located in or around the paratopes. (b) Positive and negative responses as results of the interaction between a paratope and an idiotope or an epitope.

From a functional point of view, if a paratope interacts with an idiotope, even in the absence of antigens, then the immune system must display a sort of eigen-behavior resulting from this interaction. This eigen-behavior makes the immune system achieve a dynamic steady state as its elements interact among themselves, and some elements decay in concentration while others emerge. As Jerne argued, a complete network theory of the immune system would require greater precision in stating the expected results of the various interactions within the network, but this was not accounted for at that moment.

The behavior of the immune network theory can be interpreted as illustrated in Figure 2.21. When the immune system is primed with an antigen, its epitope is recognized (with various degrees of specificity) by a set of different paratopes, called p_1. These paratopes occur on antibodies and receptor molecules together with certain idiotopes, so that the set p_1 of paratopes is associated with a set i_1 of idiotopes. The symbol p_1i_1 denotes the total set of recognizing antibody molecules and potentially responding lymphocytes with respect to the antigen (Ag). Within the immune network, each paratope of the set p_1 recognizes a set of idiotopes, and the entire set p_1 recognizes an even larger set of idiotopes. The set i_2 of idiotopes is called the *internal image* of the epitope (or antigen) because it is recognized by the same set p_1 that recognized the antigen. The set i_2 is associated with a set p_2 of paratopes occurring on the molecules and cell receptors of the set p_2i_2. Furthermore, each idiotope of the set p_1i_1 is recognized by a set of paratopes, so that the entire set i_1 is recognized by an even larger set p_3 of paratopes that occur together with a set i_3 of idiotopes on antibodies and lymphocytes of the anti-idiotypic set p_3i_3. Following this scheme, we come to ever-larger sets that recognize or are recognized by previously defined sets within the network. Besides the recognizing set p_1i_1 there is a parallel set p_xi_1 of antibodies that display idiotopes of the set i_1 in molecular association with combining sites that do not fit the foreign epitope. The arrows indicate a stimulatory effect when idiotopes are recognized by paratopes on cell receptors and a suppressive effect when paratopes recognize idiotopes on cell receptors (Jerne, 1974).

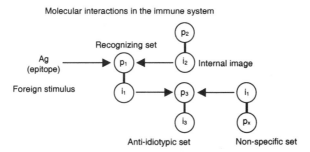

Figure 2.21.   Molecular interactions in the immune system according to the idiotypic network theory. The internal image has a stimulatory effect towards the recognizing set, while the anti-idiotypic set has an inhibitory effect (reproduced with permission from [Jerne, 1974]. © *Institut Pasteur, 1974*).

2.11.1.   Immune Learning and Memory

According to the clonal selection theory, learning in the immune system involves increasing the size and antigenic affinity of specific antibody sub-populations responsible for recognizing invading antigens. These larger antibody sub-populations with high antigenic affinities are then kept in a sort of resting state and act more efficiently in subsequent attacks by the same or slightly different antigens. This constitutes the basis of the immune learning and memory mechanisms as proposed by clonal selection.

In the immune network paradigm, different strategies are suggested to be responsible for the learning and memory of the immune system. In this case, the network acts as an autonomous system whose behavior is a consequence of regulatory mechanisms aimed at maintaining the network within a specific range of activity. This is achieved by modifying the current population of cells and molecules (antibodies) and their antigenic affinities in an continuous manner. A continuous production of novel elements might be necessary to discover and to reinforce the beneficial ones which are able to bind with the unpredictable invaders. The idea of a self-regulated system suggests that the immune memory may be more firmly deposited in a persistent network modulation; a pattern of behavior inherent to homeostatic systems (Chapter 5), i.e., a system capable of maintaining its own internal steady state. Note that such a network is continuously adapting itself to the presence of foreign substances as well as novel elements that appear and might be incorporated in the existing network.

To formally describe the network activity, F. Varela and collaborators (Varela *et al.*, 1988) introduced three important concepts: *structure*, *dynamics*. and *metadynamics*:

- *Structure*: the network structure describes the types of interaction among its molecular and cellular components without reference to the functional consequences that they might have. It corresponds to how the elements of the immune systems are structured around the idiotypic network of interactions, i.e., their patterns of connectivity. This might be represented under the form of a matrix of connectivity, for example. The network structure is strongly related to the immune memory, for it reflects the results of the interactions of the active elements of the immune system among themselves and also with the environment in which they are inserted.
- *Dynamics*: the immune network dynamics accounts for the variations with time in concentration and affinities of the cells and molecules composing the immune system. Most early network models accounted only for the variations in concentration of antibodies. Nevertheless, more recent (and biologically appealing) models are taking into account the variation in affinity of antibody molecules due, mainly, to the affinity maturation of immune responses. Thus, the immune network dynamics describes how the network *adapts* to itself and to the environment, which takes into consideration the interactions with other immune cells and molecules and with foreign antigens. It composes one of the elements responsible for the learning and maintenance of the network memory.

- *Metadynamics*: a unique property of the immune system that goes beyond the network dynamics is the continuous production and recruitment of novel cells and molecules. Any possible new element, even if newly synthesized, can interact with the working immune system; it is said to be complete. As these new elements are potentially capable of interacting with the working immune system, this might cause a constant renewal of the network structure via recruitment into activity of these newly formed elements and the death of non-stimulated or self-reactive elements. The immune network metadynamics, also named the *immune recruitment mechanism*, allows for the selection of new elements into the network according to the global state of the system, that is, according to the network sensitivity for this new element. This sensitivity is usually measured by the affinity this element has with the actual elements already present in the immune network. Metadynamics is also important for the network to cover new portions of the space of antigens and, thus, to be able to adapt itself to a wide range of unknown invaders.

As a summary, the central characteristic of the immune network theory is the definition of the molecular identity of the individual because natural tolerance, learning, and memory are global properties that cannot be reduced to the existence or activity of single clones, as proposed by clonal selection. They emerge from a germ-line encoded network organization expressed early in the development, followed by the ontogenic learning of the molecular composition of the environment where the system develops by dynamic and metadynamic recruitment of the useful cells and molecules. The network organization imposes an autonomous dynamic pattern for the behavior of the immune system that is distinct from the immune responses to external antigens but that is also influenced by their recognition. Actually, such dynamic patterns are perfectly compatible with the maintenance of memory that is not localized in memory cells, but distributed as a pattern in a sort of population-based memory.

2.12 Chapter Summary

The immune system is a remarkable natural defense mechanism. It exhibits capabilities such as learning, memory, and adaptation. For these reasons, and many others, the immune system can be viewed as a mechanism of vast potential for inspiration in a variety of domains.

This chapter examined a number of fundamental characteristics and principles of the immune system. Its anatomy and architecture were first discussed, giving an overview of the location of its primary components coupled with the various layers of protection offered. The immune system can be thought of as acting based upon two distinct but interacting mechanisms: the innate immune response and the adaptive immune response. The innate immune system was described, focusing on the ability of the immune system to extract molecular information via MHC molecules to be presented to T-cells. The adaptive immune system was then examined, primarily focusing on the creation of antibodies to fight the infection. Within the adaptive immune response, it can be clearly seen that there are many interesting natural processes occurring. A number of theories on how the immune system *learns* and maintains *memory* were examined, in particular the clonal selection principle and the more controversial immune network theory.

It is hoped that this chapter has served to convince the reader that the immune system is worthy of study from a computational point of view. The incredible ability of the vertebrate immune systems to protect our bodies from infection makes it an exciting and rich source of inspiration for computer scientists and the like. The goal of AIS is to extract what can be considered to be inspiration from the components and processes from the immune system to create effective and powerful computational systems. The following chapter will explore how it is possible to extract such *metaphors* and propose a whole framework for the construction of artificial immune systems.

2.12.1. Important Concepts

A great number of concepts studied in this chapter are currently being used in the development of artificial immune systems. These concepts are listed below, and if you are not sure about the terminology below, please refer to Appendix I or review the corresponding sections of this chapter:

- Bone marrow and Thymus;
- B-cell and BCR or antibody;
- T-cell and TCR;
- Antigen;
- Epitope, Idiotope, and Paratope;
- Self and Nonself antigen;
- Affinity;
- Positive and Negative selection;
- Clonal selection: theory used to explain how the immune system copes with a nonself antigen;
- Clonal expansion and Affinity maturation;
- Cross-reactivity;
- Potential, Available, and Actual repertoire;
- Network Structure, Dynamics, and Metadynamics.

References

Abbas, A. K. & Janeway, C. A. (2000), "Immunology: Improving on Nature in the Twenty-First Century", *Cell*, **100**, pp. 129-138.

Allen, D. et al. (1987), "Timing, Genetic Requirements and Functional Consequences of Somatic Hypermutation During B-cell Development", *Imm. Rev.*, **96**, pp. 5-22.

Banchereau, J. & Steinman, R. M. (1998), "Dendritic Cells and the Control of Immunity", *Nature*, **392**, pp. 245-252.

Berek, C. & Ziegner, M. (1993), "The Maturation of the Immune Response", *Imm. Today*, **14**(8), pp. 400-402.

Burnet, F. M. (1959), *The Clonal Selection Theory of Acquired Immunity*, Cambridge University Press.

Cohen, J. J. (1993), "Apoptosis", *Imm. Today*, **14**(3), pp. 126-130.

Darwin, C. (1859), *On the Origin of Species By Means of Natural Selection*, 6th Edition, [Online Book] www.literature.org/authors/darwin.

George, A. J. T. & Gray, D. (1999), "Receptor Editing During Affinity Maturation", *Imm. Today*, **20**(4), pp. 196.

Germain, R. N. (1995), "MHC-Associated Antigen Processing, Presentation, and Recognition Adolescence, Maturity and Beyond", *The Immunologist*, **3/5-6**, pp. 185-190.

Germain, R. N. (1994), "MHC-Dependent Antigen Processing and Peptide Presentation: Providing Ligands for T Lymphocyte Activation", *Cell*, **76**, pp. 287-299.

Hofmeyr S. A. & Forrest, S. (2000), "Architecture for an Artificial Immune System", *Evolutionary Computation*, **7**(1), pp. 45-68.

Hood, L. E., Weissman, I. L., Wood, W. B. & Wilson, J. H. (1984), *Immunology*, 2nd Ed., The Benjamin/Cummings Publishing Company, Inc.

Inman, J. K. (1978), "The Antibody Combining Region: Speculations on the Hypothesis of General Multispecificity", *Theoretical Immunology*, (eds.) G. I. Bell, A. S. Perelson & G. H. Pimbley Jr., Marcel Dekker Inc., pp. 243-278.

Janeway, C. A., P. Travers, Walport, M. & Capra, J. D. (1999), "Immunobiology: The Immune System in Health and Disease", 4th Ed., Garland Publishing.

Jerne, N. K. (1974), "Towards a Network Theory of the Immune System", *Ann. Immunol.* (Inst. Pasteur) **125C**, pp. 373-389.

Kepler, T. B. & Perelson, A. S. (1993a), "Somatic Hypermutation in B Cells: An Optimal Control Treatment", *J. theor. Biol.*, **164**, pp. 37-64.

Kepler, T. B. & Perelson, A. S. (1993b), "Cyclic Re-enter of Germinal Center B Cells and the Efficiency of Affinity Maturation", *Imm. Today*, **14**(8), pp. 412-415.

Kruisbeek, A. M. (1995), "Tolerance", *The Immunologist*, **3/5-6**, pp. 176-178.

Langman, R. E. & Cohn, M. (1986), "The 'Complete' Idiotype Network is an Absurd Immune System", *Imm. Today*, **7**(4), pp. 100-101.

McConkey, D. J., Orrenius, S. & Jondal, M. (1990), "Cellular Signalling in Programmed Cell Death (Apoptosis)", *Imm. Today*, **11**(4), pp. 120-121.

Nossal, G. J. V. (1993), "Life, Death and the Immune System", *Scientific American*, **269**(3), pp. 21-30.

Nussenzweig, M. C. (1998), "Immune Receptor Editing; Revise and Select", *Cell*, **95**, pp. 875-878.

Oprea, M. (1999), *Antibody Repertoires and Pathogen Recognition: The Role of Germline Diversity and Somatic Hypermutation*, Ph.D. Dissertation, University of New Mexico, Albuquerque, New Mexico, EUA.

Perelson, A. S. & Weisbuch, G. (1997), "Immunology for Physicists", *Rev. of Modern Physics*, **69**(4), pp. 1219-1267.

Rensberger, B. (1996), "In Self-Defense", In *Life Itself*, B. Resenberger, Oxford University Press, pp. 212-228.

Schwartz, R. S. & Banchereau, J. (1996), "Immune Tolerance", *The Immunologist*, 4/6, pp. 211-218.

Scroferneker, M. L. & Pohlmann, P. R. (1998), *Basic and Applied Immunology*, (in Portuguese) Sagra Luzzatto.

Tarlinton, D. (1998), "Germinal Centers: Form and Function", *Current Opinion in Imm.*, 10, pp. 245-251.

Taylor, R. J. (1984), *Predation*, Chapman and Hall, New York.

Tizard, I. R. (1995), *Immunology An Introduction*, 4th Ed, Saunders College Publishing.

Tonegawa, S. (1983), "Somatic Generation of Antibody Diversity", *Nature*, 302, pp. 575-581.

Varela, F. J. & Coutinho, A. (1991), "Second Generation Immune Networks", *Imm. Today*, 12(5), pp. 159-166.

Varela, F. J., Coutinho, A. Dupire, E. & Vaz, N. N. (1988), "Cognitive Networks: Immune, Neural and Otherwise", *Theoretical Immunology*, Part II, A. S. Perelson (ed.), pp. 359-375.

Weissman, I. L. & Cooper, M. D. (1993) "How the Immune System Develops", *Scientific American*, 269(3), pp. 33-40.

Zinkernagel, R. M. (2000), "Immunity 2000", *Imm. Today*, 21(9), pp. 422-423.

Further Reading

Textbooks on Immunology

Abbas, A. K., Lichtman, A. H. & Pober, J. S. (1998), *Cellular and Molecular Immunology*, W. B. Saunders Company.

Barret, J. T. (1983), *Textbook of Immunology An Introduction to Immunochemistry and Immunobiology*, 4th Ed., The C. V. Mosby Company.

Bell, G. I., Perelson, A. S. & Pimbley Jr., G. H. (eds.) (1978), *Theoretical Immunology*, Marcel Dekker Inc.

Benjamini, E., Sunshine, G. & Leskowitz, S. (1996), *Immunology A Short Course*, 3rd Ed., Wiley-Liss.

Coleman, R. M., Lombard, M. F. & Sicard, R. E. (1992), *Fundamental Immunology*, 2nd Ed., Wm. C. Brown Publishers.

Dreher H. (1995), *The Immune Power Personality*, Penguin Books.

Hood, L. E., Weissman, I. L., Wood, W. B. & Wilson, J. H. (1984), *Immunology*, 2nd Ed., The Benjamin/Cummings Publishing Company, Inc.

Janeway, C. A., P. Travers, Walport, M. & Capra, J. D. (1999), "Immunobiology: The Immune System in Health and Disease", 4th Ed., Garland Publishing.

Klein, J. (1990), *Immunology*, Blackwell Scientific Publications.

Paul, W. E. (ed.) (1999), *Fundamental Immunology*, 4th Ed., Lippincott-Raven Publishers.

History of Immunology

Bell, G. I. & Perelson, A. S. (1978), "An Historical Introduction to Theoretical Immunology", In *Theoretical Immunology*, (eds.) G. I. Bell, A. S. Perelson & G. H. Pimbley Jr., Marcel Dekker Inc., pp. 3-41.

Cambrosio, A., Keating, P. & Tauber, A. I. (1994), *Immunology as a Historical Ob*

ject, Special Issue of the Journal of the History of Biology, 27(3).

Cziko, G. (1995), "The Immune System: Selection by the Enemy", *Without Miracles*, G. Cziko, A Bradford Book, The MIT Press, pp. 39-48.

Piatelli-Palmarini, M. (1986), "The Rise of Selective Theories: A Case Study and Some Lessons from Immunology", In *Language Learning and Concept Acquisition*, Demopoulos, W. & Marros, A. (eds.), Ablex Publishing.

Silverstein, A. M. (1985), "History of Immunology", *Cellular Immun.*, **91**, pp. 263-283.

Innate and Adaptive Immunity

Carol, M. C. & Prodeus, A. P. (1998), "Linkages of Innate and Adaptive Immunity", *Current Opinion in Imm.*, **10**, pp. 36-40.

Colaco, C. (1998), "Acquired Wisdom in Innate Immunity", *Imm. Today*, **19**(1), pp. 50.

Fearon, D. T. & Locksley, R. M. (1996), "The Instructive Role of Innate Immunity in the Acquired Immune Response", *Science*, **272**, pp. 50-53.

Janeway Jr., C. A. (1992), "The Immune System Evolved to Discriminate Infectious Nonself from Noninfectious Self", *Imm. Today*, **13**(1), pp. 11-16.

Lo, D., Feng, L., Li, L. et al. (1999), "Integrating Innate and Adaptive Immunity in the Whole Animal", *Imm. Rev.*, **169**, pp. 225-239.

Malhotra, R., Merry, T. & Ray, K. P. (2000), "Innate Immunity: A Primitive System in Humans", *Imm. Today*, **21**(11), pp. 534-535.

Medzhitov, R. & Janeway Jr., C. A. (1998), "Innate Immune Recognition and Control of Adaptive Immune Responses", *Seminars in Imm.*, **10**, pp. 351-353.

Medzhitov, R. & Janeway Jr., C. A. (1997), "Innate Immunity: Impact on the Adaptive Immune Response", *Current Opinion in Imm.*, **9**, pp. 4-9.

Medzhitov, R. & Janeway Jr., C. A. (1997), "Innate Immunity: The Virtues of a Nonclonal System of Recognition", *Cell*, **91**, pp. 295-298.

Parish, C. R. & O'Neill, E. R. (1997), "Dependence of the Adaptive Immune Response on Innate Immunity: Some Questions Answered but New Paradoxes Emerge", *Imm. and Cell Biol.*, **75**, pp. 523-527.

Clonal Selection

Ada, G. L. & Nossal, G. J. V. (1987), "The Clonal Selection Theory", *Scientific American*, **257**(2), pp. 50-57.

Adams, D. (1996), "How the Immune System Works and Why it Causes Autoimmune Diseases", *Imm. Today*, **17**(7), pp. 300-302.

Ahmed, R. & Sprent, J. (1999), "Immunological Memory", *The Immunologist*, **7/1-2**, pp. 23-26.

Allen, D. et al. (1987), "Timing, Genetic Requirements and Functional Consequences of Somatic Hypermutation During B-cell Development", *Imm. Rev.*, **96**, pp. 5-22.

Burnet, F. M. (1978), "Clonal Selection and After", In *Theoretical Immunology*, (eds.) G. I. Bell, A. S. Perelson & G. H. Pimbley Jr., Marcel Dekker Inc., pp. 63-85.

George, A. J. T. (2000), "Jumping or Walking: Which is Better", *Imm. Today*, **21**(1), pp. 56.

Hodgkin, P. D. (1998), "Role of Cross-Reactivity in the Development of Antibody Responses", *The Immunologist*, **6/6**, pp. 223-226.

Mason, D. (1998), "Antigen Cross-Reactivity: Essential in the Function of TCRs", *The Immunologist*, **6/6**, pp. 220-222.

Nossal, G. J. V. (1993), "The Molecular and Cellular Basis of Affinity Maturation in the Antibody Response", *Cell*, **68**, pp. 1-2.

Perelson, A. S., Mirmirani, M. & Oster, G. F. (1978), "Optimal Strategies in Immunology II. B Memory Cell Production", *J. Math. Biol.*, **5**, pp. 213-256.

Perelson, A. S., Mirmirani, M. & Oster, G. F. (1976), "Optimal Strategies in Immunology I. B-Cell Differentiation and Proliferation", *J. Math. Biol.*, **3**, pp. 325-367.

Smith, D. J. (1997), "The Cross-Reactive Immune Response: Analysis, Modeling and Application to Vaccine Design", Ph.D. Dissertation, Computer Science, The University of New Mexico.

Sprent, J. (1994), "T and B Memory Cells", *Cell*, **76**, pp. 315-322.

Storb, U. (1998), "Progress in Understanding the Mechanisms and Consequences of Somatic Hypermutation", *Immun. Rev.*, **162**, pp. 5-11.

Self/Nonself Discrimination

Anderson, G., Hare, K. J. & Jenkinson, E. J. (1999), "Positive Selection of Thymocytes: the Long and Winding Road", *Imm. Today*, **20**(10), pp. 463-468.

Fink, P. J. & McMahan, C. J. (2000), "Lymphocytes Rearrange, Edit and Revise Their Antigen Receptors to be Useful Yet Safe", *Imm. Today*, **21**(11), pp. 561-566.

Kruisbeek, A. M. (1995), "Tolerance", *The Immunologist*, **3/5-6**, pp. 176-178.

Mannie, M. D. (1999), "Immunological Self/Nonself Discrimination", *Immunological Research*, **19**(1), pp. 65-87.

Nossal, G. J. V. (1994), "Negative Selection of Lymphocytes", *Cell*, **76**, pp. 229-239.

Parijs, L. V. & Abbas, A. K. (1998), "Homeostasis and Self-Tolerance in the Immune System: Turning Lymphocytes Off", *Science*, **280**, pp. 243-248.

von Boehmer, H. (1994), "Positive Selection of Lymphocytes", *Cell*, **76**, pp. 219-228.

Zinkernagel, R. M. & Kelly, J. (1997), "How Antigen Influences Immunity", *The Immunologist*, **4/5**, pp. 114-120.

Immune Networks: Experimental Evidence

Bersini, H. & Varela, F. J. (1994), "The Immune Learning Mechanisms: Reinforcement, Recruitment and Their Applications", In *Computing with Biological Metaphors*, R. Paton (ed.), Chapman & Hall.

Garcia, K. C., Desiderio, S. V. Ronco, P. M., Verrout, P. J. & Amzel, L. M. (1992), "Recognition of Angiostensin II: Antibodies at Different Levels of an Idiotypic Network are Superimposable", *Science*, **257**, pp. 528-531.

Iverson, G. M. & Dresser, D. W. (1970), "Immunological Paralysis Induced by an Idiotypic Antigen", *Nature*, **227**, pp. 274.

Lundkvist, I, Coutinho, A., Varela, F. & Holmberg, D. (1989), "Evidence for a Functional Idiotypic Network Among Natural Antibodies in Normal Mice", *Proc. Natl. Acad. Sci. USA*, **86,** pp. 5074-5078.

Souza, A. R. et al. (1998), "Evidence of Idiotypic Modulation in the Immune Response to gp43, the Major Antigenic Component of *Paracoccidioides brasiliensis* in both Mice and Humans", *Clinical & Experimental Immunology*, **114**(1), pp. 40-49.

Varela, F. J., Anderson, A., Dietrich, G., Sundblad, A., Holmberg, D., Kazatchkine, M. & Coutinho, A. (1991), "Population Dynamics of Antibodies in Normal and Autoimmune Individuals", *Proc. Natl. Acad. Sc. USA*, **88**, pp. 5917-5921.

Immune Networks: Theoretical Aspects and Models

Atlan, H. & Cohen, I. R. (1989), *Theories of Immune Networks*, Springer-Verlag.

Bernardes, A. T. & dos Santos, R. M. Z. (1997), "Immune Network at the Edge of Chaos", *J. theor. Biol.*, **186**, pp. 173-187.

Bersini, H. & Calenbuhr, V. (1997), "Frustrated Chaos in Biological Networks", *J. theor. Biol.*, **188**, pp. 187-200.

Bonna, C. A. & Kohler, H. (eds.) (1983), "Immune Networks", *Annals of the New York Academy of Sciences*, **418**.

Calenbuhr, V., Bersini, H., Stewart, J. & Varela, F. J. (1995), "Natural Tolerance in a Simple Immune Network", *J. theor. Biol.*, **177**, pp. 199-213.

Carneiro, J., Coutinho, A. & Stewart, J. (1996b), "A Model of the Immune Network with B-T Cell Co-Operation. II – The Simulation of Ontogenesis", *J. theor. Biol.*, **182**, pp. 531-547.

Coutinho, A. (1995), "The Network Theory: 21 Years Later", *Scand. J. Imm.*, **42**, pp. 3-8.

Coutinho, A. (1989), "Beyond Clonal Selection and Network", *Imm. Rev.*, **110**, pp. 63-87.

Coutinho, A., Forni, L., Holmberg, D., Ivars, F. & Vaz, N. (1984), "From an Antigen-Centered, Clonal Perspective of Immune Responses to an Organism-Centered, Network Perspective of Autonomous Activity in a Self-Referential Immune System", *Imm. Rev.*, **79**, pp. 152-168.

de Boer, R. J. & Perelson, A. S. (1991), "Size and Connectivity as Emergent Properties of a Developing Immune Network", *J. theor. Biol.*, **149**, pp. 381-424.

de Boer, R. J. (1989), "Information Processing in Immune Systems: Clonal Selection Versus Idiotypic Network Models", *Cell to Cell Signalling: From Experiments to Theoretical Models*, Academic Press Limited, pp. 285-302.

Detours, V., Sulzer, B. & Perelson, A. S. (1996), "Size and Connectivity of the Idiotypic Network are Independent of the Dis-

creteness of the Affinity Distribution", *J. theor. Biol.*, **183**, pp. 409-416.

Hoffmann, G. W. (1975), "A Theory of Regulation and Self-Nonself Discrimination in an Immune Network", *Eur. J. Imm.*, **5**, pp. 638-647.

Jerne, N. K. (1985), "The Generative Grammar of the Immune System", *Science*, **229**, pp. 1057-1059.

Jerne, N. K. (1984), "Idiotypic Networks and Other Preconceived Ideas", *Imm. Rev.*, **79**, pp. 5-24.

Jerne, N. K. (1974), "Clonal Selection in a Lymphocyte Network". *Cellular Selection and Regulation in the Immune Response*, G. M. Edelman (ed.), Raven Press, N. Y., p. 39.

Jerne, N. K. (1973), "The Immune System", *Scientific American*, **229**(1), pp. 52-60.

Perelson, A. S. (1988), "Towards a Realistic Model of the Immune System", *Theoretical Immunology*, Part Two, A. S. Perelson (ed.), pp. 377-401.

Perelson, A. S. (1989), "Immune Network Theory", *Imm. Rev.*, **110**, pp. 5-36.

Richter, P. H. (1978), "The Network Idea and the Immune Response", *Theoretical Immunology*, G. I. Bell, A. S. Perelson & G. H. Pimbley Jr. (eds.), Marcel Dekker Inc., pp. 539-569.

Richter, P. H. (1975), "A Network Theory of the Immune System", *Eur. J. Imm.*, **5**, pp. 350-354.

Segel, L. & Perelson, A. S. (1988), "Computations in Shape Space: A New Approach to Immune Network Theory", In *Theoretical Immunology*, Part II, A. S. Perelson (ed.), pp. 321-343.

Stewart, J. & Varela, F. J. (1991), "Morphogenesis in Shape-space. Elementary Meta-Dynamics in a Model of the Immune Network", *J. theor. Biol.*, **153**, pp. 477-498.

Varela, F. J. & Stewart, J. (1990), "Dynamics of a Class of Immune Networks. I.

Global Stability of Idiotypic Interactions", *J. theor. Biol.*, **144**, pp. 93-101.

Varela, F. J. & Stewart, J. (1990), "Dynamics of a Class of Immune Networks II. Oscillatory Activity of Cellular and Humoral Components", *J. theor. Biol.*, **144**, pp. 103-115.

Chapter 3

A Framework for Engineering Artificial Immune Systems

...it had become clear to all that there was a substantial common basis of ideas between the workers in the different fields, that people in each group could already use notions which had better developed by the others, and that some attempt should be made to achieve a common vocabulary

– N. Wiener

3.1 Introduction

When compared to other well-established computational intelligence paradigms such as artificial neural networks, evolutionary algorithms, and fuzzy systems, the field of artificial immune systems (AIS) is still in its infancy. In order to enable a more rigorous development of the field, it is beneficial to introduce a set of formal processes and algorithms that can be used as a general framework with which to create artificial immune systems.

The questions that still lie behind this new and exciting area of research are various and wide-ranging. Typically, the first question raised when one intends to study artificial immune systems, is "What is exactly an artificial immune system?" or "What characterizes an AIS?" Once this has been established, the natural question to follow tends to be "When the field emerged: what were the landmarks that established the research in AIS?" Once arriving at a consensus of what is an AIS and what were the landmarks of its research history, questions tend to go deeper. For example, questions like "How do I design an AIS for my particular application?" or "Which types of problems are suitable to be solved with an AIS?" are very common within the scientific and industrial communities interested in assessing this novel paradigm.

There are works in the literature that attempt to introduce an architecture for the construction of artificial immune systems (e.g., Hofmeyr & Forrest, 2000), a formal model for AIS (e.g., Tarakanov & Dasgupta, 2000), or even a physical model for it (e.g., Zak, 2000). Nevertheless, these works are usually either too restricted to a particular school or application, or they do not cover enough immune principles and components to provide a general framework in which to engineer an AIS. There has been another recent attempt to provide such a general-purpose framework. In a Ph.D. thesis (de Castro, 2001), the author concatenated several algorithms from theoretical immunology and AIS literature in order to introduce what was termed *immune engineering* (IE). Immune engineering was defined as a meta-synthesis process used to extract ideas from the immune system in order to build novel computational tools to solve complex problems. It presented a discussion on what can be considered to be an AIS and when it can be said to have emerged. A process of engineering an AIS was proposed from fundamental principles. The proposed process initially took the literature on theoretical immunology and AIS and used it to search for modeling schemes for the several types of immune cells and molecules. Then, some influential computational algorithms of immune principles, theories, and processes were reviewed and brought together into a single framework. It is the basis of this work that this chapter intends to explore, as it is felt to be a good foundation on which to build. These ideas will be reviewed and extended in order to introduce a more complete generic framework with which to engineer an AIS.

Contrary to what some readers might be thinking, neither this chapter nor the immune engineering processes are polarized by a particular school, application, or viewpoint. As will be discussed, an effort has been made to maintain the ideas decentralised from any particular work or application domain. The following chapter reviews several applications of artificial immune systems, and it will be demonstrated that the framework introduced here is indeed of general purpose and could have been used to engineer most of the AIS reviewed.

This chapter is organized as follows. Section 3.2 summarizes several features of the vertebrate immune system with the purpose of providing motivation to the research on artificial immune systems. Section 3.3 proposes a definition of what can be considered to be an AIS. Section 3.4 gives a general idea of the scope of AIS. In Section 3.5, general forms of modelling the several types of immune cells and molecules and mechanisms to evaluate their interactions, are introduced. In addition, some influential works from the literature used to simulate specific immune principles, algorithms, and processes are reviewed. These algorithms can be considered more general purpose; some of their variations have been used as a basis for the development of a great number of AIS in the literature. This section also describes algorithms focused on the immune network theory. Continuous immune network models (based on ordinary differential equations) will be presented separately from the discrete immune network models (based on difference equations). Section 3.6 proposes a consensual birth date for the field and presents a brief history of the major landmarks in terms of events and publications on AIS. The chapter is concluded in Section 3.7 proposing general guidelines for engineering AIS. These guidelines are based upon all the modeling schemes, principles, and algorithms described previously.

3.2   Why the Immune System?

Chapter 2 reviewed the fundamentals of the biological immune system, its architecture, main components, principles, and theories used to explain in part some of its functioning. The focus was on a high level information processing perspective, where the immune system was viewed as an independent entity within the body, with different elements acting in a distributed and complementary fashion.

Initially, it is possible to list and discuss several immune properties that are highly appealing from a computational perspective. It is hard to find another biological system that embodies such a powerful and diverse set of features. The reader is guided to the specific chapters and sections where each of these features are discussed in more detail:

- *Pattern recognition*: cells and molecules of the immune system have several ways of recognizing patterns. For example, there are surface molecules that can bind to an antigen or recognize molecular signals (e.g., lymphokines) and there are intra-cellular molecules (e.g., MHC) that bind to specific proteins and present them in the cell surface to other immune cells (Section 2.8; Section 5.4);

- *Uniqueness*: each individual possesses its own immune system, with its particular vulnerabilities and capabilities (Chapter 2; Section 5.4);

- *Self identity*: the uniqueness of the immune system gives rise to the fact that any cell, molecule and tissue that is not native to the body can be recognized and eliminated by the immune system (Section 2.10);

- *Diversity*: there exist varying types of elements (cells, molecules, proteins, etc.) that together, perform the role of identifying the body and protecting it from malefic invaders and malfunctioning cells. Additionally, there are different lines of defense, such as innate and adaptive immunity (Chapter 2);

- *Disposability*: no single cell or molecule is essential for the functioning of the immune system. These cells and molecules are constantly dying and being replaced by new ones, though some of them have long life spans as memory cells (Sections 2.9 and 2.11);

- *Autonomy*: there is no central "element" controlling the immune system; it does not require outside intervention or maintenance. It acts by autonomously classifying and eliminating pathogens and it is capable of partially repairing itself by replacing damaged or malfunctioning cells (Chapters 2 and 5);

- *Multilayered*: multiple layers of different mechanisms that act cooperatively and competitively are combined to provide a high overall security, as summarized in Figure 2.5 (Section 2.5);

- *No secure layer*: any cell of the organism can be attacked by the immune system, including those of the immune system itself (Section 2.10);

- *Anomaly detection*: the immune system can recognize and react to pathogens that the body has never encountered before (Sections 2.8, 2.10, and 2.11);

- *Dynamically changing coverage*: as the immune system cannot maintain large enough repertoires of cells and molecules to detect all existing pathogens, a trade-off has to be made between space and time. It maintains a circulating repertoire of lymphocytes constantly being changed through cell death, production, and reproduction (Chapter 2);

- *Distributivity*: the immune cells, molecules, and organs are distributed all over the body and, most importantly, are not subject to any centralized control (Section 2.5);

- *Noise tolerance*: an absolute recognition of the pathogens is not required; the system is tolerant to molecular noise (Section 2.8);

- *Resilience*: although disturbances might reduce the functioning of the immune system it is still capable of persisting despite these disturbances. When the organism is exhausted or malnourished, its immune system is less effective as more energy is required for recovery and maintenance of the organism (Chapter 2; Section 5.4);
- *Fault tolerance*: if an immune response has been built up against a given pathogen and the responding cell type is removed, this degeneracy in the immune repertoire will make other cell types to respond to this pathogen. In addition, the complementary roles performed by several immune components also allow the re-allocation of tasks to other elements in case any of them fails (Chapter 2);
- *Robustness*: the sheer diversity and number of immune cells and molecules, together with their distributivity are greatly responsible for the robustness of the immune system (Chapter 2);
- *Immune learning and memory*: the molecules of the immune system can adapt themselves, structurally and in number, to the antigenic challenges. These adaptation mechanisms are followed by a strong selective pressure, which allows the most adapted individuals to remain in the immune repertoire for long periods of time. These highly adapted cells with long life spans are called memory cells and promote faster and more effective responses to the same (or a slightly similar) antigenic challenge. Additionally, immune cells and molecules can recognize each other, and this endows the immune system with an autonomous eigen-behavior (Sections 2.9 and 2.11);
- *Predator-prey pattern of response*: the vertebrate immune system replicates cells to deal with replicating pathogens, otherwise these pathogens would quickly overwhelm the immune defenses. When the number of pathogens increases, so does the number of immune cells and molecules to cope with these pathogens. When the pathogens are eliminated, the repertoires of immune cells return to a steady state. If the number of pathogens is too large, they can overwhelm the immune system leading to the death of the organism (Sections 2.9 and 5.7);
- *Self-organization*: when an antigenic pattern interacts with the immune system, there is no information of how the immune cells and molecules should be adapted to cope with this antigen. Clonal selection and affinity maturation are responsible for selecting and expanding the most adapted cells to be maintained as long living memory cells (Section 2.9);
- *Integration with other systems*: although the introduction to the immune system presented in Chapter 2 has described it as an independent system, the immune system also communicates with other parts of the body influencing and being influenced by their behaviors. This will be discussed in Chapter 5.

These appealing computational processing features, together with a good knowledge of how the immune system works, are excellent motivations for the development of computational tools. The advances in the biological sciences including medicine and cellular and molecular biology, have contributed greatly to a good understanding of the mechanisms of the body's defenses. There are several reasons that led to search for these mechanisms, such as the necessity to avoid graft tissue rejection and to combat infectious diseases.

All the processes presented in the previous chapter emerged as a result of several years of research on the immune system. A direct benefit of this research for human beings comes as a better life quality and expectancy. Although some of the processes presented might be controversial, such as the immune network theory, these controversies are not critical from a computational perspective. This might sound a strange statement to make, but as this chapter unfolds, hopefully the reader will appreciate why this is the case. With the development of AIS, the benefits from the research on the immune system has left the level of direct human life quality, to a more abstract computational level.

3.3   What is an Artificial Immune System?

Although immunology as a science dated back to the early 1800s with Jenner's successful immunization technique against smallpox, this vaccination process had little impact on the treatment or understanding of any other disease for nearly 100 years. This was primarily due to the lack of theoretical concepts of the causes and nature of infectious diseases.

In the 20th century, various controversies on theoretical immunology were apparent, such as instructive versus selective theories of antibody formation, and clonal versus network models of repertoire activities. The majority of immune theories have been almost entirely conceptual or non-mathematical in nature. However, mathematical analysis of immune phenomena has been making an important contribution to the science of immunology. The results that can be expected from the application of mathematical analysis and models to immune phenomena are various:

- Through modeling and identification theory, it is possible to provide a deeper and more quantitative description of the immune system and its corresponding experimental results;
- Aid in the critical analysis of hypotheses and in the understanding of the biological mechanisms;
- Assist in the prediction of behaviors and the design of experiments;
- Stimulate new and more satisfactory approaches to vaccination policies, treatment of diseases, and control of graft and transplant rejections; and
- Allow the recovery of information from experimental results.

An *experiment* can be considered as a procedure performed in a controlled environment for the purpose of gathering observations, data, or facts, demonstrating known facts or theories, or testing hypotheses or theories. Immunological experiments are usually made *in vivo*, within a living organism (e.g., mice), or *in vitro*, in an artificial environment outside the living organism (e.g., a test tube). By contrast, a *simulation* attempts to predict aspects of the behavior of some system by creating an approximate (theoretical) model of that system. This can be achieved by physical modeling, by writing a special-purpose computer program, or by using a more general simulation package that is probably still aimed at a particular kind of simulation. Thus, there is a significant conceptual difference between experiment and simulation.

Mathematical theoretical immunology and artificial immune systems both deal with examining the immune system, with the difference residing on the expected goals of each technique and on their potential applicability. In an attempt to define the field of artificial immune systems, several authors have proposed definitions for it. Three examples of attempts are:

Definition 3.1   *"Artificial immune systems are data manipulation, classification, representation and reasoning methodologies which follow a biologically plausible paradigm, that of the human immune system" (Starlab).*

Definition 3.2   *"An artificial immune system is a computational system based upon metaphors of the natural immune system" (Timmis, 2000).*

In an edited book exclusively dedicated to artificial immune systems, the editor suggests that:

Definition 3.3   *"Artificial immune systems are intelligent methodologies inspired by the immune system toward real-world problem solving" (Dasgupta, 1999).*

To stretch even further the distinction between mathematical theoretical immunology and AIS, we can propose a single general concept for an AIS that complements, incorporates, and summarizes the definitions already presented:

Definition 3.4   *Artificial immune systems (AIS) are adaptive systems, inspired by theoretical immunology and observed immune functions, principles and models, which are applied to problem solving.*

It is important to remark that in this definition, theoretical immunology refers to all mathematical and non-mathematical mechanisms, principles, models, and theories used to describe the functioning of the immune system. This includes, but is not restricted to, pattern recognition mechanisms, innate and adaptive immune responses, self/nonself discrimination algorithms, and immune network models.

Definition 3.4 implies that the significant difference between AIS and theoretical immunology models concerns their rationales. Artificial immune systems are applied to solve problems in many domain areas, whilst theoretical immunology is intended to simulate, complement, and/or improve experimental analyses of the immune system. It should be noted however, that artificial immune systems are not only related to the creation of abstract or metaphorical models of the biological immune system, they also include those mathematical theoretical immunology models being applied to tasks such as optimization, control, and autonomous robot navigation. Nevertheless, it must be said that the majority of AIS make use of only a few ideas and high levels of abstractions of the immune system.

According to Definition 3.4, for a system to be characterized as an AIS it has to embody, as the minimum, a basic model of an immune component (e.g., cell, molecule, organ), it has to have been designed by incorporating ideas from theoretical and/or experimental immunology, and it has to be aimed at problem solving.

Therefore, simply attributing "immunological terminology" to a given system is not sufficient to characterize it as an AIS. For example, naming a set of input patterns as antigens and another set of patterns as antibodies does not qualify a system to be an AIS. There has to be a minimal level of immunology involved, such as a model to perform pattern matching, an incorporated immune principle such as a clonal and/or negative selection algorithm, or an immune network model.

Other types of systems that belong to the class of artificial immune systems, but were not covered by Definition 3.4, are the hybrids of computational intelligence methodologies (e.g., genetic algorithms, artificial neural networks, and fuzzy systems) with theoretical immunology models. As will be seen in Chapter 6, several computational intelligence (CI) paradigms can be hybridized with AIS and theoretical immunology models to build more powerful computational systems. Under this perspective, the pure computer simulations of the immune system do not qualify as AIS. Even if these simulations involve CI paradigms such as in the cellular automata models of the immune system proposed by Celada and Seiden (1992, 1996), as the goals of these models are significantly different from those of AIS.

3.4 Scope of Artificial Immune Systems

At a first sight, the immune system can be mistakenly seen simply as a pattern recognition system responsible for identifying and eliminating harmful elements. As a consequence, the scope of artificial immune systems could be thought to be restricted to pattern recognition tasks, with particular emphasis to computer security.

Nevertheless, the large amount of interesting computational features of the immune system suggests an almost limitless range of applications. Starting from a computational intelligence perspective features like immune learning and memory and self-organization are good indicators that the immune system offers a new paradigm to machine-learning and self-organizing systems. From a computer science and software engineering perspective immune properties such as multilayer structure, anomaly detection, fault tolerance, distributivity, and robustness present viable alternative ideas to parallel computation and the security of information systems. Features like the predator-prey pattern of response and natural integration with other systems suggest that the research on the immune system, thus artificial immune systems, might be very fruitful for the development of computational hybrid systems. Furthermore, the biological sciences can also benefit from the research on AIS by using them as tools to study, model, and even aid in the comprehension of their own problems; just as done by theoretical immunology models.

Applications of artificial immune systems are various and will be reviewed in Chapters 4, 6 and 7. These include, but are not restricted to:

- Pattern recognition;
- Fault and anomaly detection;
- Data analysis (data mining, classification, etc.);
- Agent-based systems;
- Scheduling;

- Machine-learning;
- Autonomous navigation and control;
- Search and optimization methods;
- Artificial life; and
- Security of information systems.

3.5   A Framework for Engineering AIS

The first issue to be taken into account in the development of an artificial immune system is related to which kind of problem it is going to be applied. Although the main roles of the immune system are to perform pattern recognition and to eliminate nonself or malfunctioning cells, all its features described in Section 3.2 suggest it has great potential to be applied to diverse domain areas. Therefore, independently of the application domain, the first step in the modeling and simulation of most biological phenomena is to devise the models for the components of the system. In the case of the immune system, these components include B-cells, T-cells, and antibodies. Initially it is necessary to provide a description of what we mean by the term *framework*.

Assume the case of other soft computing approaches inspired by biology, such as ANN and EAs. A set of artificial neurons can be arranged together so as to form an artificial neural network. In order to acquire some knowledge, these neural networks suffer an adaptive process, named learning or training, which alters (some of) their free parameters. Thus, in a simplified form, a framework to design an ANN is composed of a set of artificial neurons, a pattern of interconnection for these neurons, and a learning algorithm.

In evolutionary algorithms, there is a set of "artificial chromosomes" representing a population of individuals that will iteratively suffer processes of reproduction, genetic variation, and selection. As a result of this adaptive process, a population of evolved artificial individuals arises. A framework, in this case, would correspond to the genetic representation of the individuals of the population, plus the procedures for reproduction, genetic variation, and selection.

Therefore, the viewpoint is taken that a framework to design a biologically inspired algorithm requires, at least, the following basic elements:

- *A representation for the components of the system*;
- *A set of mechanisms to evaluate the interaction of individuals with the environment and each other*. The environment is usually simulated by a set of input stimuli, one or more fitness function(s), or other mean(s) and;
- *Procedures of adaptation* that govern the dynamics of the system, i.e., how its behavior varies over time.

This is the basis of the proposed framework to design artificial immune systems as well: a representation to create abstract models of immune organs, cells, and molecules; a set of functions, termed affinity functions, to quantify the interactions of these "artificial elements", and a set of general purpose algorithms to govern the dynamics of the AIS.

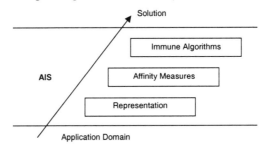

Figure 3.1. Layered Framework for AIS

The framework can be thought of as a layered approach (Figure 3.1). The basis of every system is the application domain. For this domain, the way in which the components of the system will be represented has to be considered. Once a suitable representation is decided, one or more affinity measures are used to quantify the interactions of the elements of the system. There are many possible affinity measures (which are partially dependent upon the representation adopted), such as Hamming and Euclidean distances. The next layer involves the use of algorithms or processes to govern the behavior (dynamics) of the system. This then gives us an engineered solution.

Based on this structure, the framework begins by reviewing a general abstract model of immune cells and molecules, named *shape-space*. After presenting the shape-space approach, the framework reviews works from the literature proposing several distinct measures to evaluate the interactions of the elements of the AIS.

The framework follows with a description of some influential works with which to abstract immune principles and theories, such as negative and clonal selection algorithms. Continuous and discrete immune network models are also reviewed. These can be utilized, for example, in machine learning, and the framework is then concluded with a set of general guidelines to be followed to design AIS.

3.5.1. Abstract Models of Immune Cells, Molecules, and their Interactions

In the previous chapter the white blood cells (leukocytes) were presented as the main operative elements of the immune system; this was divided into adaptive and innate immune system. The adaptive immunity is mediated by lymphocytes, and the innate immune system is mediated by granulocytes and macrophages, all of them belonging to the major class of leukocytes. From a pattern recognition perspective, the main characteristic of leukocytes is the presence of surface receptor molecules capable of recognizing and binding to molecular patterns. In cells of the innate immune system, the surface receptor molecules recognize common molecular patterns, named PAMPs that are only found in microorganisms. In contrast, the molecular patterns that can be recognized by the surface receptors on lymphocytes are named antigens.

    The receptor molecules on the surface of leukocytes are not entirely dedicated to the task of recognizing patterns. A portion of them is attached to the cell surface and can have an effector function with another portion being responsible for recognizing and binding to a molecular pattern. For example, in the case of antibodies and TCRs, the V-region binds with antigens while the C-region is attached to the cell surface. To make the terminology compact and comprehensible, the portion of a surface receptor molecule on a leukocyte that binds with a specific molecular pattern will be generally termed an *antibody*, and the molecular pattern recognized by this antibody will be termed *antigen*. It is important to bear in mind that under this assumption, an antibody corresponds to the portion of any leukocyte capable of recognizing a molecular pattern, and an antigen is equivalent to any pattern that can be recognized by this antibody. For example, in lymphocytes an antibody corresponds to the V-region of a B-cell or a T-cell receptor, and an antigen is an epitope or an idiotope. Remember, that as an idiotope can be found in and/or around an antibody molecule, an antigen can be a foreign antigen or (a portion of) an antibody, i.e., a self-antigen. Finally, the strength of binding between an antigen and an antibody is termed their *affinity*, or *degree of match*.

    By performing a theoretical study on clonal selection, Perelson and Oster (1979) introduced the concept of a *shape-space* (*S*) to quantitatively describe the interactions between molecules of the immune system and antigens. The basic aspect studied addressed the question of how large an immune repertoire has to be in order for the immune system to function reliably as a protective system. Under this perspective, the immune system was seen basically as a pattern (molecular) recognition system that was especially designed to identify *shapes*.

    Although the shape-space approach was presented as a formal description to model and evaluate interactions between antigens and antibodies, it can also be applied to study the binding between any type of cell receptor and the molecules they bind with. This is another reason why the general terminology of antigen and antibody has been adopted here and also why the choice was made to propose and extend the shape-space as a general framework to represent abstract models of immune cells and molecules. Additionally, shape-spaces have been widely employed by the theoretical immunology community to model and study interactions within the immune system, mainly in immune network models.

Shape-Spaces

The affinity between an antibody and an antigen involves several processes, such as short-range noncovalent interactions based on electrostatic charge, hydrogen binding, van der Waals interactions, etc. In order for an antigen to be recognized, the molecules (antigen and antibody) must bind complementary with each other over an appreciable portion of their surfaces. Therefore, extensive *regions of complementarity* between the molecules are required, as illustrated in Figure 3.2. The shape and charge distributions, as well as the existence of chemical groups in the appropriate complementary positions, can be considered as properties of antigens and antibodies that are important to determine their interactions. This set of features is called the *generalized shape* of a molecule.

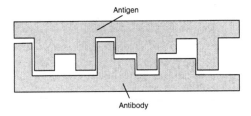

Figure 3.2. Recognition via regions of complementarity.

Assume that it is possible to adequately describe the generalized shape of an antibody by a set of L parameters (e.g., the length, width, and height of any bump or groove in the combining site, its charge, etc.). Thus, a *point* in an L-dimensional space, called shape-space S, specifies the generalized shape of an antigen binding region of the molecular receptors on the surface of immune cells with regard to its antigen binding properties. Also, assume that a set of L parameters can be used to describe an antigenic determinant, though antigens and antibodies do not necessarily have to be of the same length. The mapping from the parameters to their real biological counterparts is not important from a computational standpoint but will be basically dictated by the application domain of the AIS.

If an animal has a repertoire of size N, i.e., N antibodies, then the shape-space for that animal contains N points. These points lie within some finite volume V of the shape-space since there is only a restricted range of widths, lengths, charges, etc. that a combining site can assume. Similarly, antigens are also characterized by generalized shapes whose complements lie within the same volume V. If the antigen (Ag) and antibody (Ab) shapes are not quite complementary, then the two molecules may still bind, but with lower affinity.

It is assumed that each antibody specifically interacts with all antigens whose complement lies within a small surrounding region, characterized by a parameter ε named the *cross-reactivity threshold*. The volume V_ε resulting from the definition of the cross-reactivity threshold ε is called the *recognition region*. As each antibody can recognize (cross-react with) all antigens whose complements lie within its recognition region, a finite number of antibodies can recognize a large number of antigens into the volume V_ε, depending on the parameter ε. If similar patterns occupy neighboring regions of the shape-space, then the same antibody shape can recognize them, so long as an adequate ε is provided. Figure 3.3 illustrates the idea of a shape-space S, detaching the antibodies, antigens, and the cross-reactivity threshold.

Mathematically, the generalized shape of any molecule m in a shape-space S can be represented as an attribute string (set of coordinates) of length L. Thus, an attribute string $m = \langle m_1, m_2, ..., m_L \rangle$ can be regarded as a point in an L-dimensional shape-space, $m \in S^L$. This string might be composed of any type of attribute, such as real values, integers, bits, and symbols. These attributes are usually driven by the problem domain of the AIS and will be important in the definition of which measure(s) will be used to quantify their interactions. Most importantly, the type of attribute will define the type of shape-space to be adopted, as follows:

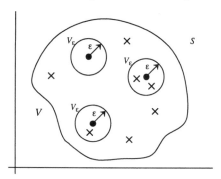

Figure 3.3.   In shape-space S, there is a volume V in which the shape of an antibody (•) and of the complement of the antigen (×) are located. An antibody can recognize any antigen whose complement lies in a volume V_ε around it.

- *Real-valued shape-space*: the attribute strings are real-valued vectors;
- *Integer shape-space*: the attribute strings are composed of integer values;
- *Hamming shape-space*: composed of attribute strings built out of a finite alphabet of length k;
- *Symbolic shape-space*: usually composed of different types of attribute strings where at least one of them is symbolic, such as a "name", a "color", etc.

Assume the general case in which an antibody molecule is represented by the set of coordinates $\mathbf{Ab} = \langle Ab_1, Ab_2, ..., Ab_L \rangle$, and an antigen is given by $\mathbf{Ag} = \langle Ag_1, Ag_2, ..., Ag_L \rangle$, where boldface letters correspond to a string. Without loss of generality, antigens and antibodies are assumed to be of same length. Under a pattern recognition perspective, the interaction of antibodies, or of an antibody and an antigen, is evaluated via a *distance measure*, also termed *affinity measure*, between their corresponding attribute strings. The affinity measure performs a mapping from the interaction between two attribute strings into a nonnegative real number that corresponds to their *affinity* or *degree of match*, $S^L \times S^L \to \mathfrak{R}^+$. Thus, the Ag-Ab (or Ab-Ab) affinity is proportional to the *degree of complementarity* (distance) between the molecules (strings).

Given an attribute string (shape) representation of an antigen and a set of antibodies, for each attribute string of an antibody molecule, one can associate a corresponding affinity with the given antigen. Thus, an *affinity landscape* can be defined on the shape-space, as illustrated in Figure 3.4.

According to the distance measure used to evaluate the affinity between the components of the AIS, real-valued shape-spaces can be of several types, including *Euclidean* and *Manhattan*. In the case of Euclidean distance, the affinity D between an antigen and an antibody is given by Equation (3.1); this corresponds to the distance between the molecules. Equation (3.2) depicts the Manhattan's distance case.

$$D = \sqrt{\sum_{i=1}^{L} (Ab_i - Ag_i)^2} \cdot \qquad (3.1)$$

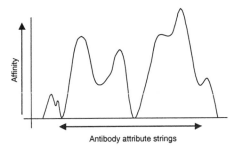

Figure 3.4. Hypothetical affinity landscape defined on an Euclidean shape-space of dimension 1. To each antibody shape in shape-space, an affinity value in relation to a given antigen is assigned; different shapes result in different affinities.

$$D = \sum_{i=1}^{L} |Ab_i - Ag_i| \cdot \tag{3.2}$$

Shape-spaces that use real-valued coordinates and that measure distance in the form of Equation (3.1) are called *Euclidean shape-spaces*. Shape-spaces that use real-valued coordinates, but Manhattan instead of Euclidean distance to evaluate the affinity between the molecules are called *Manhattan shape-spaces*. Although no report of the latter has yet been found in the literature, the Manhattan distance constitutes an interesting alternative to Euclidean distance, mainly for parallel (hardware) implementation of algorithms based on the shape-space formalism. Nevertheless, though the Manhattan distance allows in most cases a more efficient hardware implementation than the Euclidean distance, it alters the shape-space topology.

Alternatives to real-valued shape-spaces are the *Hamming shape-spaces*. In this case, antigens and antibodies are represented as sequences of symbols over a finite alphabet of length k. Equation (3.3) depicts the Hamming distance measure used to evaluate the affinity between two attribute strings of length L in a Hamming shape-space. If binary strings, termed bitstrings $k \in \{0,1\}$, are used to represent the molecules, then one has a *binary Hamming shape-space*, or a *binary shape-space*. If ternary strings, i.e., $k = 3$, are used to represent the molecules, then one has a *ternary Hamming shape-space*, or *ternary shape-space*; and so on.

$$D = \sum_{i=1}^{L} \delta_i, \text{where} \quad \delta_i = \begin{cases} 1 & \text{if } Ab_i \neq Ag_i \\ 0 & \text{otherwise} \end{cases}. \tag{3.3}$$

Depending on the problem under study, an *Integer shape-space* might also be employed. In this type of shape-space, the attributes correspond to variables that assume integer values. Note that an Integer shape-space can be viewed as a particular case of a Hamming shape-space. This type of shape-space is broadly used in tasks such as the traveling salesman problem or in scheduling applications.

Equations (3.1) to (3.3), show the basic expressions to determine the affinities between molecules in Euclidean, Manhattan, and Hamming shape-spaces, respectively. In order to study cross-reactivity, it is still necessary to define the relation between the distance D and the recognition region V_ε proportionally to the *cross-reactivity threshold* ε. If the affinity (distance or complementarity) between the molecules is larger than or equal to the cross-reactivity threshold ε, then it is assumed that a recognition event occurred between the molecules, i.e., if $D \geq \varepsilon$, the antibody recognizes the antigen. Notice that, in a Hamming shape-space, ε is directly proportional to the number of antigens an antibody can recognize and, similarly to the cell receptor, it might have a specific value for each antibody. In other shape-spaces, the behavior tends to depend on whether the space is finite or not. In addition, it is important to notice that the cross-reactivity threshold is equivalent to a *recognition threshold*, an *affinity threshold*, or an *activation threshold*, once it corresponds to the minimal degree of complementary (interaction) necessary to promote a response in the AIS.

Finally and additionally to all the shape-spaces described so far, it is also possible to identify *Symbolic shape-spaces*. In this type of shape-space, the attribute strings that represent the components of the artificial immune system are composed of at least one symbolic attribute. Figure 3.5 illustrates a Symbolic shape-space containing two antibodies that represent a database of trips.

The strings in Figure 3.5 have mixed symbolic, integer, and real-valued attributes. A simple form of evaluating the degree of interaction of the components of this AIS is to perform their match in a one by one basis. This allows the straightforward application of any affinity measure for Hamming shape-spaces. Another option is to weight the attributes according to pre-specified degrees of importance, what will require alternative forms of evaluating affinities. Specific affinity measures can be devised according to the given domain of application.

	Description	Date	Flight	Country	From	To	Price (£)
Antibody (Ab₁):	Business	1996	212	Brazil	Campinas	Greece	546.78
Antibody (Ab₂):	Holiday	2000	312	U.K.	London	Paris	102.35
Antigen (Ag):	Holiday	2000	212	U.K.	London	Greece	546.78
Match Ag – Ab₁:	0	0	1	0	0	1	1
Match Ag – Ab₂:	1	1	0	1	1	0	0

Figure 3.5. Example of a Symbolic shape-space in which some attributes are symbolic and some are numeric.

Some Philosophical and Practical Remarks

Although each B-cell has about 10^5 antibodies attached to its surface, these antibodies are monospecific; this means that all of them present the same "shape". The monospecificity property is also true for the T-cell receptors. Therefore, most artificial immune systems do not make any distinction between an immune cell and its corresponding surface receptor. An antibody corresponds to a B-cell, and a TCR to a T-cell. There are cases however, especially in immune network models, in which the cells are more complex elements than the receptor molecules; these usually contain the receptor(s) as part of their genetic information. Examples will be discussed further while presenting some discrete immune network models.

The expression "affinity" is usually adopted to quantify recognition. Nevertheless, it is possible to view affinity as a general term that relates the quality of an element of the immune system with relation to the environment in which it is placed. For example, if one is applying an AIS to solve a function optimization problem, then an antibody might correspond to a point that specifies a value for the function being optimized, and its affinity is related to the value of the function when evaluated for this individual. This is equivalent to the concept of *fitness* in an evolutionary algorithm, with the difference relying on what is the environment. In evolutionary algorithms, the environment is usually modeled as an objective or fitness function that would correspond to the affinity function in this case. On the other hand, it is important to be careful when assuming fitness equivalent to affinity. There are cases, for example when an immune network is used to quantify interactions of individuals of the population, where it is possible to have both concepts embodied in the same algorithm. In this situation, the affinity of a network cell might correspond to its degree of interaction with other cells in the network (internal environment), and the fitness of a cell might correspond to the value of this cell when evaluated for a given objective function (external environment). AIS containing both concepts of affinity and fitness will be reviewed in the next chapter.

Although it is not fully in accordance with the biological concept of shape complementarity, the affinity in shape-spaces where the variables assume integer or real values (the interval has to be finite) and in which the distance is Euclidean, could be defined as being proportional to the distance between an antibody and an antigen without reflecting or complementing it. In this case, there will be a geometric region of points in the shape-space such that all the antigens in this region present the same affinity to a given antibody, as illustrated in Figure 3.6 for the case of real-valued attributes. Indeed, in most practical applications of AIS, similarity measures are used in the place of complementarity measures, though the latter is more plausible from a biological perspective. In such cases, the goal is to search for antigens and antibodies with more similar shapes instead of more complementary shapes. This was the approach adopted in the original proposal of shape-space, but that was not pursued in this book.

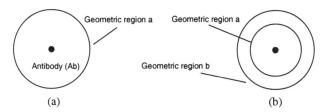

(a) (b)

Figure 3.6. Affinity through shape similarity. (a) Geometric region where all antigens present the same affinity with the given antibody. (b) The antigens lying in region b have higher affinity with the antibody than those present in region a.

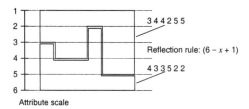

Figure 3.7. Reflection in cases of non-complementary strings.

In the shape-spaces studied here, the coordinates of an antigen are represented as the complement of their attributes. This way, when the distance between an antibody and the complement of an antigen is minimal, the molecules present maximal affinity. If the affinity between the molecules is not maximal, it becomes necessary to use the norms defined in each space, so that it becomes possible to evaluate their interactions. However, if we adopt the original antigen coordinates in shape-space, instead of their complement, then the affinity will be higher for larger distances, at least in the binary Hamming shape-spaces. To other types of norms and alphabets, the concepts of *reflection pattern* discussed by Suzuki and Yamamoto (1998) can be adopted; the antigen image must be reflected in a mirror before its affinity to a given antibody can be determined, as illustrated in Figure 3.7.

The affinity measures presented in Equations (3.1) to (3.3) assume that there is only one possible alignment in which two molecules may react. Nevertheless, from a biological perspective, the molecules are allowed to interact with each other in different alignments: this can be modeled in several forms. For example, assume that two molecules can interact over all possible alignments. Thus, the total affinity can be calculated by summing the affinity of each possible alignment, as follows:

$$D = \sum_{k=1}^{L} D_k,$$
(3.4)

where D_k is given by any of the Equations (3.1) to (3.3) when the molecules are in a given alignment k. This process is illustrated in Figure 3.8 for two binary strings of length $L = 8$.

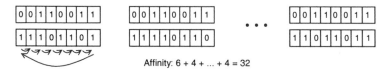

Affinity: 6 + 4 + ... + 4 = 32

Figure 3.8. Affinity for bitstrings considering different alignments. One string is fixed and the other flipped (rotated) from left to right (or from right to left) and the Hamming distance applied to each possible alignment. This process is repeated until the flipping string returns to its original configuration. The affinity might then be taken as the sum of the match of each alignment. This strategy can be used with strings of different lengths.

Another possibility for Figure 3.8 is to determine all possible alignments and to take the alignment that presents the largest (or the average) match to correspond to the affinity between the molecules. Other approaches, such as determining the affinity for a set of possible alignments and choosing the largest one, can be applied according to the necessity or application domain. It is important to bear in mind that rotating an attribute string corresponds to changing its relative position in shape-space in relation to the other attribute strings. This might have undesired effects to some applications and must be carefully analyzed before implemented.

As can be noted from the affinity measures presented, they only take into account the strength of interaction between pairs of strings. In some applications however, it might be interesting to consider other parameters, such as the *number* of antigens recognized by a given antibody. In such cases, a new criterion named *stimulation level* is defined to quantify the interactions of the components of the AIS, taking into account more than simply recognition between antigens and antibodies. The stimulation level is commonly addressed in immune network models. Basically, it includes parameters such as the number of antigens recognized and the degree of interaction of an antibody with other antibodies and with antigens, and to some extent it dictates the survival of a cell within the network.

There is an important conceptual distinction between the expressions *match* and *affinity*. This sometimes causes confusion in those interested in developing and studying AIS. *To perform a match between two strings means to evaluate how they interact with each other.* In contrast, *the affinity between two strings is the result of their match.* For example, in Figure 3.5 the match between the antigen Ag and the antibodies Ab_1 and Ab_2 is presented. If the affinity is measured via the Hamming distance between the molecules, then the affinity Ag-Ab_1 corresponds to 3, and the affinity Ag-Ab_2 is equal to 4.

Finally, although the shape-space approach was introduced to quantify shape interactions between antibodies and antigens, its extensions presented here allow it to be adopted as a general formalism to model any type of immune cell and molecule. The fact that some molecules interact more strongly chemically (or through any other(s) form) than via shape interactions is not a barrier to abstractly employ a "shape-space" to model these elements. In addition, the suggestion that affinity is related to the quality of an individual to its environment, not only to the strength of match between molecules, contribute to the generality of the approach. As will be seen, the extended shape-space proposed is appropriate to describe most of the AIS developed so far and reviewed in Chapter 4. Other shape-spaces could also be proposed based on this general idea; an example will be given in Section 6.6 with the so-called DNA shape-space.

Affinities in Hamming Shape-Space

Hamming shape-spaces are, to date, the most frequently employed in artificial immune systems and also in theoretical immune network models. Thus, this section is exclusively dedicated to this particular class of shape-space.

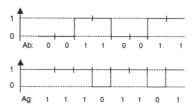

Figure 3.9.   Graphical interpretation of the interactions between two bitstrings of length $L = 8$.

Within the Hamming shape-spaces, the binary case is the most popular. This is due to several reasons, such as the easy manipulation of binary attribute strings and their straightforward graphic interpretation, as depicted in Figure 3.9. In addition to the Hamming distance presented in Equation (3.3), there are several other affinity measures proposed in the literature for binary Hamming shape-spaces.

The Hamming distance between an antibody bitstring and an antigen bitstring can be simply computed by applying the exclusive-or operator (XOR) between these strings, as depicted in Figure 3.10(a). The expected affinity between two randomly chosen bitstrings is equal to half of their length (if they are of same length).

Shape-spaces that measure the number of r-contiguous complementary symbols (Percus *et al.*, 1993), named r-contiguous bit rule, are more biologically appealing and can also be used, as depicted in Figure 3.10(b).

Extensive complementary regions might be interesting for the detection of similar characteristics in symmetric portions of the molecules, and can be useful to perform specific tasks, such as pattern recognition. An affinity measure that privileges regions of complementarity was proposed by Hunt and his collaborators (Hunt *et al.*, 1995) and is given by:

$$D = D_H + \sum_i 2^{l_i} , \qquad (3.5)$$

where D_H is the total Hamming distance given by Equation (3.3), and l_i is the length of each complementary region i with 2 or more consecutive complementary bits, as illustrated in Figure 3.10(c). We termed this equation the *multiple contiguous bit rule*.

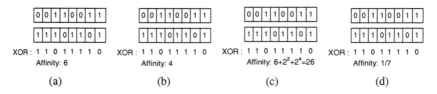

Figure 3.10.   Different affinity measures for binary Hamming shape-spaces. (a) Hamming distance: total number of complementary bits (Equation (3.3)). (b) r-contiguous bit rule. (c) Multiple contiguous bits rule (Equation (3.5)). (d) Affinity measure of Rogers and Tanimoto (Equation (3.6)).

Harmer and Lamont (2000) used the similarity measure of Rogers and Tani-moto, described in Equation (3.6), to evaluate the affinity between two bitstring molecules. The authors suggested that this measure is more selective than the Hamming distance and less than the r-contiguous bit rule.

$$D = \frac{a+d}{a+d+2(b+c)},$$

$$a = \sum_{i=1}^{L} \zeta_i, \quad \zeta_i = \begin{cases} 1 & Ab_i = Ag_i = 1 \\ 0 & \text{otherwise} \end{cases}$$

$$b = \sum_{i=1}^{L} \xi_i, \quad \xi_i = \begin{cases} 1 & Ab_i = 1, Ag_i = 0 \\ 0 & \text{otherwise} \end{cases} \qquad (3.6)$$

$$c = \sum_{i=1}^{L} \gamma_i, \quad \gamma_i = \begin{cases} 1 & Ab_i = 0, Ag_i = 1 \\ 0 & \text{otherwise} \end{cases}$$

$$d = \sum_{i=1}^{L} \varphi_i, \quad \varphi_i = \begin{cases} 1 & Ab_i = Ag_i = 0 \\ 0 & \text{otherwise} \end{cases}$$

In Hamming shape-spaces, the potential repertoire, i.e., the total number N of different molecules that can be generated, is given by

$$N = k^L, \qquad (3.7)$$

where k is the size of the alphabet and L the string length. A given antibody mole-cule recognizes some set of antigens and therefore covers some portion of the shape-space (see Figure 3.3). The cross-reactivity threshold ε determines the *coverage* provided by each single antibody molecule. If $\varepsilon = L$, i.e., a perfect match is re-quired, an antibody can only recognize the antigen that is its exact complement. The number of antigens covered by a single antibody increases as ε decreases according to the following expression

$$C = \sum_{i=0}^{L-\varepsilon} \binom{L}{i} = \sum_{i=0}^{L-\varepsilon} \frac{L!}{i!(L-i)!}, \qquad (3.8)$$

where C is the coverage of the antibody, L the length of its bitstring representation, and ε the cross-reactivity threshold.

Based on Equation (3.8), a given bitstring of length L and a cross-reactivity threshold ε, the minimum number of antibody molecules (N_m) necessary to cover the whole shape-space can be calculated by

$$N_m = ceil\left(\frac{N}{C}\right), \qquad (3.9)$$

where N is the potential repertoire given by Equation (3.7), C is the coverage of each antibody given by Equation (3.8), and *ceil* the operator that rounds the value in parenthesis towards its upper nearest integer. Table 3.1 exemplifies the shape-space coverage for binary strings of variable lengths as a function of their coverage and the affinity threshold.

Table 3.1.   Antigenic coverage C of each antibody, and minimal repertoire size N_m for binary strings ($k = 2$) of different lengths L and cross-reactivity threshold ε.

L	2^L	$\varepsilon = L$ C	N_m	$\varepsilon = L-1$ C	N_m	$\varepsilon = L-2$ C	N_m	$\varepsilon = L-3$ C	N_m
2	4	1	4	3	2	4	1	-----	-----
3	8	1	8	4	2	7	2	8	1
4	16	1	16	5	4	11	2	15	2
6	64	1	64	7	10	22	3	42	2
8	256	1	256	9	29	37	7	93	3
16	65536	1	65536	17	3856	137	479	697	95
32	4.30×10^9	1	4.30×10^9	33	1.30×10^8	529	8.12×10^6	5489	7.82×10^5
64	1.84×10^{19}	1	1.84×10^{19}	61	2.84×10^{17}	2081	8.86×10^{16}	43745	4.22×10^{14}

As one last aspect to be addressed in Hamming shape-spaces, one can consider the possibility of determining gradual degrees of affinity between molecules. In the discussion presented so far, an antigen was assumed to be recognized by an antibody if their affinity was greater than or equal to the cross-reactivity threshold, $D \geq \varepsilon$. This is illustrated in Figure 3.11(a), where $D \geq \varepsilon$ results in a *binding value b* of 1, $b = 1$.

To define a gradual binding value between two molecules proportionally to their affinity D, several *binding functions* can be adopted, such as the *sigmoid binding function* illustrated in Figure 3.11(b). In this case, for example, $\varepsilon = 5$ corresponds to the inflection point of the sigmoid. Thus, the binding between the two molecules has a strength $b = 0.5$. The decay of the squashing function of Figure 3.11(b) implies that a match score greater than the cross-reactivity threshold $\varepsilon = 5$ produces a high binding value, while a match score of 3, for example, corresponds to a binding value of approximately zero.

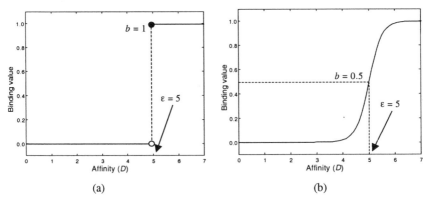

(a)   (b)

Figure 3.11.   Trade-off between the binding value and the affinity D for attribute strings of length $L = 7$ and cross-reactivity threshold $\varepsilon = 5$. (a) Threshold binding function. (b) Sigmoid binding function.

It is worth saying at this point, that the binding value is not necessarily limited to Hamming shape-spaces. If the affinity measure between two molecules is in a normalized range, this technique could be applied to Integer shape-spaces as well. In the case of real-valued shape-spaces, the result of the application of an affinity measure to a pair of strings is already a gradual ('fuzzy') number.

3.5.2. Algorithms and Processes

Given a suitable representation for the immune cells and molecules, and how to evaluate their interactions, it is now possible to present some general-purpose immune algorithms that model specific aspects of the immune system. This section outlines some computational procedures used to model varying immune mechanisms and theories that can be used as building blocks for engineering AIS. These algorithms are generic and can be applied to problem solving in different settings. Among them, it is possible to remark models of two major components (bone marrow and thymus) and of two distinct theories (clonal selection and immune network):

- *Bone marrow models*: used to generate repertoires of cells and molecules (Section 2.5);
- *Thymus models*: used to generate repertoires of cells and molecules capable of performing self/nonself discrimination (Section 2.10);
- *Clonal selection algorithms*: used to control how the components of the immune system interact with the external environment or antigens (Section 2.9); and
- *Immune network models*: used to simulate immune networks, including their structure, dynamics and metadynamics (Section 2.11).

The algorithms will be described in a high-level, outlining how the immune metaphors were used in their development, i.e., the mapping from the biological immune process to the computer algorithm. In Appendix II, pseudocode for the implementation of these algorithms are provided.

Bone Marrow Models

The bone marrow is the site responsible for the generation of all blood cells, including the lymphocytes. Bone marrow algorithms are considered to be the ones used to generate populations of immune cells and/or cell receptors for artificial immune systems.

The simplest bone marrow model simply generates attribute strings with length L using a (pseudo) random number generator. In the case of real-valued shape-spaces, one has to determine the interval in which m is going to be defined, e.g., $m \in [0,1]^L$. In the case of Hamming shape-spaces, the string that represents the molecule m must be randomly generated from elements belonging to a pre-defined alphabet, e.g., $m \in \{0,1\}$ for binary strings (bitstrings). In the case of Integer shape-spaces, an algorithm to perform a random permutation of L elements can be used.

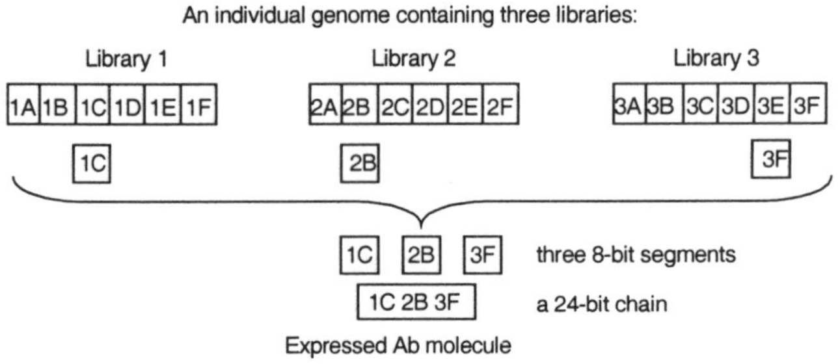

An individual genome containing three libraries:

Library 1	Library 2	Library 3
1A 1B 1C 1D 1E 1F	2A 2B 2C 2D 2E 2F	3A 3B 3C 3D 3E 3F
1C	2B	3F

1C 2B 3F   three 8-bit segments

1C 2B 3F   a 24-bit chain

Expressed Ab molecule

Figure 3.12. Construction/expression of an antibody molecule from gene libraries.

The most complex, and biologically appealing, bone marrow models demand the use of gene libraries from which the immune cells and molecules will be rearranged or evolved. In the case of antibodies, five libraries store the genes used to encode a molecule. Two of these libraries are used to generate the variable region of the light chain (V_L) and three libraries are used to generate the variable region of the heavy chain (V_H). The production of an antibody molecule occurs through the concatenation of different gene components randomly selected from each of the gene libraries.

Hightower *et al.* (1995), Perelson *et al.* (1996), and Oprea (1999) used a genetic algorithm to study the effects of evolution in the genetic encoding of antibody molecules. One characteristic of this encoding is that not all genes existent in the *genotype* (total collection of genes) are expressed in the *phenotype* (expressed antibody molecules). In these models, bitstrings representing the genotype of an individual are divided into libraries of gene segments to the generation of antibody molecules, as illustrated in Figure 3.12. In this example, each library contains six elements, represented by binary strings of length 8, such that each individual genome contains a total of 144 (48×3) bits. The expressed antibodies present a total length $L = 24$ ($3 \times 8 = 24$).

Similar models can be employed to simulate the bone marrow in the processes of repertoire generation. The number of libraries, the size of each gene segment, and the final length L of the molecules, may be user-defined and problem dependent. It is important to stress however, that the use of gene libraries inherently imposes a certain structure in the repertoire, like the kind of data being used (e.g., numeric, symbolic), and their domain (e.g., [1..10], {Monday, Tuesday,...}). If one component c is taken from each library, an AIS containing l libraries with c components each can produce c^l different antibody molecules (if each component has length 1), i.e., the potential antibody repertoire is composed of c^l molecules.

Thymus Models

As a primary lymphoid organ, the thymus plays an important role in the maturation of T-cells. Naïve (or immature) T-cells are originated in the bone marrow and migrate to the thymus where some of them differentiate into immunocompetent cells (positive selection), and others are purged from the repertoire due to a strong recognition of self-peptides/MHC complexes (negative selection). These processes of thymic positive and negative selection have to guarantee that the population of T-cells that leaves the thymus and goes to the periphery does not contain cells that recognize self-peptides at the same time that it is ready to be stimulated by a peptide presented by a self-MHC molecule.

Positive Selection Algorithms

The positive selection of T-cells stimulates and allows for the maturation of only those T-cells capable of recognizing the self-MHC molecules. This process generates MHC restriction, i.e., the property by which T-cells recognize antigens only if they are presented in the context of self-MHC molecules.

Seiden and Celada (1992) proposed a cellular automaton model to perform computer simulations of the immune system. This work was aimed basically at simulating an immune response, thus it does not qualify as an AIS according to the definition proposed in this book (Definition 3.4). However, it is felt that the positive selection algorithm proposed has interesting properties from a computational perspective.

Several types of components of the immune system were used in their simulations, such as B-cells, T-cells and antigen presenting cells (APCs). A T-cell was composed of a single binary attribute string (bitstring) of length L, representing its receptor. A B-cell contained a bitstring of length L representing its receptor, plus another bitstring of length L representing its MHC complex. The antigen presenting cells possessed only an MHC molecule. Examples of a B-cell, a T-cell, and an APC are illustrated in Figure 3.13. The role of the MHC molecules of APCs and B-cells was to present peptides (antigens) to T-cells. The MHC molecules were of same length as the receptors on B-cells and T-cells.

The idea of the algorithm is simple. T-cells can only recognize antigenic peptides presented by self-MHC molecules. Given the set of self-MHCs, named self-set **S**, the T-cell receptors will have to be tested for their capability of binding with these self-MHCs. If a T-cell cannot recognize at least one of the self-MHCs it is discarded, else it is selected as an immunocompetent cell and enters the available repertoire **A**.

The positive selection algorithm is illustrated in Figure 3.14 and can be summarized as follows:

1. *Initialization*: generate the *potential repertoire*, **P**, of immature T-cells. Assuming all molecules (receptors and MHCs) represented as binary strings of same length L, 2^L distinct cells are generated;
2. *Affinity evaluation*: determine the affinity of all elements in **P** with all elements of the self set **S**;

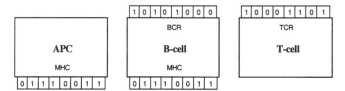

Figure 3.13.   Examples of an APC, a B-cell, and a T-cell for bitstrings of length $L = 8$.

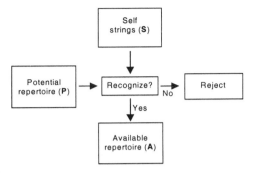

Figure 3.14.   The positive selection algorithm.

3. *Generation of the available repertoire*: if the affinity of an element of **P** with at least one MHC molecule is greater than or equal to a given cross-reactive threshold ε, then the T-cell recognizes this MHC, is positively selected and introduced into the system (available repertoire **A**); else the T-cell is eliminated.

Negative Selection Algorithms

The negative selection of T-cells is responsible for eliminating the T-cells whose receptors are capable of binding with self-peptides presented by self-MHC molecules. This process guarantees that the T-cells that leave the thymus do not recognize any self-cell or molecule.

Forrest *et al.* (1994) proposed a change detection algorithm inspired by the negative selection of T-cells within the thymus. This procedure was named *negative selection algorithm,* and its original application was in computational security. A single type of immune cell was modeled: T-cells represented as bitstrings of length *L*.

Like the positive selection algorithm of Seiden and Celada, the negative selection algorithm of Forrest and collaborators is simple. Given a set of self-peptides, named self-set **S**, the T-cell receptors will have to be tested for their capability of binding the self-peptides. If a T-cell recognizes a self-peptide it is discarded, else it is selected as an immunocompetent cell and enters the available repertoire **A**. The negative selection algorithm is illustrated in Figure 3.15 and can be summarized as follows:

1. *Initialization*: randomly generate strings and place them in a set **P** of immature T-cells. Assume all molecules (receptors and self-peptides) represented as binary strings of same length *L*;
2. *Affinity evaluation*: determine the affinity of all T-cells in **P** with all elements of the self set **S**;
3. *Generation of the available repertoire*: if the affinity of an immature T-cell (element of **P**) with at least one self-peptide is greater than or equal to a given cross-reactive threshold ε, then the T-cell recognizes this self-peptide and has to be eliminated (negative selection); else the T-cell is introduced into the available repertoire **A**.

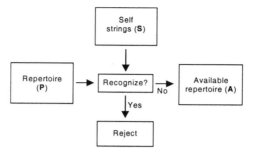

Figure 3.15.   The negative selection algorithm (reproduced with permission from [Forrest *et al.*, 1994]. © *IEEE 1994*).

Some Remarks on the Thymus Models

The algorithms presented have the property of being used to define an *available repertoire* of T-cells (attribute strings) to perform pattern recognition. In the positive selection case, the purpose of the algorithm is to recognize a set of known patterns. By contrast, in the negative selection case the algorithm aims at recognizing patterns that do not belong to a known set of patterns. This is an interesting aspect of the negative selection algorithm, once it performs pattern recognition by storing information about the complement set of the known patterns. Note that the difference between both algorithms is only philosophical; the set **S** of positive selection is composed of strings representing self-MHCs, while the set **S** of negative selection is composed of strings corresponding to self-peptides presented by self-MHCs.

In its original formulation, the positive selection algorithm evaluated recognition according to a cross-reactive threshold ε of the Hamming distance between strings, while the negative selection was based upon ε for the *r*-contiguous bit rule. Given an affinity measure, a pattern was assumed recognized if its affinity with at least one element of **P** was greater than or equal to ε for the affinity measures chosen. Although both mechanisms employed a binary Hamming shape-space and specific affinity measures, it is possible to use different types of shape-spaces and/or affinity measures.

The process of generating the available repertoire in the negative selection algorithm was termed *censoring phase* by the authors. The algorithm is also composed of a *monitoring phase*. In the monitoring phase, a set **S*** of protected strings is matched against the elements of the available repertoire **A**. The set **S*** might be the own set **S**, a completely new set, or composed of elements of **S**. If a recognition occurs, then a nonself pattern (string) is detected. This procedure can also be used as a second step in the positive selection algorithm of Seiden and Celada. In this case, the pattern detected corresponds to a self-element (self-MHC), instead of a nonself. Figure 3.16 illustrates the generic censoring phase for the thymus models, as introduced by Forrest *et al.* (1994).

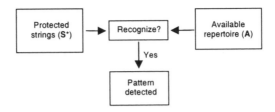

Figure 3.16.   The generic monitoring phase for the thymic positive and negative selection algorithms (reproduced with permission from [Forrest *et al.*, 1994]. © *IEEE, 1994*).

In the positive selection algorithm, the authors suggested the generation of the whole *potential repertoire*, which corresponds to 2^L elements for binary strings, in the set **P**. This is only feasible, from a computational perspective, because the authors used bitstrings of length $L = 8$ in their implementations. In real-valued shape-spaces, for example, the potential repertoire is of infinite size. In contrast, the negative selection algorithm suggests the random generation of strings, until an available repertoire **A** of appropriate size is generated. This approach could be adopted in both algorithms.

Even the random generation of the repertoire **P** results in algorithms with some drawbacks. First, this approach results in an exponential cost to generate the available repertoire **A** in relation to the number of self strings in **S**. Second, randomly generating **P** does not account for any adaptability in the algorithm and neither any information contained in the set **S**.

In order to alleviate the exponential cost of generating **A**, D'haeseleer *et al.* (1996) proposed two novel detector-generating algorithms that run in linear time with respect to the size of the self set. The authors also discussed how to set parameters for the algorithms, such as repertoire sizes, probabilities of match and failure in change detection, and other practical issues. Another approach to the generation of **A** was presented by Wierzchón (2000a,b).

Dasgupta and Niño (2000) compared the performance of the negative selection algorithm with a positive selection algorithm. Nevertheless, the system they proposed to perform positive selection was simply an ART neural network. No specific positive selection algorithm was introduced. Under their perspective, any algorithm that models (or approximates) the input patterns can be considered a positive selection algorithm. As examples it is possible to suggest artificial neural networks and fuzzy models as positive selection algorithms.

This approach, although lacking the immune inspiration, is none the less interesting. This is because it addresses the second problem of the random generation of **P**: the adaptability and use of information contained in **S**. It is possible to suggest, however, adaptive strategies that do not rely upon other computational intelligence approaches (such as ANN). For example, one can generate a set **P** of a given size and match the elements of **P** against those of **S**. Assume as the stopping criterion a pre-defined number of elements in **A**. If positive selection is being simulated, the algorithm could run as follows:

1. Select the elements of **P** that do not recognize any element of **S** and place them in a set **U** of unmatched elements;
2. For each element of **U**, perform a guided mutation (see next section for mutation) such that its affinity with the unrecognized element of **S** that best matches it is increased;
3. When their affinity is greater than the cross-reactive threshold, add this new element of **U** to the set **A** and return to Step 2.

With few modifications, this algorithm can also be used in combination with negative selection.

Finally, the positive selection algorithm presented, though based upon a model that contains different types of cells and molecules, does not account for this variety. The algorithm summarized in Figure 3.14 assumes a single type of cell, such as in the negative selection case. However, the use of different cell types, such as APCs, B-cells, and T-cells, gives the algorithm an enhanced flexibility. For example, if the B-cells and T-cells models presented in Figure 3.13 were used, two different types of pattern recognizers would be available: a B-cell type and a T-cell type. The B-cells would have receptors capable of recognizing any pattern (free antigen) and also, to present specific patterns to T-cells. As the T-cells will suffer positive selection in thymus, which will restrict them to the MHCs of the B-cells (self-MHCs), the T-cells would only be capable of recognizing specific patterns that match the MHCs of B-cells. This way, B-cells would be more general cells to recognize antigens and to present peptides to T-cells, while the T-cells would be capable of recognizing specific patterns (peptides).

Seiden and Celada (1992) also proposed a negative thymic selection algorithm for their cellular automata model of the immune system. This algorithm was implemented in conjunction with the positive selection described previously, but as it involved the presentation of self-peptides by MHC molecules, it will not be discussed here. In essence, it works exactly in the same way as the negative selection algorithm presented.

Clonal Selection Algorithms

Clonal selection is the name of the theory used to explain how the adaptive immune system copes with pathogenic microorganisms. It is valid for B- and T-cells, with the difference that B-cells suffer somatic hypermutation during proliferation and T-cells do not. As the B-cells' case involves adaptability via mutation, it is the one usually modeled by the AIS community and, thus, will be discussed here.

In brief, when a B-cell receptor (antibody) recognizes a nonself antigen with a certain affinity, it is selected to proliferate, and it produces antibodies in high volumes. Proliferation in the case of immune cells is asexual, a mitotic process; the cells divide themselves (there is no crossover). During reproduction, the B-cell progenies (clones) undergo a mutation process with high rates (*hypermutation*) that, together with a strong selective pressure, result in B-cells with antigenic receptors presenting higher affinities with the selective antigen (mutation will be discussed in the next section). This whole process of mutation and selection is known as *affinity maturation of the immune response* and is analogous to the natural selection of species, as will be discussed in Section 5.6. In addition to differentiating into antibody producing cells, the activated B-cells with high antigenic affinities are selected to become memory cells with long life spans. These memory cells are pre-eminent in future responses to this same antigenic pattern, or a similar one. Important features of clonal selection from the viewpoint of computation are:

- An antigen selects several immune cells to proliferate. The proliferation rate of each immune cell is proportional to its affinity with the selective antigen: the higher the affinity, the higher the number of offspring generated, and vice-versa;
- The mutation suffered by each immune cell during reproduction is inversely proportional to the affinity of the cell receptor with the antigen: the higher the affinity, the smaller the mutation, and vice-versa.

Some authors (e.g., Forrest *et al.*, 1993) have argued that a genetic algorithm (Section 6.3) without crossover is a reasonable model of clonal selection. However, the standard genetic algorithm does not account for the two important immune properties listed above: affinity proportional reproduction and mutation. Other authors (de Castro & Von Zuben, 2000a) proposed a clonal selection algorithm, named CLONALG, to fulfill these basic processes involved in clonal selection. This algorithm is evolutionary in nature, and it was initially proposed to perform pattern recognition and then adapted to solve multi-modal function optimization tasks. Given a set of patterns to be recognized (**S**), the basic steps of the CLONALG algorithm are as follows:

1. *Initialization*: create an initial random population of individuals (**P**);
2. *Antigenic presentation*: for each antigenic pattern, do:
   - 2.1. *Affinity evaluation*: present it to the population **P** and determine its affinity with each element of the population **P**;
   - 2.2. *Clonal selection and expansion*: select n_1 highest affinity elements of **P** and generate clones of these individuals proportionally to their affinity with the antigen: the higher the affinity, the higher the number of copies, and vice-versa;
   - 2.3. *Affinity maturation*: mutate all these copies with a rate inversely proportional to their affinity with the input pattern: the higher the affinity, the smaller the mutation rate, and vice-versa. Add these mutated individuals to the population **P** and re-select the best individual to be kept as the memory **m** of the antigen presented;
   - 2.4. *Metadynamics*: replace a number n_2 of individuals with low affinity by (randomly generated) new ones;
3. *Cycle*: repeat Step 2 until a certain stopping criterion is met.

The elements of matrix **M**, composed of all **m**, are part of the set **P** (**M** $\subseteq$ **P**) with the difference that they are only replaced by elements of higher affinity. This process, together with the affinity proportional mutation, promotes a greedy search of the affinity landscape.

One difference between the pattern recognition (PR) and the optimization (OPT) versions of the clonal selection algorithm is that the PR version assumes a set **S** of patterns to be recognized, while the OPT version assumes a function $f(\cdot)$ to be optimized; each element of **P** corresponds to a value of the function $f(\cdot)$.

The authors suggested that this algorithm can naturally solve multi-modal optimization tasks by simply selecting all elements of **P** to proliferate with equal probability, $n_1 = N$, where N is the number of cells in the repertoire. The proliferation rate in this situation is not proportional to affinity, only the mutation rate. This procedure gives all the peaks of the affinity landscape equal opportunities to be climbed and alleviates the computational cost of the algorithm by eliminating Step 3.

Some Remarks on the Clonal Selection Algorithm

By comparing CLONALG with the evolutionary algorithms (EAs), to be described in Section 6.3, it is possible to note that the main steps composing the EAs are embodied in CLONALG, allowing it to be characterized as an evolutionary-like strategy. However, while evolutionary algorithms use a vocabulary borrowed from natural genetics and inspired by the neo-Darwinian theory of evolution, the clonal selection algorithm described makes use of the shape-space formalism, along with immunological terminology, to describe antigen-antibody interactions and cellular evolution. The CLONALG performs its search through the mechanisms of somatic mutation (Step 4) and receptor editing (Step 6), balancing the exploitation of the best solutions with the exploration of the search-space. Essentially, its encoding scheme is not different from that of evolutionary algorithms; this will depend on the shape-space adopted.

Another important aspect of CLONALG, when compared with the EAs, is the fact that it takes into account the cell affinity, corresponding to the fitness of the individuals, in order to define the proliferation and mutation rates to be applied to each member of the population. The *evolution strategies* and *evolutionary programming* (see Chapter 6) techniques also employ self-adapting parameters, but based on a mathematical framework they are very distinct from the immunologically inspired mechanism used by CLONALG. Nevertheless, CLONALG is indeed a particular type of evolutionary algorithm, but inspired by the immune clonal selection principle.

Affinity Maturation

The process of affinity maturation plays an important role in an adaptive immune response. It is responsible for the selection and genetic variation of those B-cells bearing receptors capable of recognizing antigenic stimuli. The receptors (antibody molecules) of the selected B-cells will have their genetic composition (shapes) altered through a process of somatic mutation with high rates or hypermutation.

Based upon the shape-space approach proposed to model the antibody molecules, the representation of an immune component is similar to the representation used for the chromosomes of an evolutionary algorithm (Section 6.3). Thus, the same mechanisms of selection and mutation can be used for both strategies. The selection procedures are general and applicable to any type of shape-space, but the mutation operators are classified according to the shape-space under study.

There is a difference between the evolutionary theory of species, which gave birth to the evolutionary algorithms, and the maturation of immune cell receptors. In the former, mutation is usually believed to be a random process with low rates, while in the latter mutation is proportional to the antibody affinity with the selective antigen, has high rates on average, and is sometimes believed to be guided by antigens. This way, the somatic hypermutation of B-cells is a controlled, instead of a random, process. Section 5.6 points out how the natural selection of species is related to the mechanisms of genetic variation plus selection in the immune system.

This section discusses some selection and mutation mechanisms commonly employed in evolutionary algorithms. For a deeper analysis and other selection and mutation procedures of evolutionary algorithms the interested reader might refer to (Bäck *et al.*, 2000). The selection procedures will be presented in a general form, and the mutation mechanisms will be classified according to the shape-space used. The section is concluded discussing some forms of implementing the affinity proportional mutation.

Selection Mechanisms

The selection of cells for cloning in the immune system is proportional to their affinities with the selective antigens. Thus, implementing an affinity proportionate selection can be performed probabilistically using an algorithm like the *roulette wheel* selection, to be discussed in Section 6.3. Other evolutionary selection mechanisms can be used, such as *elitist selection, rank-based selection, bi-classist selection*, and *tournament selection*. These can be implemented as follows.

In *elitist selection*, the best or a number of best individuals (B-cells and/or antibodies) are always maintained in the repertoire. *Rank-based selection* assigns a reproduction (cloning) or survival probability to each individual proportionally to the rank ordering of the individuals in the current repertoire. In the *bi-classist selection*, a number $b\%$ of the best individuals and a number $w\%$ of the worst individuals of the repertoire are selected; the remaining individuals are selected randomly. Finally, in the *tournament selection* a group of q individuals are selected randomly from the repertoire. This group takes part in a tournament; that is, a winning individual is determined depending on its affinity. The best individual having the highest affinity is usually chosen deterministically and inserted in the repertoire of the next generation. This process is repeated a number of times.

Somatic Mutation for Hamming, Integer, and Symbolic Shape-Spaces

Somatic hypermutation has two important roles in an adaptive immune response. First, it is responsible for promoting and maintaining repertoire diversity. Second, associated with a strong selective process, it increases the affinity of the B-cell receptors (antibodies) in relation to the selective stimuli. Somatic hypermutation is only observed in B-cell receptors and not in TCRs.

In the case of Hamming shape-spaces, a position in the string can be randomly chosen, and its element changed for another one from the alphabet k. Figure 3.17 illustrates single- and multi-point mutations for bitstrings and strings from an alphabet of size $k = 4$. This type of mutation is called *random mutation* because it allows the random choice of an element of the set of possible attributes for the alphabet k and inserts it in the place of the current attribute value.

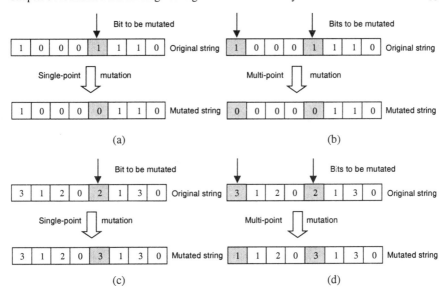

Figure 3.17.　Examples of specific mutations for Hamming shape-spaces. (a) Single-point mutation for binary strings. (b) Multi-point mutation for binary strings. (c,d) Single-point and multi-point mutations, respectively, for a Hamming shape-space with $k = \{0,1,2,3\}$. The values on the mutated strings were chosen randomly from the set k.

An Integer shape-space may be treated as a Hamming shape-space in cases where the size of the alphabet is reduced. If the elements of the strings suffer any sort of restriction, e.g., they cannot be repeated in the string, it is possible to propose specific mutation operators. For example, when an attribute cannot be repeated, one might choose pairs of attributes and inverse their positions, as illustrated in Figure 3.18. This process is called *inversive mutation* and might occur between one or more pairs of attributes. An attribute in the start (at the end) of the string might also be changed by the attribute at the end (in the start) of the string.

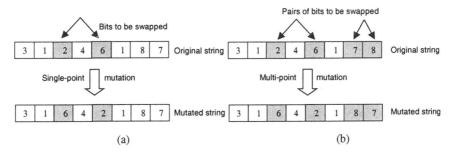

Figure 3.18.　Mutations for the Integer shape-space. (a) Single-point inversive mutation. (b) Multi-point inversive mutation.

The Symbolic shape-spaces can be dealt with in a similar manner as an Integer shape-space, with the difference lying in the types of each attribute and their respective boundaries. Assume the shape-space of Figure 3.5 as an example. This shape-space is composed of the following attributes: *description, date, flight, country, from, to,* and *price.* Each of these attributes might have its value bounded by a given domain. Suppose the attribute *country* was selected to be mutated and that the domain of this attribute is composed of the following elements {Brazil, U.K., U.S.A.}. If antibody Ab_1 is going to be mutated, then its attribute country might be changed to U.K. or U.S.A.

Somatic Mutation for Real-Valued Shape-Spaces

Mutating real-valued attribute strings (vectors) has the same essence as mutating the other types of strings, i.e., a change is made in one or more of the attributes, but it has to respect the upper and lower limits of each attribute (vector coordinate).

In *inductive mutation,* a random number to be added to a given attribute is generated. A common mutation operator for real-valued vectors in evolutionary algorithms is *Gaussian mutation.* The Gaussian mutation alters all the attributes of a string according to the following expression:

$$m' = m + \alpha(D)\, N(0,\sigma), \tag{3.10}$$

where $m = \langle m_1, m_2, ..., m_L \rangle$ is the attribute string, m' its mutated version, $\alpha(D)$ is a function that accounts for the affinity proportional mutation (see next section), and $N(0,\sigma)$ is a vector of independent Gaussian random variables of zero mean and standard deviation σ.

In the *uniform mutation* case, an attribute m_a, $a \in \{1,...,L\}$, of the string $m = \langle m_1,...,m_a,...,m_L \rangle$, is chosen randomly and a new string $m' = \langle m_1,...,m_a',..., m_L \rangle$ is generated. The new attribute m_a' is a random number (with uniform probability distribution) sampled over the interval $[LB,UB]$, where LB and UB are the lower and upper bounds of the variable m_a, respectively.

Affinity Proportional Mutation Rates

From the viewpoint of evolution, a remarkable characteristic of the affinity maturation process is its controlled nature. That is to say the hypermutation rate to be applied to every immune cell receptor is proportional to its antigenic affinity. By computationally simulating this process, one can produce powerful algorithms that perform a search akin to local search around each candidate solution. The previously reviewed mutations borrowed from evolutionary algorithms do not account for this important aspect of the mutation in the immune system: it is inversely proportional to the antigenic affinity.

As an example, assume an artificial immune system to perform multi-modal function optimization was developed. Each candidate solution (an attribute string in a given shape-space) has an independent mutation rate in proportion to its affinity with the optima solutions. Thus, candidates in higher peaks of the affinity landscape will be subject to smaller mutation rates while candidates located far from optima solutions will suffer larger mutation rates. One problem with this approach is that, usually, nothing is known a priori about the optima solutions of a problem. In this case, one can evaluate the relative affinity of each candidate solution by scaling (normalizing) their affinities. The inverse of an exponential function can be used to establish a relationship between the hypermutation rate $\alpha(\cdot)$ and the normalized affinity D^*, as described in Equation (3.11) and depicted in Figure 3.19. In some cases it might be interesting to re-scale α to an interval such as $[0..0.1]$.

$$\alpha(D^*) = \exp(-\rho D^*), \tag{3.11}$$

where ρ is a parameter that controls the smoothness of the inverse exponential, and D^* is the normalized affinity, that can be determined by $D^* = D/D_{max}$.

If complementarity is being taken into account, that is if higher affinities correspond to higher distances, then any function that determines the mutation rate α as being inversely proportional to the affinity can be used in its calculation.

In Section 2.9 it was illustrated that learning according to clonal selection involves raising the population (clone) size and affinity of the antibodies that are selected by a given antigen. Based upon this fact, Kepler and Perelson (1993a,b) proposed a control strategy for the affinity maturation of an immune response. They suggested that the maturation of the humoral immune response by somatic hypermutation is marked by a rapid and dramatic increase in affinity for the eliciting antigen. An optimal mutation schedule would be the one in which periods of rapid mutation alternate with periods of mutation free growth. In their optimal solution, the population is allowed to grow as quickly as possible without mutation until the clone size is large enough to ensure the appearance of one advantageous mutation, and then it is turned off, so that the new high affinity mutants can grow in size. Figure 3.20 depicts a hypothetical simulation behavior of a controlling schedule for the mutation rate, similar to the one proposed by Kepler and Perelson (1993a,b). Notice that in this picture the iterations correspond to a time scale that could be the order of hours or days. The quantitative events are not relevant for the development of AIS, but the qualitative behavior is.

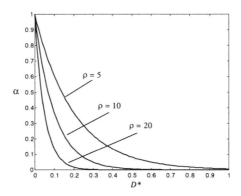

Figure 3.19. Trade-off between the normalized antibody affinity D^* and its mutation rate α, according to Equation (3.11), for different values of ρ.

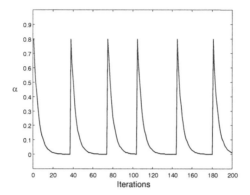

Figure 3.20.   Hypothetical schedule of the mutation rate (normalized over the [0,0.8] interval) similar to the process proposed by Kepler and Perelson (1993a,b).

3.5.3. Immune Network Models

There is a distinguishing difference between the clonal selection principle and the immune network theory. The former proposes an immune system originally at rest and only stimulated when invaded by a foreign antigen, and the latter suggests that the immune system presents a dynamic behavior (activity) even in the absence of external stimulus. The immune network theory is based on the premise that the B-cell receptors (antibodies) have some portions, called idiotopes, that can be recognized by other free antibodies or receptors attached to cells. This capability of recognizing and being recognized by other elements of the immune system endows it with an intrinsic dynamic behavior.

When Jerne proposed the philosophical aspects of the functioning of an immune network (Jerne, 1974a), no formal model of its behavior was presented. As argued by himself "The weakness of this incipient network theory lies in its lack of precision". Several issues remained open, such as how to define if the interaction of two elements is going to be suppressive or stimulatory. After little time, he proposed the first model for his network theory (Jerne, 1974b). Following his work, several other attempts originated from the theoretical immunology community in order to model the network proposal. Among these theoretical models, two are the most relevant for the research on artificial immune systems: the model by Farmer and collaborators (Farmer *et al.*, 1986) that marked the beginning of the field and the model by Varela and Coutinho (1991) that attempted to describe network features such as structure, dynamics, and metadynamics.

These *continuous network models* based on differential equations were successfully applied to several complex problems like autonomous navigation, optimization, and automatic control. They also served as good sources of inspiration for the development of the *discrete immune network models*, based upon a set of difference equations or iterative procedures of adaptation. The following sections review some influential works of both classes of networks: continuous and discrete.

Continuous Models

The Pioneer Model of N. K. Jerne

In his pioneer model, Jerne (1974b) attempted to put his theoretical network proposal into mathematical terms. A differential equation was constructed to describe the dynamics of a set of identical lymphocytes. Identical lymphocytes correspond, in this case, to cells that are indistinguishable with respect to their states of differentiation, as well as to their receptors (antibodies). The identical lymphocytes were called lymphocytes of type i, and c_i, $i = 1,...N_1$, denoted the concentration (number) of lymphocytes of this type. Lymphocytes of type i interact with other types of cells and molecules, e.g., lymphocytes of type j, and antibodies of type j via idiotopes and combining sites. Similarly, lymphocytes of type j interact with other types of lymphocytes and these with others and so on. These interactions could be either excitatory or inhibitory. It was argued that the interaction of different types of lymphocytes would naturally result in a dynamic network of lymphocytes. Jerne proposed the following equation to control the rate at which lymphocytes of a particular type vary in number

$$\frac{dc_i}{dt} = c_i \sum_{j=1}^{N_1} f(E_j, K_j, t) - c_i \sum_{j=1}^{N_2} g(I_j, K_j, t) + k_1 - k_2 c_i, \qquad (3.12)$$

where k_1 is the rate at which lymphocytes enter the set i, and k_2 is the rate (per lymphocyte) at which the lymphocytes die or leave the set. The functions $f(\cdot)$ and $g(\cdot)$ are used to track the excitatory and inhibitory signals produced within the network. The first sum is over all excitatory signals generated by idiotopes in the sets E_j that are recognized with association constants K_j by the combining sites on lymphocytes of type i. The second sum is over the inhibitory interactions generated by lymphocytes in sets I_j whose combining sites recognize idiotopes on cells of type i.

An important aspect of this model is that a further term would be required to account for an external invader (antigen). A differential equation of the type of Equation (3.12) was needed for each network element (lymphocytes and antibodies) and would be responsible for governing the number of excitatory and inhibitory lymphocytes in each set. Thus, no antigen was required for the network to present a dynamic behavior.

The Model of J. D. Farmer and Collaborators

Farmer *et al.* (1986, 1987) proposed bitstring models for the immune network theory. Their works are of extreme importance, as they constituted the first attempts to bring together mathematical theoretical immunology and computational intelligence paradigms. As in Jerne's work, their model consisted of a set of differential equations to quantify the dynamics of the components of the immune network.

In this model, immune cells and molecules were represented as binary strings of various lengths in a Hamming shape-space, as illustrated in Figure 3.21. An antibody molecule was represented by its *epitope* (*e*) and *paratope* (*p*) concatenated into a single bitstring. As the epitope is the portion of the antibody molecule that can be recognized by its paratope, this is termed *idiotope* (*i*) within the immune network context.

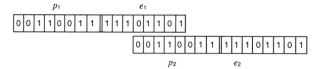

Figure 3.21.   Bitstrings represent the epitope (or idiotope) and paratope of antibody molecules.

Strings were allowed to match complementarily in any possible alignment, modeling the fact that two molecules may react in more than one way. Equation (3.13) specifies the *matrix of matching specificities* $m_{i,j}$ (compare Equation (3.13) with Equation (3.4), and refer to Figure 3.8).

$$m_{i,j} = \sum_k G\left(\left(\sum_n e_i(n+k) \wedge p_j(n)\right) - \varepsilon + 1\right), \qquad (3.13)$$

where $e_i(n)$ is the n-th bit of the i-th epitope, $p_j(n)$ is the n-th bit of the j-th paratope, $\wedge$ corresponds to the Hamming distance between $e_i(\cdot)$ and $p_j(\cdot)$, given by Equation (3.3), and ε corresponds to the cross-reactivity threshold. The parameter k corresponds to a given alignment between a paratope and an epitope. If matches occur in more than one alignment, their strengths are summed, as in the case of Figure 3.10. This includes the case of strings with different lengths. The function $G(\cdot)$ measures the strength of a possible reaction between an epitope and a paratope as given by Equation (3.14).

$$G(x) = \begin{cases} x & x > 0 \\ 0 & \text{otherwise} \end{cases}. \qquad (3.14)$$

Note that what the authors defined as the matrix of specificities is a function of the affinity measure evaluated over the interactions of all the components of the system. In this model, the recognition of an epitope by a paratope results in the reproduction of the antibody with the paratope (stimulation), and the probabilistic elimination of the antibody with the epitope (suppression). No distinction between B-cell receptors and free antibodies was made.

To model the network dynamics, it was assumed N antibody types with concentrations, $\{c_1,...,c_N\}$ and M antigens with concentrations $\{y_1,...,y_M\}$. The rate of change of antibody concentration is given by

$$\frac{dc_i}{dt} = k_1\left[\sum_{j=1}^{N} m_{j,i}c_ic_j - k_2\sum_{j=1}^{N} m_{i,j}c_ic_j + \sum_{j=1}^{M} m_{j,i}c_iy_j\right] - k_3c_i, \qquad (3.15)$$

where the first term represents the stimulation of the paratope of an antibody type i by the epitope of an antibody type j. The second term represents the suppression of antibody of type i when its epitope is recognized by the paratope of type j. The parameter k_1 is a rate constant that depends on the number of collisions per unit time and the rate of antibody production stimulated by a collision. Constant k_2 represents a possible inequality between stimulation and suppression. The third term of Equation (3.15) models the antigen concentrations and the last term models the tendency of cells to die (natural death rate, k_3). An expression to quantify change in antigen concentration was given in (Farmer *et al.*, 1987) according to Equation (3.16). This equation describes the elimination of antigens from the system.

$$\frac{dy_i}{dt} = -k_4 \sum_{j=1}^{M} m_{j,i} c_j y_i,$$

(3.16)

where k_4 is an arbitrary constant.

Equations (3.12) to (3.16) are used to control the dynamics (adaptability) of the system. This is in the sense that antibodies that recognize antigens or other antibodies are amplified, whereas antibodies that do not are eliminated. Additionally, antigens that are recognized are also eliminated. The production of novel antibodies provides the system with the ability to cope with unexpected (or unseen) antigens.

An essential characteristic of this model is its metadynamics. That is the repertoires of antibodies and antigens are dynamic, changing as new elements are added to or removed from the network. To perform this, the authors used a minimum threshold on all concentrations, so that an element is eliminated when its concentration falls below the threshold. The new antibody types were generated by applying genetic operators to the bitstrings, such as crossover, inversion, and point mutations.

The Model of F. Varela and A. Coutinho

The model proposed by F. Varela and A. Coutinho (1991) was named *second-generation immune network*. The authors emphasized three remarkable characteristics of the immune networks: their structure, dynamics, and metadynamics. The network *structure* describes the patterns of connectivity among the network elements. The immune *dynamics* account for the variation with time of the concentrations and affinities of cells and molecules comprising the network. The *metadynamics* property of the immune system addresses the continuous production and recruitment of novel elements and death of non-stimulated or self-reactive elements.

The mathematical formulation of a second-generation immune network model can be described as follows. Each of the N types of elements in the repertoire is indexed by i. Each idiotype exists either cell-bound $b_i(t)$ or free in amounts $f_i(t)$. The affinity between an idiotype of type i and an idiotype of type j is denoted by $m_{i,j}$, and the network sensitivity (σ_i) for the i-th idiotype is given by

$$\sigma_i(t) = \sum_{j=1}^{N} m_{j,i} f_j.$$

(3.17)

Free antibodies are produced as a result of the maturation of specific B-cells. The probability of B-cell maturation depends on the degree of connectivity of a given idiotype with the current network configuration, i.e., it depends on its sensitivity (Equation (3.17)), according to a double threshold function, as the one illustrated in Figure 3.22. Note the similarity with the function presented in Figure 2.19.

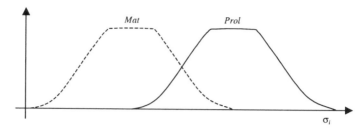

Figure 3.22. Maturation (*Mat*) and proliferation (*Prol*) functions.

A differential equation is proposed to describe the dynamics of the free molecules, i.e., change in the antibody concentration, as follows:

$$\frac{df_i}{dt} = k_1 b_i Mat(\sigma_i) + k_2 f_i \sigma_i - k_3 f_i, \tag{3.18}$$

where k_1, k_2 and k_3 are arbitrary constants, b_i represents the bound molecules, and $Mat(\cdot)$ is the lymphocyte maturation function that assumes a shape similar to the one depicted in Figure 3.22.

Correspondingly, the change in concentration of the molecules attached to B-cells b_i decays at a given rate and proliferates to an extent that depends on their degree of network connectivity. This is also a double-threshold function $Prol(\cdot)$ shifted from the one that regulates the probability of maturation, as illustrated in Figure 3.22. A last term $Meta[i]$ is added to include cells that are recruited from a resting pool into the active network:

$$\frac{db_i}{dt} = k_4 b_i Prol(\sigma_i) + Meta[i] - k_5 b_i. \tag{3.19}$$

The maturation $Mat(\cdot)$ and proliferation $Prol(\cdot)$ functions are bell-shaped in order to simulate low-zone and high-zone tolerance, suggesting that both insufficient and excessive receptor interactions lead to the retention of the cell in the inactive state, i.e., network tolerance.

Some Philosophical and Practical Remarks

The models of N. Jerne and F. Varela do not take into account the presence of foreign perturbation in the system, i.e., foreign antigens. In contrast, the model proposed by Farmer introduces not only a term in the differential equation describing the network dynamics, but also proposes an independent term to simulate the dynamics of the antigen population. This might be due to the fact that Jerne's and Varela's aims were mainly related to issues like pre-immune repertoire selection, internal lymphocyte activities, tolerance, and self/nonself discrimination. Their theories were supposed to complement clonal selection, used mainly to explain immune responses to foreign antigens. The Farmer's network model, on the other hand, was more of a computational intelligence paradigm. Thus, it addressed an immune system capable of interacting with the internal and external environments under the format of a network.

In terms of notation, Farmer's model was the only one to explicitly propose a specific representation (binary Hamming shape-space) for the components of the immune system. The other models presented the equations of motion but did not specify any type of representation. In essence, the lymphocyte types of Jerne's network, the antibody types of Farmer's model, and the idiotypes of Varela's network are equivalent. In all cases the terminology is related with the portions of the surface receptor molecules (bound as cell receptors or free as antibodies) that can recognize and/or be recognized by other molecules.

The network approach is particularly interesting for the development of computational tools because it naturally provides an account of emergent properties such as learning, memory, self-tolerance, size and diversity of cell populations, and network interactions with the environment and the self components. In general terms, the structure of most network models can be described similarly to the way suggested by Perelson (1989):

$$\begin{matrix} \text{Rate of} \\ \text{population} \\ \text{variation} \end{matrix} = \begin{matrix} \text{Network} \\ \text{stimulation} \end{matrix} - \begin{matrix} \text{Network} \\ \text{suppression} \end{matrix} + \begin{matrix} \text{Influx} \\ \text{of new} \\ \text{elements} \end{matrix} - \begin{matrix} \text{Death of} \\ \text{unstimulated} \\ \text{elements} \end{matrix} \qquad \textbf{(3.20)}$$

The first two terms of Equation (3.20) are related to the immune network dynamics, while the last two terms correspond to the immune metadynamics. The network activation embodies the stimulation of a paratope by an idiotope on another antibody or an antigenic epitope. The network suppression is a result of an idiotope being recognized by a paratope.

Discrete Models

In contrast to the continuous models, the discrete immune networks are based upon difference equations and/or iterative procedures of adaptation that govern the behavior of the network. These models were mainly developed as artificial immune systems and, as such, were aimed at problem solving. Continuous immune network models, however, are based on ordinary differential equations (ODEs) designed to simulate the immune system. These ODEs have the difficulty that it is not always possible to find an analytical solution for them, and often, numerical integration has to be used to study the behavior of the system.

Two other important features can be highlighted when comparing discrete with continuous network models. The discrete networks are usually adaptive not only in their number of elements, but also in the structure of these elements. This means that the cells and molecules of a discrete immune network can increase or decrease in number and also can change their 'shapes' (attribute strings), in shape-space, in order to improve their affinities. The other feature is that as the discrete networks are aimed at problem solving, they naturally address the interactions with the external environment (antigens), while some of the continuous models simply disregard antigenic stimulation.

Here, the learning algorithms for two discrete immune network models are discussed. They were originally developed for pattern recognition, data clustering, and data compression. However, these learning algorithms are generic and can be applied to other domains such as optimization, control, and robotics. In order to describe these generic learning algorithms, the descriptions will be restricted to the pattern recognition case, continually reflecting on the immune network metaphor.

According to the network theory proposed by Jerne (1974a) the immune system is composed of a network whose dynamics is disturbed by foreign antigens. This interaction with foreign antigens results in a network that corresponds to an *internal image* of the universe of antigens. Within the immune networks, groups of cells and molecules correspond to antigenic groups. There are basically two levels of interactions in the network: 1) the interaction with the environment (foreign antigens) and 2) the interaction with other network elements.

The two network learning algorithms to be presented constitute distinct approaches aimed at capturing the basic features of the immune network theory from a computational intelligence perspective. Each learning algorithm can be used to construct an artificial immune network capable of extracting information from a set of input patterns that corresponds to the antigenic universe. For both algorithms, B-cells and antibodies (Ab) are the main elements of the immune networks, and antigens (Ag) correspond to the input patterns.

The Algorithm of J. Timmis and Collaborators

Timmis (2000) proposed an immune network learning algorithm named RAIN (*Resource limited Artificial Immune Network*). Each network element corresponds to a B-cell composed of an antibody (e.g., an attribute string in an Euclidean shape-space), a stimulation level, and a record of the number of *resources* held. A resource allocation mechanism is used to control B-cell population and will be discussed later. The network antibodies are initialized by randomly taking a sub-section of the input patterns (Ag), and the stimulation level and record of resources are all initialized to zero.

The next stage is the presentation of the antigenic patterns. Each pattern is presented to each network cell and the stimulation level s_i is determined after presenting all antigens to the cell i, according to Equation (3.21).

$$s_i = \sum_{j=1}^{M}(1 - D_{i,j}) + \sum_{k=1}^{n}(1 - D_{i,k}) - \sum_{k=1}^{n}D_{i,k}, \qquad (3.21)$$

where M is the number of antigens, n is the number of connected B-cells, $D_{i,j}$ is the Euclidean distance (Equation (3.1)) between each antigen j and the B-cell i, and $D_{i,k}$ is the Euclidean distance between the cell i and a B-cell k to which it is connected. Note that $(1 - D_{i,j})$ corresponds to the affinity of a B-cell with antigens or other B-cells in the network. In this case, affinity is inversely proportional to distance.

The stimulation level determines which cells are selected for expansion (*clonal expansion*) and which cells are removed from the network (*metadynamics*). In order to decide which cells are to be maintained within the network, a resource allocation mechanism is employed. There are a predefined maximum number of resources in the network, for which each B-cell must compete. Each B-cell is allocated a number of resources in proportion to its stimulation level: the higher the stimulation level, the higher the number of resources allocated. If the number of resources allocated is greater than the maximum number allowed, then the B-cells that hold the least number of resources are removed from the network. This is repeated until the number of resources allocated is less than or equal to the maximum number allowed.

Some of the remaining network cells will be selected for clonal expansion based upon their stimulation level: the higher the stimulation the higher the probability of cloning. Those cells selected for cloning also reproduce in proportion to their stimulation level: the higher the stimulation level the higher the number of clones to be produced.

Affinity maturation allows selected network cells to adapt their antibodies to the antigenic pattern presented. Each antibody is mutated inversely proportional to its B-cell stimulation level: the higher the stimulation the lower the mutation rate. Finally, the mutated clones are matched against all network cells and their affinity is calculated. If their affinity falls below a given threshold, they are linked together.

These processes are repeated until either a fixed number of iterations is performed, or the network reaches a period of stability, i.e., the number of network B-cells remains constant over a given period of time.

The network learning algorithm can be summarized as follows:

1. *Initialization*: create an initial network out of a sub-section of the antigens;
2. *Antigenic presentation*: for each antigenic pattern, do:
    2.1 *Clonal selection and network interactions*: for each network cell, determine its stimulation level according to Equation (3.21);
    2.2 *Metadynamics*: eliminate network cells with low stimulation level via the resource allocation mechanism;
    2.3 *Clonal expansion*: select the most stimulated network cells and reproduce them proportionally to their stimulation;
    2.4 *Somatic hypermutation*: mutate each clone inversely proportional to its stimulation level;
    2.5 *Network construction*: select mutated clones to incorporate into the network;
3. *Cycle*: Repeat Step 2 until a stopping criterion is met.

The Model of L. N. de Castro and F. J. Von Zuben

In the immune network learning algorithm proposed by (de Castro & Von Zuben, 2000b), named aiNet (*Artificial Immune NETwork*), the network is initialized with a small number of elements randomly generated. Each network element corresponds to an antibody molecule, i.e an attribute string represented in an Euclidean shape-space.

The next stage is the presentation of the antigenic patterns. Each pattern is presented to each network cell and their affinity is determined according to Equation (3.1). A number of high affinity antibodies are selected and reproduced (*clonal expansion*) according to their affinity: the higher the affinity, the higher the number of clones to be produced. The clones generated undergo somatic mutation inversely proportional to their antigenic affinity: the higher the affinity, the lower the mutation rate. A number of high affinity clones is selected to be maintained in the network, constituting what is defined as a clonal memory.

The affinity between all remaining antibodies is determined. Those antibodies whose affinity is less than a given threshold are eliminated from the network (*clonal suppression*). All antibodies whose affinity with the antigen is less than a given threshold are also eliminated from the network. Additionally, a number of new randomly generated antibodies are incorporated into the network (*metadynamics*).

The remaining antibodies are incorporated into the network, and their affinity with the existing antibodies is determined. All but one antibody whose affinity is less than a given threshold are eliminated.

The aiNet learning algorithm can be summarized as follows:

1. *Initialization*: create an initial random population of network antibodies;
2. *Antigenic presentation*: for each antigenic pattern, do:
    2.1 *Clonal selection and expansion*: for each network element, determine its affinity with the antigen presented. Select a number of high affinity elements and reproduce (clone) them proportionally to their affinity;
    2.2 *Affinity maturation*: mutate each clone inversely proportional to affinity. Re-select a number of highest affinity clones and place them into a clonal memory set;
    2.3 *Metadynamics*: eliminate all memory clones whose affinity with the antigen is less than a pre-defined threshold;
    2.4 *Clonal interactions*: determine the network interactions (affinity) among all the elements of the clonal memory set;
    2.5 *Clonal suppression*: eliminate those memory clones whose affinity with each other is less than a pre-specified threshold;
    2.6 *Network construction*: incorporate the remaining clones of the clonal memory with all network antibodies;
3. *Network interactions*: determine the similarity between each pair of network antibodies;
4. *Network suppression*: eliminate all network antibodies whose affinity is less than a pre-specified threshold;
5. *Diversity*: introduce a number of new randomly generated antibodies into the network;
6. *Cycle*: repeat Steps 2 to 5 until a pre-specified number of iterations is reached.

Some Philosophical and Practical Remarks

Although both algorithms may seem rather similar, there are major differences between them in several levels, such as basic network element, immune network interaction, population control mechanism, and interpretation.

In RAIN, the basic element is a B-cell comprised of an antibody attribute string, a stimulation level, and a resource allocation indicator, whereas in aiNet the basic element is primarily an antibody attribute string. However, the same way that the stimulation level is part of a B-cell in RAIN, the antibody affinity with antigens and other antibodies could also be viewed as parameters contained within a B-cell in aiNet.

To determine the stimulation level of each network B-cell, RAIN employs a difference equation version of the differential equation proposed by Farmer and collaborators (Farmer *et al.*, 1986). This stimulation level takes into account antigenic stimulation and network interactions, thus dictating B-cell survival and repro-duction. Similarly, aiNet uses an affinity measure to quantify the degree of anti-genic recognition and the degree of interaction with other network antibodies. How-ever, this is performed in different time scales during learning and not combined in a single equation as in RAIN.

To prevent an exponential growth of the network population, both algorithms employ different population control strategies. In RAIN, a resource allocation mechanism encourages B-cells of high stimulation to survive in the network. This promotes the control of the network size and the creation of a representative internal image of the antigenic universe. In contrast, aiNet attempts to reduce redundancy by eliminating similar antibodies, based upon their degree of similarity (affinity) with other network antibodies. This has the effect of controlling the population size.

Finally, what network results from the learning algorithm? The RAIN learning algorithm produces a topological representation of the antigenic patterns. This al-lows the identification of important features contained within the antigenic uni-verse, such as clusters and inter-relationships between data items. A special tool has been designed to visualize the network structure (Timmis, 2001). In aiNet, a re-duced discrete set of antibodies is constructed so as to follow the spatial distribution of the antigenic universe. In order to interpret the resultant aiNet various graph con-cepts and hierarchical clustering techniques can be utilized (de Castro & Von Zu-ben, 2001), such as minimum spanning trees and dendrograms.

As general comments for both learning algorithms, it is important to note that these networks also follow the same structure as the continuous networks, according to Equation (3.20). The behavior of the population of network cells is a function of the antigenic and network interactions, added to the metadynamics effects, i.e., in-flux of new elements and death of unstimulated ones. In addition, although both algorithms were originally implemented using real-valued vectors in an Euclidean shape-space, they are not necessarily restricted to this shape-space; others could be used.

3.5.4. Guidelines for the Design of AIS

The framework to engineer artificial immune systems is based upon a formalism to create abstract models of the components of the system and a set of algorithms to determine the interactions (dynamics and metadynamics) of these components. The question that still remains is how to use this framework in order to design an AIS. Although the answer to this question is rather intuitive and might be problem de-pendent, it is the intent here to present some guidelines to engineer artificial im-mune systems for any domain. Taking into account the layered approach outlined in Section 3.5, a simple process can be followed:

1. **Problem description**

Describing the problem to be resolved corresponds to identifying all elements to be part of the AIS. This includes variables, constants, agents, functions, and parameters necessary to appropriately describe and solve the problem. These are not always known a priori and new components might have to be included in the system at later design stages.

2.   Deciding the immune principle(s) to be used for problem solving

The models, algorithms, and processes presented in Section 3.5 are generic and can be used in different settings. New algorithms can be proposed based upon variations of these ones, other theoretical aspects presented in Chapter 2, and even other immune processes not described in this book. A discussion about potential immune components and/or theories not yet modeled will be presented in Chapter 8.

3.   Engineering the artificial immune system

Engineering the AIS involves several aspects, such as deciding which immune components are going to be used, how to create the abstract models of these components, and the application of the immune principles (algorithms) that will control the behavior (dynamics and metadynamics) of the system. (Note that Step 2 could be part of the engineering process).

3.1   Defining the types of immune components to be used

Most of the applications use a single cell type (usually a B-cell or an antibody) and an antigen. However, any type of immune component like T-cells, lymphokines, bone marrow, thymus, etc., can be employed. Examples of systems that simultaneously take into account many different components of the immune system and the most common metaphors used are given in Chapters 4 and 7.

3.2   Defining the mathematical representation for the elements of the AIS

The shape-space formalism is suitable to mathematically represent immune cells and molecules.

3.3   Applying immune principle(s) to problem solving

Application of the principles and/or algorithms chosen in Step 2.

3.4   The metadynamics of an AIS

The immune system is metadynamic in the sense that some cells and molecules are constantly being recruited into the system while others die and are removed. This metadynamics, though proposed for a specific immune network model, can be viewed as a general principle that governs the recruitment of new components into and elimination of useless elements of an AIS. This process is responsible for the double-plasticity of artificial immune systems, i.e., their capability of dynamically changing their own structure in addition to other free parameters (Step 3.3).

4.   Reverse mapping from AIS to the real problem

After resolving the problem, it is sometimes necessary to interpret (or decode) the results presented by the artificial immune system into the original problem domain.

A Simple Example for Pattern Recognition

To illustrate how to use the framework and guidelines proposed, consider the simple problem of developing an artificial immune system to recognize the binary patterns illustrated in Figure 3.23.

Step 1: Problem Description

The problem corresponds to generate a system capable of learning to identify the numbers 1 and 4 represented using a bitmap according to Figure 3.23. The picture is binary with its pixels corresponding to 0 (white pixels) or 1 (dark pixels). Two main elements can be identified: the patterns to be recognized and the element(s) of the AIS to be used as recognizers, or pattern recognizers.

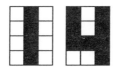

Figure 3.23.   Patterns corresponding to the numbers 1 and 4.

Step 2: Deciding the Immune Principles

To make the explanation more comprehensive, two AIS will be developed for solving this problem. In the first AIS, the negative selection algorithm will be used to create a set of elements that do not recognize the patterns corresponding to the numbers 1 and 4. The idea is to have an AIS that recognizes patterns considered to be anomalies in relation to the patterns 1 and 4. The second AIS will employ the clonal selection algorithm to evolve an antibody repertoire capable of recognizing only the patterns 1 and 4 (or small variations of them).

Step 3: Engineering the AIS

This main step is responsible for implementing the immune metaphors taken, representing the components of the AIS in a suitable shape-space, and applying an immune algorithm to govern the behavior of the system.

Step 3.1: Defining the Immune Components

CASE 1: The Negative Selection Algorithm

The goal of the negative selection algorithm is to generate an available repertoire **A** that recognizes patterns that do not correspond to the numbers 1 and 4 (protected strings). Thus, the strings to be protected will compose the set **S** and another set **P** of strings will have to be generated and compared to the strings in **S**, so that those strings of **P** that do not recognize any string of **S** will compose the set **A** (Figure 3.15).

In this case, the strings in **S** correspond to the self, the strings in **P** correspond to naïve T-cells, and the strings in **A** are equivalent to tolerant T-cells, i.e., T-cells that do not react with any self cell.

CASE 2: The Clonal Selection Algorithm

The goal of the clonal selection algorithm is opposite to negative selection. Clonal selection will evolve a repertoire of cells that recognize the two patterns. Each pattern of the set **S** to be recognized corresponds to an antigen while each pattern recognizer of the set **P** is equivalent to an antibody or a B-cell receptor.

Step 3.2: Mathematical Representation

Due to the intrinsic binary characteristic of the patterns, a binary Hamming shape-space is a natural abstract model of their 'shapes'. Assume that the elements of **S** and **P** are represented in the same shape-space S^L. Each character is a picture containing 12 bits, 4 rows with 3 bits each, that can be represented as a single attribute string of length $L = 12$. This way, a matrix **S** with 2 rows and 12 columns can be used to represent the patterns, where row 1 corresponds to the number 1 and row 2 corresponds to the number 4, as follows:

$$\mathbf{S} = \begin{bmatrix} s_1 \\ s_2 \end{bmatrix} = \begin{bmatrix} 0 & 1 & 0 & 0 & 1 & 0 & 0 & 1 & 0 & 0 & 1 & 0 \\ 1 & 0 & 1 & 1 & 0 & 1 & 1 & 1 & 1 & 0 & 0 & 1 \end{bmatrix}$$

Step 3.3: Applying Immune Principles

If each component of the AIS has length $L = 12$ and belongs to a binary Hamming shape-space ($k = 2$), then according to Equation (3.7) the potential repertoire that can be generated has a size $N = 2^{12} = 4096$.

Assume that the recognition of an antigen by an antibody is measured via the Hamming distance given by Equation (3.3). Assume also that an element of **S** will be considered recognized by an element of **P** when their Hamming distance is $D = L - \varepsilon$, where ε is the cross-reactivity threshold. This means that affinity is measured via complementarity between two bitstrings, and the maximal affinity corresponds to L (maximal Hamming distance between two strings).

Let's take $\varepsilon = 1$. Thus, when there is up to one bit in common between two strings they are said to match. Both algorithms, negative and clonal selection, will start with the matrix **P** shown below representing the patterns illustrated in Figure 3.24. Note that the first two patterns of **P** are the exact complement of patterns 1 and 4, respectively. Note also that this situation is very unlikely to happen with a random initialization procedure.

$$\mathbf{P} = \begin{bmatrix} p_1 \\ p_2 \\ p_3 \\ p_4 \\ p_5 \end{bmatrix} = \begin{bmatrix} 1 & 0 & 1 & 1 & 0 & 1 & 1 & 0 & 1 & 1 & 0 & 1 \\ 0 & 1 & 0 & 0 & 1 & 0 & 0 & 0 & 0 & 1 & 1 & 0 \\ 1 & 1 & 0 & 0 & 1 & 0 & 0 & 1 & 0 & 0 & 1 & 0 \\ 1 & 0 & 1 & 0 & 0 & 1 & 1 & 0 & 1 & 1 & 0 & 1 \\ 1 & 1 & 1 & 1 & 0 & 1 & 1 & 1 & 1 & 0 & 0 & 1 \end{bmatrix}$$

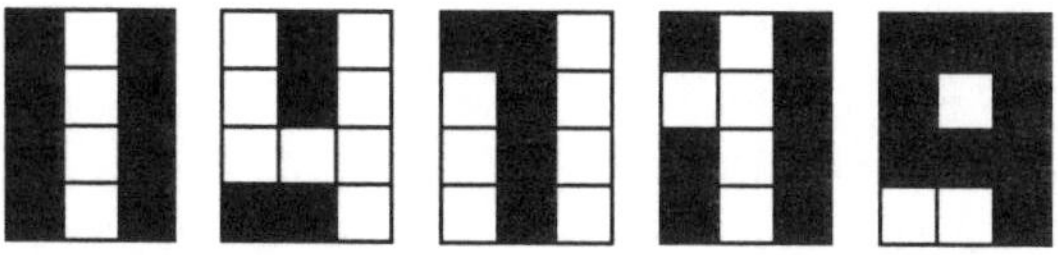

Figure 3.24. Patterns composing the set **P**.

By using Equation (3.3) to determine the affinity between all elements of **P** in relation to the elements of **A**, we can determine the matrix **M** of affinities, where $m_{1,1}$ corresponds to the affinity of the first element of set **S** in relation to the first element of the set **P**, $m_{1,2}$ corresponds to the affinity of the first element of the set **S** in relation to the second element of the set **P**, and so on.

$$\mathbf{M} = \begin{bmatrix} 12 & 2 & 1 & 11 & 9 \\ 2 & 12 & 9 & 3 & 1 \end{bmatrix}$$

According to the cross-reactivity threshold adopted, $\varepsilon = 1$, the elements 1 and 4 of **P**, p_1 and p_4, recognize the pattern 1 ($m_{1,1}$ and $m_{1,4}$), and the element 2 of **P**, p_2, recognizes the pattern corresponding to number 4 ($m_{2,2}$).

CASE 1: The Negative Selection Algorithm

To run the negative selection algorithm (Figure 3.15) means to generate a set of patterns **P** and to match them against the patterns in **S**, and those elements of **P** that match the elements of **S** are eliminated; the remaining ones compose the available repertoire **A**.

In our example, we will assume that the set **P** is fixed as defined a priori. The elements p_1 and p_4 recognize the string s_1 and thus are rejected, and the element p_2 recognizes the string s_2 and is also rejected. So, the available repertoire **A** is composed only of elements p_3 and p_5.

During the monitoring phase (Figure 3.16), any pattern that is recognized by an element of **A** is signaled as an anomaly, i.e., nonself. Note that in practical applications the available repertoire would be composed of a much larger number of elements.

CASE 2: The Clonal Selection Algorithm

To illustrate how CLONALG works, we will run its first iteration for the first element of **S**, s_1. Steps 1 and 2 are already completed; the population **P** is defined and the affinities presented in matrix **M** calculated. Assume now the following parameters for the algorithm: $n_1 = 3$, and $n_2 = n_3 = 1$.

Step 3: for the first element of **S**, s_1, the $n_1 = 3$ highest affinity elements of **P** are p_1, p_4 and p_5 ($m_{1,1}$, $m_{1,4}$ and $m_{1,5}$), respectively. Assume that the highest affinity element of **P**, p_1, generates 3 offspring, p_4 generates 2 offspring, and p_5 generates a single offspring, as illustrated in Figure 3.25(a). This implements the affinity proportional reproduction; the higher the affinity, the higher the number of clones (copies).

Step 4: in this step, the clones generated previously are mutated; the higher the affinity, the smaller the mutation rate. Assume that the clone that is the exact complement of s_1 (have maximal affinity – clone 1) do not suffer any mutation at all, the clone with Hamming distance 11 (clone 2) suffers a one bit mutation, and the clone with Hamming distance 9 (clone 3) suffers a three bit mutation. Hypothetical mutated clones are illustrated in Figure 3.25(b). Note that the second element of clone 2 improved its affinity with s_1 while the first element reduced its affinity. Clone 3 also improved its affinity with s_1.

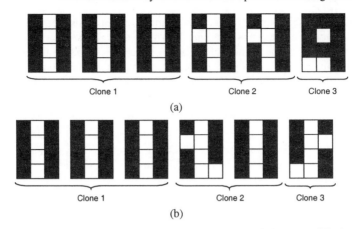

Figure 3.25.   CLONALG. (a) Clones generated for the selected elements of **P**. (b) Mutated clones.

Steps 5 and 6: any of the mutated elements that have maximal affinity with s_1 can be selected to be kept as a memory of the system for the pattern s_1. The first element of clone 2 or clone 3 is going to be replaced by a randomly generated individual, as they have the lowest affinities in relation to s_1.

The same steps apply to the second pattern of **S**, s_2.

Step 3.4: Metadynamics

Metadynamics here is embodied in Step 5 of CLONALG and is not accounted for in the negative selection algorithm.

Step 4: Reverse Mapping

As we are working with the Hamming distance between the elements of **S** and **P**, we can complement the resultant elements of **P** such that they represent explicit copies of the patterns in **S**, instead of their complements (compare the two patterns on the left of Figure 3.24 with those of Figure 3.23).

3.6   Landmarks in the History of AIS

Now that the area in question has been defined, it is possible to discuss a "consensual birth date" for the field of AIS. This however, is not as simple as it sounds. It is hard to find a record of the first time the term "artificial immune system" was used, or when and by whom it was coined. To the authors' knowledge, the first reference identified in the literature proposing the name "artificial immune system" was presented by H. Sieburg and collaborators in 1990 (Sieburg *et al.*, 1990). In this paper however, the authors coined the term to describe an immune system model that does not fit the proposed Definition 3.4.

Another important point to make is that the expression "artificial immune system" is not the single term in use to describe the field. Other names such as *immu-*

nological computation, immunocomputing, computational immunology, or *immune-based systems* have also been employed as synonyms to AIS. Thus, it is important at this stage to specify a unique denomination for the field. There is mounting evidence to suggest that the scientific community is reaching a natural and implicit agreement for it to be *artificial immune systems* (AIS). Henceforth, AIS is adopted in this text as a synonym to all the remaining terminology.

By examining the literature, and given the definition of AIS proposed, it is suggested that the field was initiated by two different works: the paper by J. D. Farmer and his collaborators, and the one by G. W. Hoffmann, both published in the mid 1980s (Farmer *et al.*, 1986; Hoffmann, 1986). In the former work, the authors proposed a dynamical model for the immune network theory whose basic form (equations of motion) could be observed in other biological systems. By representing *classifier systems* (Section 6.6) in the form of dynamical systems, the authors illustrated remarkable similarities between the two systems. Classifier systems belong to the major field of computational intelligence and may incorporate other approaches like a genetic algorithm. By indicating these similarities, the authors argued that artificial (computational) intelligence could benefit from the study of the immune system and suggested that there may be certain universal approaches to the design of efficient learning systems. As a matter of fact, the authors were right about their predictions. The immune network model proposed was widely used and modified by the computational intelligence community and applied in such areas as data analysis, autonomous navigation, and optimization.

In the papers presented by Hoffmann (Hoffmann, 1986; Hoffmann *et al.*, 1986), the authors explored the similarities and differences between the nervous and immune system (Section 5.4) in order to formulate a novel neural network model. This model has the peculiarity that learning does not involve adaptations in the connection strengths among neurons; it only alters the strength of the stimuli being presented. In contrast to the work proposed by Farmer and collaborators, the model introduced by Hoffmann did not have many applications in the computational intelligence field. The ideas of exploring the similarities and differences between both systems however, served as inspiration for the study and proposal of several novel network models, such as the early works on AIS introduced by Y. Ishida (1990, 1993) and F. T. Vertosick and R. H. Kelly (1989, 1991).

Works by H. Bersini and F. J. Varela (Bersini & Varela, 1990, 1991; Bersini, 1991) are the first known applications of immune algorithms to problem solving. Based upon their own immune network model, the authors assessed the performance of these algorithms when applied to problems such as machine learning, optimization, and adaptive control. Analogies with classifier systems, genetic algorithms, and reinforcement learning strategies were also discussed.

Research on using the immune system models followed in the early 1990s with the use of genetic algorithms to study the pattern recognition capabilities of binary immune system models (Forrest & Perelson, 1991; Forrest *et al.*, 1993). With the increase in use of immune models by the computer science community, researchers soon realized the potential of employing some of these ideas and abstract models of the immune system to develop *computer immune systems* in the so called *computer immunology.* Computer immune systems are basically simplified and abstract models of the immune system designed to protect computers, or networks of computers, from unauthorized invasions (e.g., viruses and network intrusions). The interest in the development of computer immune systems became more widespread within the scientific community, and major computer companies like IBM began to take an interest, with the development of their own immune based anti-virus software. The earliest works on computer immunology were undertaken by S. Forrest and collaborators at the University of New Mexico and J. O. Kephart and collaborators at IBM (Forrest *et al.*, 1994, 1997; Kephart, 1994; Kephart *et al.*, 1997a,b). This area of research is still highly active, and it is our belief that computer systems still have much to gain with the artificial immune system techniques.

Nevertheless, the domain of artificial immune systems has not had an exclusive hold on the development of computer immune systems. Since 1995, work has began to diversify significantly (see Chapter 4 for different applications) and to attract interest from major companies such as IBM, Sun Microsystems, US Navy, and the British Postal service to apply AIS to their particular problems.

3.6.1. Events and Major Publications on AIS

Since 1996 there has been a realization of several workshops, special tracks, presentations, and tutorials concerning artificial immune systems. Table 3.1 summarizes the main events up to the end of 2001. As can be seen from this table, a wide variety of conferences have attracted interest for AIS. These range from the IEEE SMC conferences (Systems, Man and Cybernetics series) to GECCO (Genetic and Evolutionary Computation Conference) and various conferences on artificial neural networks.

In early 1998 Y. Ishida and collaborators edited the first book on "Immunity-Based Systems – Intelligent Systems by Artificial Immune Systems" (in Japanese). The first edited book in English) was launched in early 1999 by D. Dasgupta, entitled "Artificial Immune Systems and Their Applications". In addition to these edited volumes, books with more general scopes also involve whole sections, collections of AIS papers, or discussions on the use of immune system metaphors. These can be identified as:

- *Computing with Biological Metaphors*, R. Paton (ed.), Chapman & Hall, 1994;
- *New Ideas in Optimization*, D. Corne, M. Dorigo, and F. Glover (eds.), McGraw-Hill, 1999;
- *Intelligent Information Systems, Series: Advances in Soft Computing*, L. Zadeh, J. Kacprzyk, 2000;
- *Digital Biology*, P. Bentley, Headline, 2001; and
- *Data Mining: A Heuristic Approach,* H. A. Abbass, R. A. Sarker, and C. S. Newton (eds.), Idea Group Publishing, 2001.

The journal IEEE Transactions on Evolutionary Computation (TEC) will bring the first special issue on Artificial Immune Systems, early 2002. For the year 2002, four major events on AIS are scheduled:

Table 3.2. Summary of major events and publications on AIS. IMBS: Immunity-Based Systems Workshop; SMC: Systems, Man and Cybernetics; GECCO: Genetic and Evolutionary Computation Congress; SBRN: Brazilian Symposium on Neural Networks; CEC: Congress on Evolutionary Computation, ICANNGA: International Conference on Neural Networks and Genetic Algorithms; BCS: International Conference on Artificial Intelligence; ICARIS: International Conference on Artificial Immune Systems.

Year	Event	Activity	Organizer/Speaker
1996	IMBS	Workshop	Y. Ishida
1997	SMC	Special Track	D. Dasgupta
1998	SMC	Special Track	D. Dasgupta
	Book	Edited book	Y. Ishida et al. (eds.)
	PI Meeting	Talk: "Computational Immunology"	M. Stillman
1999	Book	Edited book	D. Dasgupta (ed.)
	SMC	Special Track / Tutorial	D. Dasgupta
2000	GECCO	Workshop	D. Dasgupta
		Talk: "Why Does a Computer Need an Immune System"	S. Forrest
	SMC	Tutorial: "Immunological Computation"	D. Dasgupta
		Special Track	
	SBRN	Tutorial: "Artificial Immune Systems and Their Applications"	L. N. de Castro
2001	CEC	Tutorial: "Artificial Immune Systems: An Emerging Technology"	J. I. Timmis
	ICANNGA	Tutorial: "An Introduction to the Artificial Immune Systems"	L. N. de Castro
	BCS	Tutorial "An Introduction to Artificial Immune Systems"	J. I. Timmis
2002	Journal (Special Issue)	IEEE-TEC: Special Issue on Artificial Immune Systems	D. Dasgupta (ed.)
	ICARIS	First International Conference on Artificial Immune Systems	J. Timmis and P. Bentley

- Workshop on Artificial Immune Systems, at the World Congress on Computational Intelligence (WCCI) to be held in Hawaii/U.S.A., 12-17 May;
- Special Session on Immunity-Based Systems, at the 6th International Conference on Knowledge-Based Intelligent Information Engineering Systems, Podere d'Ombriano, Crema, Italy, 16-18 September.

- Special Session on Artificial Immune Systems and Their Applications at ICONIP (International Conference on Neural Information Processing), SEAL (Asia-Pacific Conference on Simulated Evolution and Learning), FSKD (International Conference on Fuzzy Systems and Knowledge Discovery), Singapore, November 18-22.
- 1st International Conference on Artificial Immune Systems (ICARIS), University of Kent at Canterbury, UK, September 9th to 11th, 2002.

Tutorials on "Immunological Computation: Theory and Applications" and "Artificial Immune Systems" are scheduled for the GECCO 2002 to be held in New York/U.S.A., 9-13 July, and the CEC 2002 to be held in Hawaii/U.S.A., 12-17 May, respectively.

3.7   Chapter Summary

Artificial immune systems can be defined as computational systems inspired by theoretical immunology and observed immune functions, principles and models, which are applied to problem solving. By utilizing the basic concepts of the immune system it is possible to construct artificial immune systems that can be applied to a myriad of computational scenarios. This chapter proposed a formal definition for AIS, traced its history in terms of major events and publications, and proposed a consensual birth date for the field by stressing some research landmarks.

There has been increasing use of this immune metaphor for creating computational systems; however the development has been a little disparate at times. To address this issue, this chapter has introduced mechanisms by which such artificial immune systems can be created in a methodical, rigorous, and standard way. Simple abstract models of basic immune components and processes have bee drawn together into a single framework for the construction of artificial immune systems. It is hoped that this framework has made the field of AIS somewhat more accessible and shaped. It should be noted, as well, that no claim is being made here that the framework proposed is complete. It has been proposed in such a way as to allow for refinement and augmentation by the community in general.

References

Bäck, T., Fogel, D. B. & Michalewicz, Z. (2000), *Evolutionary Computation 1 Basic Algorithms and Operators*, Institute of Physics Publishing (IOP), Bristol and Philadelphia.

Bersini, H. (1991), "Immune Network and Adaptive Control", *Proc. of the First European Conference on Artificial Life*, MIT Press, pp. 217-226.

Bersini, H. & Varela, F. J. (1990), "Hints for Adaptive Problem Solving Gleaned from Immune Networks", *Parallel Problem Solving from Nature*, pp. 343-354.

Bersini, H. & Varela, F. J. (1991), "The Immune Recruitment Mechanism: A Selective Evolutionary Strategy", *Proc. of the Int. Conference on Genetic Algorithms*, pp. 520-526.

Celada, F. & Seiden, P. E. (1996), "Affinity Maturation and Hypermutation in a Simulation of the Humoral Immune Response", *Eur. J. Imm.*, **26**, pp. 1350-1358.

de Castro, L. N. & Von Zuben, F. J. (2001), "aiNet: An Artificial Immune Network for Data Analysis", in *Data Mining: A Heuristic Approach*, Hussein A. Abbass, Ruhul A. Sarker, and Charles S. Newton (eds.), Idea Group Publishing, USA, Chapter XII, pp. 231-259.

de Castro, L. N. & Von Zuben, F. J. (2000a), "The Clonal Selection Algorithm with Engineering Applications", *Proc. of the Genetic and Evolutionary Computation Conference*, Workshop on Artificial Immune Systems and Their Applications, pp. 36-37.

de Castro, L. N. & Von Zuben, F. J. (2000b), "An Evolutionary Immune Network for Data Clustering", *Proc. of the IEEE Brazilian Symposium on Artificial Neural Networks*, pp. 84-89.

Dasgupta, D. (1999), "Information Processing Mechanisms of the Immune System", In *New Ideas in Optimization*, D. Corne, M. Dorigo & F. Glover (eds.), McGraw Hill, London, pp. 161-165.

Dasgupta, D. & Niño, F. (2000), "A Comparison of Negative and Positive Selection in Novel Pattern Detection", *Proc. of the Congress on Evolutionary Computation*, pp. 125-130.

D'haeseleer, P., Forrest, S. & Helman, P. (1996), "An Immunological Approach to Change Detection: Algorithms, Analysis and Implications", *Proc. of the IEEE Symposium on Computer Security and Privacy*, IEEE Computer Society Press, Los Alamitos, CA, pp. 110-119.

Farmer, J. D., Kauffman, S. A. Packard, N. H. & Perelson, A. S. (1987), "Adaptive Dynamic Networks as Models for the Immune System and Autocatalytic Sets", *Ann. of the N. Y. Acad. of Sci.*, **504**, pp. 118-131.

Farmer, J. D., Packard, N. H. & Perelson, A. S. (1986), "The Immune System, Adaptation, and Machine Learning", *Physica 22D*, pp. 187-204.

Forrest, S., Hofmeyr S. A. & Somayaji A. (1997), "Computer Immunology", *Communications of the ACM*, **40**(10), pp. 88-96.

Forrest, S., A. Perelson, Allen, L. & Cherukuri, R. (1994), "Self-Nonself Discrimination in a Computer", *Proc. of the IEEE Symposium on Research in Security and Privacy*, pp. 202-212.

Forrest, S., Javornik, B., Smith, R. E. & Perelson, A. S. (1993), "Using Genetic Algorithms to Explore Pattern Recognition in the Immune System", *Evolutionary Computation*, **1**(3), pp. 191-211.

Forrest, S. & A. Perelson (1991), "Genetic Algorithms and the Immune System", *Proc. of the Parallel Problem Solving form Nature*, H-. P. Schwefel & R. Manner (eds.), Springer-Verlag.

Harmer, P. K. & Lamont, G. B. (2000), "An Agent Based Architecture for a Computer Virus Immune System", *Proc. of the Genetic and Evolutionary Computation Conference*, Workshop on Artificial Immune Systems and Their Applications, pp. 45-46.

Hightower R. R., Forrest, S. A & Perelson, A. S. (1995), "The Evolution of Emergent Organization in Immune System Gene Libraries", *Proc. of the 6th Int. Conference on Genetic Algorithms*, L. J. Eshelman (ed.), Morgan Kaufmann, pp. 344-350.

Hoffmann, G. W. (1986), "A Neural Network Model Based on the Analogy with the Immune System", *J. theor. Biol.*, **122**, pp. 33-67.

Hoffmann, G. W., Benson, M. W., Bree, G. M. & Kinahan, P. E. (1986), "A Teachable Neural Network Based on an Unorthodox Neuron", *Physica 22D*, pp. 233-246.

Hofmeyr S. A. & Forrest, S. (2000), "Architecture for an Artificial Immune System", *Evolutionary Computation*, **7**(1), pp. 45-68.

Hunt, J. E., Cooke, D. E. & Holstein, H. (1995), "Case Memory and Retrieval Based on the Immune System", *1st Int. Conference on Case-Based Reasoning*, Published as Case-Based Reasoning Research and Development, Manuela Weloso and Agnar Aamodt (eds.), Lecture Notes in Artificial Intelligence, **1010**, pp 205 -216.

Ishida, Y. (1993), "An Immune Network Model and Its Applications to Process Diagnosis", *Systems and Computers in Japan*, **24**(6), pp. 646-651.

Ishida, Y. (1990), "Fully Distributed Diagnosis by PDP Learning Algorithm: Towards Immune Network PDP Model", *Proc. of the Int. Joint Conf. on Neural Networks*, pp. 777-782.

Ishida, Y., Hirayama, H., Fujita, H., Ishiguro, A. & Mori, K. (eds.) (1998), *Immunity-Based Systems - Intelligent Systems by Artificial Immune Systems*, Corona Pub. Co. Japan (in Japanese).

Jerne, N. K. (1974a), "Towards a Network Theory of the Immune System", *Ann. Immunol.* (Inst. Pasteur) **125C**, pp. 373-389.

Jerne, N. K. (1974b), "Clonal Selection in a Lymphocyte Network". *Cellular Selection and Regulation in the Immune Response*, G. M. Edelman (ed.), Raven Press, N. Y., p. 39.

Kephart, J. O., Sorkin, G. B. & Swimmer, M. (1997a), "An Immune System for Cyberspace", *Proc. of the IEEE Systems, Man, and Cybernetics Conference*, pp. 879-884.

Kephart, J. O., Sorkin, G. B., Swimmer, M. & White S. R. (1997b), "Blueprint for a Computer Immune System", *Presented at the International Conference Virus Bulletin*.

Kephart, J. O. (1994), "A Biologically Inspired Immune System for Computers", R. A. Brooks & P. Maes (eds.), *Artificial Life IV Proceedings of the Fourth International Workshop on the Synthesis and Simulation of Living Systems*, MIT Press, pp. 130-139.

Kepler, T. B. & Perelson, A. S. (1993a), "Somatic Hypermutation in B Cells: An Optimal Control Treatment", *J. theor. Biol.*, **164**, pp. 37-64.

Kepler, T. B. & Perelson, A. S. (1993b), "Cyclic Re-enter of Germinal Center B Cells and the Efficiency of Affinity Maturation", *Imm. Today*, **14**(8), pp. 412-415.

Oprea, M. (1999), *Antibody Repertoires and Pathogen Recognition: The Role of Germline Diversity and Somatic Hypermutation*, Ph.D. Dissertation, University of New Mexico, Albuquerque, New Mexico, EUA.

Percus, J. K., Percus, O. E. & Perelson, A. S. (1993), "Predicting the Size of the T-cell Receptor and Antibody Combining Region from Consideration of Efficient Self-Nonself Discrimination", *Proc. Natl. Acad. Sci. USA*, **90**, pp. 1691-1695.

Perelson, A. S. (1989), "Immune Network Theory", *Imm. Rev.*, **110**, pp. 5-36.

Perelson, A. S., Hightower, R. & Forrest, S. (1996), "Evolution and Somatic Learning in V-Region Genes", *Research in Immunology*, **147**, pp. 202-208.

Perelson, A. S. & Oster, G. F. (1979), "Theoretical Studies of Clonal Selection: Minimal Antibody Repertoire Size and Reliability of Self-Nonself Discrimination", *J. theor.Biol.*, **81**, pp. 645-670.

Seiden, P. E. & Celada, F. (1992), "A Model for Simulating Cognate Recognition and Response in the Immune System", *J. theor. Biol.*, **158**, pp. 329-357.

Sieburg, H., McCutchan, H., Clay, O., Caballero, L. & Ostlund, J. (1990), "Simulation of HIV-infection in Artificial Immune Systems", *Physica D*, **45**, pp. 208-228.

Starlab, users.pandora.be/richard.wheeler1/ais/inn.html.

Suzuki, J. & Yamamoto, Y. (1998), "The Reflection Pattern in the Immune System", *Proc. of the OOPSLA'98, workshop on Non-Software Examples of Software Architecture*, CD-ROM.

Tarakanov A., Dasgupta, D. (2000), "A Formal Model of An Artificial Immune System", *BioSystems*, **55**(1-3), pp. 151-158.

Timmis, J. (2001), "aiVIS: Artificial Immune Network Visualisation", *Proc. of EuroGraphics*, University College London, pp. 61-69.

Timmis, J. & Neal, M. (2000), "Investigating the Evolution and Stability of a Resource Limited Artificial Immune System", *Proc. of the Genetic and Evolutionary Computation Conference*, Workshop on Artificial Immune Systems and Their Applications, pp. 40-41.

Varela, F. J. & Coutinho, A. (1991), "Second Generation Immune Networks", *Imm. Today*, **12**(5), pp. 159-166.

Vertosick, F. T. & Kelly, R. H. (1991), "The Immune System as a Neural Network: A Multi-epitope Approach", *J. theor. Biol.*, **150**, pp. 225-237.

Vertosick, F. T. & Kelly, R. H. (1989), "Immune Network Theory: A Role for Parallel Distributed Processing?", *Immunology*, **66**, pp. 1-7.

Wierzchón, S. T. (2000a), "Discriminative Power of the Receptors Activated by *k*-Contiguous Bits Rule", *J. of Computer Science and Technology*, **1**(3), pp. 1-13.

Wierzchón, S. T. (2000b), "Generating Optimal Repertoire of Antibody Strings in an Artificial Immune System", *Intelligent Information Systems*, M. A. Klopotek, M. Michawicz & S. T. Wierzchon (eds.), Physica-Verlag, Berlin-Heidelberg-NY, pp. 119-134.

Zak, M (2000), "Physical Model of Immune Inspired Computing", *Information Sciences*, **129**, pp. 61-79.

Further Reading

3.7.1. Reviews on Mathematical Theoretical Immunology

Bell, G. I., Perelson, A. S. & Pimbley Jr., G. H. (eds.) (1978), *Theoretical Immunology*, Marcel Dekker Inc.

Mohler, R. R., Bruni, C. & Gandolfi, A. (1980), "A Systems Approach to Immunology", *Proc. of the IEEE*, **68**(8), pp. 964-989.

Perelson, A. S. & Weisbuch, G. (1997), "Immunology for Physicists", *Rev. of Modern Physics*, **69**(4), pp. 1219-1267.

Perelson, A. S. (ed.) (1988), *Theoretical Immunology: The Proceedings of the Theoretical Immunology Workshops*, Part I and II, Addison-Wesley.

Přikrylová, D., Jílek, M., & Waniewski, J. (1992), *Mathematical Modeling of the Immune Response*, CRC Press, Boca Raton, Fla.

3.7.2. The Framework

Bezzi, M., Celada, F., Ruffo, S. & Seiden, P. E. (1997), "The Transition Between Immune and Disease States in a Cellular Automaton Model of Clonal Immune Response", *Physica A*, **245**(1-2), pp. 145-163.

Celada, F. & Seiden, P. E. (1992), "A Computer Model of Cellular Interaction in the Immune System", *Imm. Today*, **13**, pp. 56-62.

de Boer, R. J., Segel, L. A. & Perelson, A. S. (1992), "Pattern Formation in One- and Two-Dimensional Shape-Space Models of the Immune System", *J. theor. Biol.*, **155**, pp. 295-333.

de Castro, L. N. & Timmis, J. (2002), "Artificial Immune Systems as A Novel Soft Computing Paradigm", *Soft Computing* (in print).

de Castro, L. N. & Timmis, J. (2002), "Artificial Immune Systems: A Novel Paradigm to Pattern Recognition", In *Artificial Neural Networks in Pattern Recognition*, J. M. Corchado, L. Alonso, and C. Fyfe (eds.), SOCO-2002, University of Paisley, UK, pp. 67-84.

de Castro, L. N. & Von Zuben, F. J. (2001), "Immune and Neural Network Models: Theoretical and Empirical Comparisons", *International Journal of Computational Intelligence and Applications*, **1**(3), pp. 1-19.

de Castro, L. N. & Von Zuben, F. J. (2002), "Learning and Optimization Using the Clonal Selection Principle", accepted for publication at the *IEEE Transaction on Evolutionary Computation*, Special Issue on AIS (in print).

D'haeseleer, P., Forrest, S. & Helman, P. (1996), "An Immunological Approach to Change Detection: Algorithms, Analysis and Implications", *Proc. of the IEEE Symposium on Computer Security and Privacy*, IEEE Computer Society Press, Los Alamitos, CA, pp. 110-119.

Farmer, J. D. (1990), "A Rosetta Stone for Connectionism", *Physica 42D*, pp. 153-187.

Farmer, J. D., Kauffman, S. A. Packard, N. H. & Perelson, A. S. (1987), "Adaptive Dynamic Networks as Models for the Immune System and Autocatalytic Sets", *Ann. of the N. Y. Acad. of Sci.*, **504**, pp. 118-131.

Forrest, S., Hofmeyr S. A., Somayaji A. & Longstaff, A. (1996), "A Sense of Self for Unix Processes", *Proc. of the IEEE Symposium on Computer Security and Privacy*.

Kim, J. & Bentley, P. (1999), "Negative Selection and Niching by an Artificial Immune System for Network Intrusion Detection", *Proc. of the Genetic and Evolutionary Computation Conference*, pp. 149-158.

Kleinstein, S. & Seiden, P. E. (2000), "Simulating the Immune System", *Computing in Sciences and Engineering*, July/August, pp. 69-77.

Knight, T. & Timmis, J. (2001) "AINE: An Immunological Approach to Data Mining", *Proc. of the IEEE International Conference on Data Mining*, pp. 297-304.

Segel, L. & Perelson, A. S. (1988), "Computations in Shape Space: A New Approach to Immune Network Theory", In *Theoretical Immunology*, Part II, A. S. Perelson (ed.), pp. 321-343.

Smith, D. J., Forrest, S., Hightower, R. R. & Perelson, S. A. (1997), "Deriving Shape Space Parameters from Immunological Data", *J. theor. Biol.*, **189**, pp. 141-150.

Stewart, J. & Varela, F. J. (1991), "Morphogenesis in Shape-space. Elementary Meta-Dynamics in a Model of the Immune Network", *J. theor. Biol.*, **153**, pp. 477-498.

Timmis, J. (2000), *Artificial Immune Systems: A Novel Data Analysis Technique Inspired by the Immune Network Theory*, Ph.D. Dissertation, Department of Computer Science, University of Wales, September.

Timmis, J & Neal, M. (2001), "A Resource Limited Artificial Immune System", *Knowledge Based Systems*, **14**(3-4), pp. 121-130.

Timmis, J., Neal, M. & Hunt, J. (2000), "An Artificial Immune System for Data Analysis", *BioSystems*, **55**, pp. 143-150

Varela, F. J., Thompson, E. & Rosch, E. (1991), *The Embodied Mind*, MIT Press.

Varela, F. J., Anderson, A., Dietrich, G., Sundblad, A., Holmberg, D., Kazatchkine, M. & Coutinho, A. (1991), "Population Dynamics of Antibodies in Normal and Autoimmune Individuals", *Proc. Natl. Acad. Sc. USA*, **88**, pp. 5917-5921.

Varela, F. J., Coutinho, A. Dupire, E. & Vaz, N. N. (1988), "Cognitive Networks: Immune, Neural and Otherwise", *Theoretical Immunology*, Part II, A. S. Perelson (ed.), pp. 359-375.

Varela, F. J. & Stewart, J. (1990), "Dynamics of a Class of Immune Networks. I. Global Stability of Idiotypic Interactions", *J. theor. Biol.*, **144**, pp. 93-101.

Varela, F. J. & Stewart, J. (1990), "Dynamics of a Class of Immune Networks II. Oscillatory Activity of Cellular and Humoral Components", *J. theor. Biol.*, **144**, pp. 103-115.

Weisbuch, G. (1990), "A Shape-Space Approach to the Dynamics of the Immune System", *J. theor. Biol.*, **143**, pp. 507-522.

Chapter 4

A Survey of Artificial Immune Systems

*The practical applications of a science often
precede the birth of the science itself*

                − N. K. Jerne

4.1   Introduction

During the early stages of research on artificial immune systems (mid 1980s to mid 1990's), there were a small number of publications and a relatively low interest from the computational intelligence research community. In the first workshop dedicated to immune-based systems, held in 1996, Y. Ishida published the first survey of the field (Ishida, 1996a). This survey contained 33 references of which around 18 of them would be classified as artificial immune systems according to Definition 3.4. The remaining references covered related topics or citations of works on theoretical immunology.

Approximately one year later, Dasgupta and Attoh-Okine (1997) published another survey of the field in a special track on artificial immune systems held at the IEEE System, Man, and Cybernetics conference. This survey contained 30 references, from among which around 18 would be classified as artificial immune systems. An extended version of this paper was presented later by Dasgupta (1999b). Surprisingly, the majority of the AIS reviewed in both works were different from the ones reviewed in Ishida's paper, indicating a natural growth of the field.

In early 2000, de Castro and Von Zuben (2000a) published a technical report which undertook a more extensive survey of the field. This report listed 93 references, of which around 83 would be classified as AIS. More recently, Dasgupta and collaborators (Dasgupta *et al.*, 2001) published a technical report with 293 references as a bibliography of artificial immune systems. Again, of all these references, only around 120 would be categorized as AIS; the authors presented a list of works related to theoretical immunology, essential as fundamentals to the design of AIS, but that are not AIS themselves.

From this development of survey papers, it can be seen that there has been a rapid growth in the interest and work undertaken in this field, particularly in the last five years. This is also reinforced by the appearance of special tracks, journal issues, and talks dedicated exclusively to AIS (refer to Table 3.2).

In a similar mould to the survey papers cited above, this chapter presents a broad review of the literature on artificial immune systems. It is hoped that this chapter will provide the reader with a list of those areas that have already been explored and a guide to the search for references to previous and related work on AIS. This attempt at performing an exhaustive survey is only possible due to the young age of the field. Whilst reviewing the field, it was estimated that there were around 180-220 papers related to the application of immune metaphors and theoretical immunology to problem solving, i.e., artificial immune systems.

When attempting to review the field of AIS, it is possible to focus on a number of aspects, such as the application domain, the results obtained, the metaphors used, the adequacy of the proposed framework to the engineering of AIS, the algorithms implemented, and so on. In this chapter each section will provide a brief description of the problem domain, with each review examining the metaphors the authors have employed, in terms of the framework.

As with all approaches that are inspired by biology or that try to extract metaphors from a different paradigm, the strength (or adequacy) of the inspiration and/or metaphors varies from one work to another. This chapter will not address this issue. Instead the chapter will attempt to present the survey in a neutral form, without giving the authors' own judgments of their quality, originality, and usefulness. In order to make the survey easy reading, the works will be classified by domain or application area, and those that do not fit into the major areas described (or where a single reference only was found in the literature) will be grouped altogether in a single closing section named Other Approaches.

Another important fact is that many artificial immune systems have been implemented in conjunction (or compared) with other computational intelligence paradigms, mainly evolutionary algorithms (EAs) and artificial neural networks (ANNs). If the reader is not familiar with these approaches, they are encouraged to read through Sections 6.2 and 6.3 before continuing with this chapter. When considering hybrids of AIS with other approaches, it is possible to distinguish two types of hybridization. One is the simple combination of the algorithms, and the other is the use of one paradigm to improve the performance of the other. Only the former case will be reviewed in this chapter. All the other hybrids aimed at combining strengths for the development of more powerful strategies will be reviewed in Chapter 6.

4.1.1. How to Read this Chapter

The sheer practicalities of providing an in-depth review of all works would result in a book chapter that had an unreasonable amount of pages and would be virtually impenetrable to the reader. Therefore, by limiting the focus of what is discussed, the reader will be provided with a brief overview of the works. A more detailed investigation into certain specific areas, in the forms of case studes, is provided in Chapter 7.

It is becoming more common to develop an algorithm and to apply and test it in several different applications. This process results in a number of publications differing basically by their applications and results. It is also common to publish progressive results of a given project or research. Thus, in order not to overload the chapter with the review of sequential works or the application of the same algorithm to several problems in various papers, a single work of a series will be reviewed. The reader will be guided to the related references from the authors, whenever they are available (or were found). This will also allow the reader to identify the major areas of interest of a specific researcher or research group, and to find out which are the potential applications of a given AIS. Contained within the text are references to the works being reviewed; the reader can find the full references for these in the references section at the end of the chapter. For those works where the metaphors are numerous or substantial, a table of how the authors mapped the immune system into the artificial immune system is provided.

This chapter is organized as follows. Sections 4.2 to 4.13 review the works on the domains of pattern recognition, computational security, anomaly detection, optimization, machine learning, robotics, control, scheduling, fault diagnosis, antibody libraries, associative memories, and ecology, respectively. Section 4.14 reviews the other approaches that did not fit into any of these other catagories. Section 4.15 presents a summary of the most important immune principles, theories, and metaphors used for the development of problem solving strategies inspired by the immune system. This section also draws general comments on the suitability of the framework proposed for the design of artificial immune systems, based upon the works reviewed.

4.2   Pattern Recognition

The pattern recognition field is the one that studies the operation and design of systems capable of identifying patterns in data. The patterns to be discovered are usually contained within groups of measurements or observations, defining points in an appropriate multi-dimensional space. Sub-disciplines such as discriminant analysis, feature extraction, error estimation, cluster analysis, grammatical inference, and parsing (sometimes called syntactical pattern recognition), are all included in the major field of pattern recognition. Important application areas are image analysis, character recognition, clustering, speech analysis, man and machine diagnosis, person identification, and industrial inspection.

4.2.1. Spectra Recognition

A general form of a chemical reaction maps a set of reactants ($\mathbf{R}$) into a set of products ($\mathbf{P}$), $\sum_m R \rightarrow \sum_n P$, where each one of them is identified by a specific spectrum. Given the two sets $\mathbf{R}$ and $\mathbf{P}$, Dasgupta *et al.* (1999) described each of the reactants and products for spectra recognition. The authors employed a binary Hamming shape-space, coupled with a hybrid model that combined an artificial immune system and a genetic algorithm. Their approach was composed of two phases: 1) the evolution of a population of specialists for each of the products, and 2) the process of spectrum recognition itself. Rather than simply using the Hamming distance to evaluate affinity, the authors proposed an affinity function that weights each bit in the string according to a spectroscopic characteristic.

In the first stage of the process, a randomly generated population of bitstrings is matched against each product (viewed as an antigen). The bitstrings that match the product with an affinity greater than a given threshold are then passed through a negative selection algorithm. This is to ensure that that they do not recognize any of the reactants in R nor a product different from the one currently presented. The bitstrings that "survive" from the negative selection phase, named antibodies, are specialists in recognizing that product. This process was performed for each one of the n products. After generating the repertoire of specialist antibodies, the recognition results in the automatic process of finding all possible products responsible for the observed spectrum. This was argued to be akin to antigenic recognition in the immune system. The immune metaphors employed are summarized in Table 4.1.

Genetic variation operators, such as crossover and mutation, were used to alter bitstrings that do not recognize a given product in the first stage of the algorithm. In the process of spectra recognition, a genetic algorithm was used to evolve a population of specialist antibodies in case a new spectrum goes undetected by the existing specialist library. This mechanism endows the system with the capability of learning new types of spectra.

Table 4.1.   Immuno-inspired approach for spectra recognition.

Immune System	Spectra Recognition
Self	Set of starting reactants **R** before chemical or photochemical reactions
Nonself	Set of products due to reaction
Antigen	Any of the products **P**
Antibody	Any evolved population that uniquely recognizes a single product
Affinity function	Measures how well two spectra match
Matching	The process of applying the affinity function to a pair of bitstrings

4.2.2. Surveillance of Infectious Diseases

Tarakanov et al. (2000) proposed an artificial immune system as an attempt to improve risk analysis and understanding the spatio-temporal dynamics of the plague in Central Asia. This work attempted to create a more rigorous mathematical model of immune system peptides, which could then be used to predict future infections. The main idea of the approach consisted in treating arbitrary patterns as a way of defining a binding energy (function) between "formal peptides". The formal peptides follow a mathematical model of interactions between proteins of the immune system and antigens, treated using a shape-space approach.

Related Works from the Authors

Tarakanov A., Dasgupta, D. (2000), "A Formal Model of An Artificial Immune System", *BioSystems*, **55**(1-3), pp. 151-158.

Tarakanov A. (1999), "Formal Peptide as a Basic Agent of Immune Networks: From Natural Prototype to Mathematical Theory and Applications", *Proc. of the 1st Int. Workshop of Central and Eastern Europe on Multi-Agent Systems*, pp. 281-292.

4.2.3. Medical Data Analysis

Carter (2000) designed a pattern recognition and classification system based on supervised learning and ideas gleaned from the immune system. His strategy, named Immunos-81, consisted of antigens, T-cells, B-cells, clones, and an amino-acid library. The components of the AIS and their respective mappings are summarized in Table 4.2. Immunos-81 was tested using two standard data sets, both from the medical field.

Immunos-81 used the T-cells to control the production of B-cells. The B-cells would in turn compete for the recognition of unknown patterns. The amino-acid library acts as a library of epitopes (or variables) currently in the system. When a new antigen is introduced into the system, its variables are entered into this library. The T-cells then use the library to create their receptors, which are used to identify the new antigen. During the recognition stage of the algorithm, T-cell paratopes are matched against the epitopes of the antigen, and a B-cell is then created, which has paratopes that match the epitopes of the antigen. T-cells and antigen binding sites were represented as binary strings in a Hamming shape-space and the affinity between an antigen and a T-cell was proportional to the number of matches (similarities) between them.

Table 4.2.   Mapping between the immune system and Immunos-81.

Immune System	Immunos-81
Antigen	Data that may consist of multiple variables of any type
T-cell	Control agent that represents a particular class and determines the sequence and types of variables within an antigen; if an antigen is known; and which clone will decide the identity of an antigen
B-cell	Entity that represents an instance of a particular class during learning
Amino-acid library	All variables encountered, which are assigned a name and type, and may be used to construct new antigens
Clone	Recognition agent; mathematical representation of a repertoire of B-cells

4.2.4. Disjunct Rule Discovery

In the area of data mining, small disjuncts correspond to rules covering a small number of examples. Work in Carvalho and Freitas (2001) proposed an immunological algorithm to discover these small-disjunct rules. The proposed system is a hybrid of an AIS with a decision tree. The decision tree algorithm is used to classify examples belonging to large disjuncts, and the AIS is used to discover rules classifying examples belonging to small disjuncts. The authors claim that decision trees have a bias towards generality and are thus suited for large disjuncts. In contrast, the immune algorithm copes more efficiently with small disjuncts.

In their AIS, a decision tree corresponds to the innate immune system, whereas the immune algorithm incorporates features of the adaptive immune system. The recognition and response to antigens (knowledge stored in a database) is performed by antibodies represented in the form of IF-THEN rules. Each antibody represents a conjunction of conditions composing the antecedent of a given rule, and each condition is an attribute-value pair.

4.3   Computational Security

Through the observations so far made on immunology, it could be seen that the immune system is very efficient in the task of recognizing and eliminating infectious microorganisms. Its capability for dynamically adapting to previously unseen disease causing agents is remarkable.

Two areas of computer security which have been of considerable interest to people researching AIS have been the elimination of computer viruses and worms and the detection of network intrusions (e.g., unauthorized users). An intuitive thought by many when considering AIS is "can the idea of the natural defense mechanism be mapped into a computational domain?" Indeed, some of the early pioneering work in AIS was undertaken in this area and is still a highly active research topic. This section will explores some of these investigations.

4.3.1. Virus Detection and Elimination

In an attempt to create a computer immune system for both computers and networks of computers, Kephart (1994) proposed a novel immune inspired approach. The proposed AIS is capable of developing antibodies to previously unknown computer viruses or worms. These antibodies are then capable of extracting information (learning) about these new viruses and remembering them so as to recognize and respond faster in future infections. The author was also concerned about minimizing the risk of an "autoimmune response" in which the computer immune system would mistakenly identify legitimate software as being undesirable (nonself).

In the implementation, a particular virus is recognized via an exact or fuzzy match to a relatively short sequence of bytes occurring in the virus, called a signature. The process by which the proposed computer immune system establishes whether new software contains a virus is split into various stages. Integrity monitors are used to check for any changes to programs and data files; they have a notion of self, that is any difference between the original and current versions of a file is flagged. However, evidence of a nonself entity is not enough to trigger a computer immune response (virus detection and elimination). Mechanisms employing the strategy of "knowing the enemies" are also brought into play. These mechanisms are based on heuristics to determine whether an anomaly can be attributed to a known virus, thus reducing the risk of an autoimmune response.

Programs carefully designed to be attractive to viruses, named decoy programs, were used to capture samples of the new viruses. This process is somewhat analogous to the ingestion of an antigen by an antigen-presenting cell. In this computer immune system, the infected decoys were then processed by another component of the immune system, called a signature extractor, so as to develop a recognizer for the virus. The computer immune system had an additional task that was not shared by its biological counterpart: it had to attempt to extract from the decoys, information about how the virus attached to its host, so that infected hosts could be repaired (if possible). Hence, the system automatically developed both a recognizer and a repair algorithm appropriate to the virus. Finally, viral self-replication was dealt with self-replication, in the sense that detection of a virus by a single computer would trigger killer signals that would propagate along the path taken by the virus.

Related Works from the Authors

Kephart, J. O., Sorkin, G. B., Swimmer, M. & White S. R. (1999), "Blueprint for a Computer Immune System", In *Artificial Immune Systems and Their Applications*, D. Dasgupta (ed.), Springer-Verlag, pp. 242-259.

Kephart, J. O., Sorkin, G. B. & Swimmer, M. (1997), "An Immune System for Cyberspace", *Proc. of the IEEE System, Man, and Cybernetics Conference*, pp. 879-884.

S. Forrest and her collaborators have also been pursuing the problem of developing a computer immune system since the early 1990s. This research started with the proposal of the negative selection algorithm described in Section 3.5, and follows up to the very recent works of S. Hofmeyr, to be fully described and referenced as one of the case studies of Chapter 7.

Somayaji *et al.* (1997) articulated a broad vision for the development of computer immune systems by using the vertebrate immune system as a source of inspiration. Given the many interesting properties of the immune system discussed in Section 3.2, the authors described several possibilities to design systems based on direct mappings between immune components and current computer system architectures, as summarized in Table 4.3 and Table 4.4. Despite the appealing source of inspiration, the authors addressed five issues that are supposed to be part of a computer security system which are not directly tackled by the immune system: confidentiality, integrity, availability, accountability, and correctness. They argued that the vertebrate immune system is primarily concerned with survival, viewed as a combination of integrity and availability. Finally, the immune system might display some kind of accountability, but not of the same kind as one typically associated with computer security. These issues were argued to be possible limitations to the use of the immune metaphor.

Table 4.3.   Mapping between the immune system and computer security architecture to protect static data.

Immune System	Network Environment
Protecting Static Data	
Self	Uncorrupted data
Nonself	Any change to self

Table 4.4. Mapping between the immune system and computer security architectures according to the elements to be protected.

Immune System	Network Environment
Protecting Active Processes on Single Host	
Cell	Active process in a computer
Multicellular organism	Computer running multiple processes
Population of organisms	Set of networked computers
Skin and innate immunity	Security mechanisms, like passwords, groups, file permissions, etc.
Adaptive immunity	Lymphocyte process able to query other processes to seek for abnormal behaviors
Autoimmune response	False alarm
Self	Normal behavior
Nonself	Abnormal behavior
Protecting a Network of Mutually Trusting Computers	
Organ in an animal	Each computer in a network environment
Cell	Each process
Individual	Network of mutually trusting computers
Innate immune system	Host-based security mechanisms combined with network security mechanisms
Adaptive immune system	Lymphocyte processes with migration to other computers in the network
Thymus	One computer from the network
Protecting a Network of Mutually Trusting Disposable Computers	
Cell	Each computer
Individual	Network of mutually trusting computers
Innate immune system	Network's defenses
Adaptive immune system	Set of lymphocyte machines

Related Works from the Authors

D'haeseleer, P., Forrest, S. & Helman, P. (1996), "An Immunological Approach to Change Detection: Algorithms, Analysis and Implications", *Proc. of the IEEE Symposium on Computer Security and Privacy*, pp. 110-119.

Forrest, S., Hofmeyr S. A. & Somayaji A. (1997), "Computer Immunology", *Communications of the ACM*, **40**(10), pp. 88-96.

Forrest, S., Hofmeyr S. A., Somayaji A. & Longstaff, A. (1996), "A Sense of Self for Unix Processes", *Proc. of the IEEE Symposium on Computer Security and Privacy*, pp. 120-128.

Forrest, S., A. Perelson, Allen, L. & Cherukuri, R. (1994), "Self-Nonself Discrimination in a Computer", *Proc. of the IEEE Symposium on Research in Security and Privacy*, pp. 202-212.

Table 4.5.   Mapping between the anti-virus system and the immune system.

Immune System	Anti-Virus System
Self	Information characterizing the host files
Antibody	Agent that monitors host files and neutralizes an infected file
Killer T-cell	Agent that removes the file altered by viruses and neutralized by antibody agents
Helper T-cell	Agent that controls the processes of the anti-virus system

Okamoto and Ishida (1999) proposed a distributed approach to computer virus detection and neutralization by using autonomous and heterogeneous agents. Unlike the other strategies discussed so far, their system detects viruses by matching "self" with the current host files. In this case, the self-information is a set of data characterizing the identity of the host file, such as the first few bytes of the head of a file, and the file size and path. Thus, a set of antibody agents containing the self-information was represented in a Symbolic shape-space. They were also responsible to neutralize a detected change by overwriting the self-information on the infected files. Some types of agents, including antibody agents, were devised inspired by the immune system. These agents along with their roles are summarized in Table 4.5.

Related Works from the Authors

Okamoto, T. & Ishida, Y. (2000), "A Distributed Approach Against Computer Viruses Inspired by the Immune System", *IEICE Trans. on Communications.*, **E83-B**(5), pp. 908-915.

Okamoto, T. & Ishida, Y. (1999), "A Distributed Approach to Computer Virus Detection and Neutralization by Autonomous and Heterogeneous Agents", *Proc. of the ISADS'99*, pp. 328-331.

In an attempt to create a more efficient computer immune system, work in Lamont *et al.* (1999) reviewed the works of Forrest and Kephart discussed above, combined, and extended some of their features to develop their own computer immune system based on intelligent agents. For example, the authors employed the strategy of decoy programs proposed by Kephart and the negative selection algorithm of Forrest. Negative selection was implemented in conjunction with a genetic algorithm to provide and maintain the diversity of the detectors. The representation used for the detectors was a set of attributes such as file size and name, directory location, and priority, suggesting a Symbolic shape-space.

Related Works from the Authors

Harmer, P. K. (2000), "A Distributed Agent Architecture for a Computer Virus Immune System", M.Sc. Thesis, Air Force Institute of Technology, WPAFB, OH.

Harmer, P. K. & Lamont, G. B. (2000), "An Agent Based Architecture for a Computer Virus Immune System", *Proc. of the Genetic and Evolutionary Computation*

Conference, Workshop on Artificial Immune Systems and Their Applications, pp. 45-46.

Marmelstein, R. E., Van Veldhuizen, D. A., Harmer, P. K. & Lamont, G. B (1999), "A White Paper on Modeling and Analysis of Computer Immune Systems Using Evolutionary Algorithms", TR 1, Air

Force Institute of Technology, WAPAFB, OH.

Marmelstein, R. E., Van Veldhuizen, D. A. & Lamont, G. B (1998), "A Distributed Architecture for an Adaptive Computer Virus Immune System", *Proc. of the IEEE Systems, Man, and Cybernetics Conference*, pp. 3838-3843.

4.3.2. Network Intrusion Detection

In Kim and Bentley (1999a), the authors reviewed and assessed the analogy between the human immune system and network intrusion detection systems. They aimed at unraveling the significant features of the immune system that would be successfully applied to the task of detecting intrusions in computer networks. Upon their analysis, they identified three fundamental requirements for the derivation of the design goals for network-based intrusion detection systems: distribution, self-organization, and being lightweight. Table 4.6 describes the components and functions of the immune system argued to satisfy these three requirements.

In a further work, Kim and Bentley (1999b) proposed a negative selection algorithm with niching in an attempt to improve on their initial ideas. The proposed negative selection with niching is a variation of the algorithm introduced in the previous chapter with the repertoire **P** of naïve antibodies being evolved towards the nonself, instead of being randomly generated. This strategy addresses the discussed lack of adaptability of the original negative selection algorithm and may indeed reduce the computational cost of generating the repertoire **P**.

The authors also suggested that a generic artificial immune system for network intrusion detection would be comprised of three distinct evolutionary stages: 1) negative selection, 2) clonal selection, and 3) gene library evolution. Table 4.7 summarizes the immune metaphors devised for their network intrusion detection system (IDS).

Table 4.6. Components of the immune system that satisfy the requirements for the development of an efficient network intrusion detection system (IDS).

Immune System	Characteristic of an IDS
Immune network	Distribution
Unique antibody sets	
Gene library evolution	
Negative selection	Self-Organization
Clonal selection	
Approximate recognition	
Memory cells	Lightweight
Gene expression	

Table 4.7. Mapping between the network intrusion detection system and the immune system.

Immune System	Network Environment
Bone marrow and thymus	Primary IDS that generates the detector sets
Secondary lymph nodes	Local hosts
Antibodies	Detectors
Antigens	Network intrusions
Self	Normal activities
Nonself	Abnormal activities

In the actual implementation of the IDS, the authors employed a Hamming shape-space with an alphabet of length $k = 10$ to model the antibodies (detectors). In light of the AIS framework, an interesting aspect of this work is that the affinity between two molecules is determined based upon a *phenotypic* instead of *genotypic* matching. The genotype corresponds to the attribute strings representing the molecules, and the phenotype is equivalent to their decoded values. All the affinity measures utilized in the reviewed work are on the genotypic level, i.e., they evaluate affinities amongst the strings themselves. A more complete discussion of genotypes and phenotypes will be presented in Section 6.3, and the possibility of extending the affinity measures to the phenotypic spaces will be assessed in Chapter 8.

Related Works from the Authors

Kim, J. & Bentley, P. J. (2001), "Investigating the Roles of Negative Selection and Clonal Selection in an Artificial Immune System for Network Intrusion Detection", *IEEE Transactions of Evolutionary Computation*, Special Issue on AIS (in print).

Kim, J. & Bentley, P. J. (2001), "Evaluating Negative Selection in an Artificial Immune System for Network Intrusion Detection", *Proc. of the Genetic and Evolutionary Computation Conference*, pp.1330 - 1337.

Kim, J. & Bentley, P. J. (2001), "Towards an Artificial Immune System for Network Intrusion Detection: An Investigation of Clonal Selection with a Negative Selection Operator", *Proc. of the Congress on Evolutionary Computation*, pp.1244-1252.

Work in Dasgupta (1999a) proposed an agent-based system for intrusion/anomaly detection and response in networked computers. In his approach, mobile agents roamed around the nodes and routers of a network of computers monitoring its situation. The author claimed that the most appealing properties of the proposed agents are mobility, adaptability, and collaboration. The immune inspired agents were able to interact freely and dynamically with the environment and each other. Table 4.8 summarizes the immune metaphors used.

Table 4.8. Mapping between the network intrusion detection system and the immune system.

Immune System	Network Environment
Lymphokines	Agents that serve as message carriers or negotiators throughout the network
Helper T-cell	Agents that reports the status of the environment to the user or display the decision report
Killer T-cell	Agent that takes a "drastic" action in case of real intrusion or malicious activity
Suppressor T-cell	Agent that suppresses the actions of other agents
Lymphocyte trafficking	Mobile agents that navigate through the network
Co-stimulation	Signal sent by agents in the network in order to confirm an anomaly

In order to detect anomalies and/or intrusions, the author proposed the monitoring of several parameters, such as type of user and user privileges, login/logout period and location, amount of free memory, and type of connection. These are spread over several levels in the network environment (user-level, system-level, process-level, and packet-level) and suggest a Symbolic shape-space representation for the AIS components. One of the detection processes was performed by determining the affinity (matching) between a current parameter value with the profile of the normal usage.

Related Works from the Author

Dasgupta, D. (2000), "An Immune Agent Architecture for Intrusion Detection", *Proc. of the Genetic and Evolutionary Computation Conference*, Workshop on Artificial Immune Systems, pp. 42-44.

Dasgupta, D. & Gonzalez, F. A. (2001), "An Immunogenetic Approach to Intrusion Detection", CS Technical Report, CS-01-001, University of Memphis.

Skormin *et al.* (2001) argued that information security systems (ISS) play an important role in the protection of information in computer networks. They explored the fundamentals of the biological immune system and assessed the potential implementation of these principles in a multi-agent ISS of networked computers. In their analogy, biological systems and computer networks are highly complex and connected systems, with extensive interaction among their components and numerous entry points. In addition, both systems are vulnerable to malicious entities (e.g., viruses or unauthorized accesses) which are composed of the same building blocks (e.g., amino-acids or macro commands). The authors also proposed a mapping between the innate, humoral and cellular immune responses when compared to computer networks, as summarized in Table 4.9.

Table 4.9. Mapping between the immune responses and computer networks.

Immune Response	Computer Network
Innate	Passwords and firewalls
Humoral	Specialized software
Cellular	Antivirus programs

Gu *et al.* (2000) proposed a detection and elimination system, called the antibody layer, against Internet hackers and viruses, termed Internet antigens. Under the AIS perspective, three major parts compose this system: 1) a data base about known Internet antigens and some of their features; 2) an evolvable antibody layer that allows the system to detect unknown antigens; and 3) an anti-antigen procedure responsible for controlling the antibody layer and to prescribing a form of antigen elimination. Table 4.10 summarizes the immune metaphors used by the authors.

Table 4.10. Mapping between the antibody layer and the immune system.

Immune System	Network Environment
Host	Computer over the Internet
Antigens	Hackers, viruses
B-cells	Scanning mechanism that searches for specific antigens
Helper T-cell	A data base containing information about known antigens, such as suspicious behaviors, that will be used to create new antigenic patterns to be presented to the B-cells
Suppressor T-cell	Host alliance that alleviates the load of the host security procedures
Anti-antigen procedure	Controls the antibody layer and provides the antibody prescription

4.4 Anomaly Detection

The normal behavior of a system is often characterized by a series of observations over time. The problem of detecting novelties, or anomalies, can be viewed as finding deviations of a characteristic behavior, or property, of the system. For computer scientists, the identification of computational viruses and network intrusions are considered very important anomaly detection tasks, and these have been widely studied by the artificial immune systems community. Works in this avenue were reviewed in the previous section.

Note that anomaly detection can be viewed as a sub-problem of pattern recognition, but due to the broad applicability of artificial immune systems to anomaly detection, it was felt appropriate to create a separate section for the topic.

4.4.1. Image Inspection

Aisu and Mizutani (1996) combined a variation of the Farmer's continuous immune network model with the negative selection algorithm in order to develop a machine learning system to detect anomalies. Their algorithm was applied to a simple image inspection problem, but was claimed to be applicable to any type of anomaly detection tasks. The authors used a binary Hamming shape-space with an additional bit incorporating the cross-reactive threshold into the genetic encoding of the detectors. The set of self-patterns to be protected was simply represented by binary strings. The affinity between two molecules was measured via Hamming distance. Genetic variation was introduced in a detector by mutating, with a given probability, one of its bits. This system also accounted for the network metadynamics by allowing the replacement of "unsuitable" detectors, i.e., those with low concentrations, measured by an equation similar to the one proposed by Farmer and collaborators.

Related Works from the Author

Aisu, H. & Mizutani H. (1996), "A Rule Acquisition for Image Processing Using Immune Mechanism", *Proc. of the 12th Fuzzy System Symposium*, pp. 75-78.

4.4.2. Image Segmentation

McCoy and Devarajan (1997) suggested that the pattern recognition task performed by the immune system has much in common with the aerial image segmentation problem. The authors used the negative selection algorithm to construct a set of detectors to perform pattern recognition. The detectors are hyperspheres in a Euclidean shape-space composed of an L^2 vector of pixels values plus a radius r. The affinity measure used was taken to be the sum of squared differences between the image and the detector pixels. A detector was activated when its affinity with an image is less than the cross-reactive threshold r^2. The authors argued that finding a repertoire of detectors that covers nonself features is easier than finding a single optimal detector, since there are many ways to arrive at an acceptable solution.

Related Works from the Authors

McCoy, D. F. & Devarajan, V. (1998), "Artificial Immune Systems for Multispectral feature Extraction", *Proc. of SPIE Conf. on Algorithms for Multispectral and Hyperspectral Imagery IV*, SPIE 3372, pp. 241-249.

4.4.3. Time Series Data

Dasgupta and Forrest (1996) applied the negative selection algorithm to detect novelties in time series data. The authors employed a binary Hamming shape-space to represent the data to be protected, and the r-contiguous bit rule to evaluate the affinities among the self-patterns and the repertoire P to be used to generate the set of detectors. They assessed the quality of this algorithm by applying it to several different data sets (in a series of papers), such as the Mackey Glass series, a simulated cutting tool dynamics in a milling process, and some sensory data.

Related Works from the Authors

Dasgupta, D. & Niño, F. (2000), "A Comparison of Negative and Positive Selection in Novel Pattern Detection", *Proc. of the Congress on Evolutionary Computation*, pp. 125-130.

Dasgupta, D. & Forrest, S. (1999), "Artificial Immune Systems in Industrial Applications", *Proc. of the Int. Conf. on Intelligent Processing and Manufac-turing of Materials*, **1**, pp. 257-267.

Dasgupta, D. & Forrest, S. (1999), "An Anomaly Detection Algorithm Inspired by the Immune System", In *Artificial Immune Systems and Their Applications*, D. Dasgupta (ed.), Springer-Verlag, pp. 262-277.

Dasgupta, D. (1996), "A New Algorithm for Anomaly Detection in Time Series Data", *Proc. of the Int. Conf. on Knowledge-Based Computer Systems*.

4.5   Optimization

Optimization may be defined as the task of making a system or designing it as effective or functional as possible. It usually consists in finding a relatively (or an absolutely) best set of admissible conditions to be achieved by a certain objective, formulated in mathematical terms. Problems in optimization arise in several areas of applications. This section presents artificial immune systems specially designed to solve constrained, multi-modal, combinatorial, and time dependent optimization problems.

Mori *et al.* (1993) developed an immune optimization algorithm hybridizing ideas from immune network theory and evolutionary algorithms. Their algorithm is based upon an entropy measure to maintain the diversity of a repertoire of antibodies. Crossover and mutation operators are used to promote genetic recombination and variation in the repertoire. The algorithm is of general purpose and will be fully described in Section 6.5 as a hybrid of an evolutionary and an immune-inspired approach. Its applications have been several, from function optimization to scheduling and will be referenced in the next sub-section.

4.5.1. Numerical Function Optimization

The immune network model proposed by Varela and collaborators introduced Equation 3.16 to describe the network sensitivity of components in the immune system. In addition, this model proposed the incorporation of a metadynamics function responsible for the recruitment of novel components and death of useless elements in the network.

Based upon these two features, network sensitivity and metadynamics, Bersini and Varela (1990) developed a search technique to be applied to function optimization tasks. The algorithm introduced has some interesting aspects, such as the combination of an affinity measure and a fitness function. The fitness function was responsible for evaluating the quality of each individual in relation to the environment, while the affinity measure was used to evaluate the degree of similarity among individuals of the population. Individual candidates suffered genetic variation through crossover and mutation, operators borrowed from evolutionary algorithms. The authors reported results on a simple problem using a binary Hamming shape-space and a normalized affinity function inversely proportional to the Hamming distance among individuals. Results comparing their algorithm with the standard genetic algorithm were also presented.

Note that the approach adopted of measuring the similarity among individuals in order to decide where and when to insert a new individual (network metadynamics) is a process similar to fitness sharing to be reviewed in Section 6.3.

Related Works from the Author

Bersini, H. & Varela, F. J. (1994), "The Immune Learning Mechanisms: Reinforcement, Recruitment and Their Applications", In *Computing with Biological Metaphors*, R. Paton (ed.), Chapman & Hall, pp. 166-192.

Bersini, H. & Varela, F. J. (1991), "The Immune Recruitment Mechanism: A Selective Evolutionary Mechanism", *Proc. of the 4th Int. Conf. on Genetic Algorithms*, R. Belew & L. Booker (eds.), Morgan Kaufmann, pp. 520-526.

Chun *et al.* (1998) applied a slightly modified version of the immune algorithm developed by Mori and collaborators (Mori *et al.*, 1993) to several function optimization problems and compared its performance with that of genetic algorithms and evolution strategies. They also compared the performance of the algorithms when applied to the design of a surface permanent magnet synchronous motor. Based upon their results, the authors claimed that the modified immune algorithm is very suitable for solving multi-modal optimization problems.

This algorithm was also applied to optimize the shape of a pole face of an electromagnet (Chun *et al.*, 1997).

Huang (2000) applied another modified version of the Mori's immune algorithm to the problem of placing capacitors in a distribution system.

4.5.2. Constrained Optimization

Hajela and Yoo (1999) took inspiration from the immune system to address several problems in design optimization: 1) how to enhance the convergence speed of a genetic algorithm (GA), 2) how to handle constraints in a GA-based search, and 3) how to adapt the GA search to large scale design problems. The authors argued that the immune system capabilities of performing pattern (schema) recognition and adaptation could be used advantageously to improve the performance of genetic algorithms in structural optimization problems. The method was applied to several tasks, including the optimal design of a 10-bar truss structure for minimum weight and with pre-defined allowable constraints on maximum stresses of tension and compression in the bar elements.

Like the majority of GA applications, they used a binary encoding for the strings representing the immune components, i.e., a binary Hamming shape-space. The antibodies corresponded to the unfeasible designs, while the antigens were equivalent to the feasible ones. The goal of the algorithm was to (co-)adapt the unfeasible designs (antibodies) to the feasible ones (antigens), so as to reduce the constraint violations of the GA-based search. The immune algorithm to handle constraints in a GA based search will be described in Section 6.5.

The fitness of an individual was determined by its ability to recognize either a specific or a broad group of antigens, given by a function that measured the number of matching bits between a pair of strings. Thus, affinity was measured via similarity instead of complementarity. However, the authors suggest that complementarity measures, such as the Hamming distance, could be employed in the place of similarity.

Related Works from the Authors

Yoo, J. & Hajela, P. (1999), "Immune Network Simulations in Multicriterion Design", *Structural Optimization*, **18**, 2/3, pp. 85-94, 1999.

Yoo, J. & Hajela, P. (1999), "Multicriterion Design of Fuzzy Structural Systems Using Immune Network Modeling", *Proc. of the AIAA/ASME/ASCE/AHS SDM Meeting*, AIAA 99-1425, pp. 1880- 1890.

Hajela, P., Yoo, J. & Lee, J. (1997), "GA Based Simulation of Immune Networks - Applications in Structural Optimization", *Engineering Optimization*, **29**, pp. 131-149.

Hajela, P., & Lee, J. (1996), "Constrained Genetic Search via Schema Adaptation: An Immune Network Solution", *Structural Optimization*, **12**(1), pp. 11-15.

4.5.3. Inventory Optimization

Joshi (1995) approached the immune system as an adaptive production system where the relation between the demand, likened to antigens, and a product, likened to antibodies, is nonlinear and probabilistic. Based upon an immune network model, the author studied the inventory (antibody) level corresponding to an immune network memory, which would help in the adaptive maintenance of response quality with minimum cost for an inventory system.

It was argued that the immune network approach gives rise to an important multiproduct inventory optimization problem. The correponding multivariate model represents a complex and general example of industrial systems where a nonlinear and probabilistic network of interactions exists between demand and products, influencing the involved cost functions. In addition, the supplies of products triggered by a single demand are associative and mutually competitive.

4.5.4. Combinatorial Optimization (n-TSP Problem)

The traveling salesman problem (TSP) is one of the most well known combinatorial optimization problems. Simply stated, the traveling salesman must visit every city in his territory exactly once and then return to the starting city. The problem is: given the cost of travel between all cities, which is the tour with smallest cost? For sake of simplicity, the reader must consider the cost as being the length of the itinerary traveled by the salesman. The n-th traveling salesman problem (n-TSP) is an extension of the traditional TSP, where n salesmen are available for finding the minimal tour. The salesmen might perform independent routes and start from the same base city. Figure 4.1 illustrates the TSP and n-TSP problems.

Toma *et al.* (1999) proposed an adaptive optimization algorithm inspired by the immune network theory and MHC peptide presentation. In their model, immune network principles were used to produce adaptive behaviors for the n-TSP agents, and antigenic presentation by MHC molecules was used to induce competitive behaviors among these agents. The agents possessed a sensor, mimicking MHC peptide presentation by macrophages. T-cells were used to control the behavior of agents, and B-cells were used to produce behaviors. Table 4.11 summarizes the proposed mapping between the n-TSP problem and the immune system.

The system operated as follows: first macrophages acquired a city number at random and presented it to the T- and B-cells. If a T-cell recognized this number, it tried to help B-cells by sending stimulatory signals. If T- and B-cells recognized the same number, the B-cell produced an antibody and traveled, then MHC was changed. The representation was based on an Integer shape-space, and the affinity of each agent with the environment was directly proportional to the distance traveled by the agent.

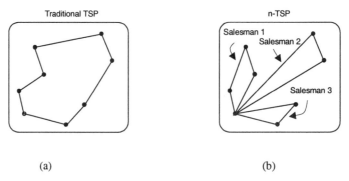

Figure 4.1.   The Traveling salesman problem. (a) Standard version. (b) n-TSP.

Table 4.11. Immune cells and molecules and their roles in the n-TSP problem solving.

Immune System	Role in the n-TSP problem
Antigen	Contains information about the cities and salesmen
Macrophage	Selects the city number that the salesman agent must visit
T-cells	Help the activation of B-cells
B-cells	Produce antibodies
Antibody	Perform the behavior of an agent

Related Works from the Authors

Toma, N., Endo, S. & Yamada, K. (**2000**), "The Proposal and Evaluation of an Adaptive Memorizing Immune Algorithm with Two Memory Mechanisms", *Journal of the Japanese Society for Artificial Intelligence*, **15**(6), pp. 1097-1106.

Endoh, S., Toma, N. & Yamada, K. (**1998**), "Immune Algorithm for n-TSP", *Proc. of the IEEE Systems, Man, and Cybernetics Conference*, pp. 3844-3849.

4.5.5. Time Dependent Optimization

The time dependent optimization problem (TDO) consists in locating successive optima of non-stationary functions. It associates, at a time t, a fitness function to each individual, defining a time dependent fitness function. TDO can be considered as 1) a problem of maintaining a viable state in a reactive, instead of convergent, GA; 2) an efficient optimization in dynamic environments; or 3) a realization of adaptive versus convergent dynamics in artificial systems.

The artificial immune system proposed by Gaspar and Collard (2000) to solve the TDO problem was composed of three phases. In the first phase, a set of B-cells was evaluated for their affinity with the environment and each other. Their affinity with the environment allowed the system to seek for the optimum solution, while the affinity with each other was used to select for reproducing those cells that are not related to the current optimum, so that the diversity of the repertoire was maintained. The second phase corresponded to the clonal selection and affinity maturation processes. The last phase, named the recruitment phase, was used to select and recruit into the repertoire the useful cells while discarding the useless ones. The B-cells were represented using binary strings in a Hamming shape-space and the affinity among cells was measured via Hamming distance.

Related Works from the Authors

Gaspar, A. & Collard, P. (**2000**), "Immune Approaches to Experience Acquisition in Time Dependent Optimization", *Proc. of the Genetic and Evolutionary Computation Conference*, Workshop on Artificial Immune Systems, pp. 49-50.

Gaspar, A. & Collard, P. (**1999**), "From GAs to Artificial Immune Systems: Improving Adaptation in Time Dependent Optimization", *Proc. of the Congress on Evolutionary Computation*, **3**, pp. 1859-1866.

4.6   Machine Learning

Learning is commonly addressed as the process of acquiring knowledge from experience and abstracting this knowledge to solve new, previously unseen problems. In order to perform learning, a system (biological or computational) usually has to adapt itself, or some of its parameters, as a result of the interactions with an environment, and it has to maintain (remember) this adaptation for some period of time. Machine learning involves the study of how to create systems (machines) that are capable of learning from experience, i.e., modifying their behavior as a result of learning and remembering the learnt subjects so as to use this acquired knowledge in the future.

The process of immunizing through vaccination is an example of an immune learning mechanism. Once a person is injected with a weakened (or dead) sample of a given pathogenic agent (e.g., a virus or a bacteria), our immune system alters the concentration and structural composition (affinity) of those specific antibodies that react with the injected pathogen, thus resulting in immunization.

4.6.1. Reinforcement Learning

In (Watkins, 2001), the author proposed a resource limited artificial immune system classifier model, using as a basis the discrete immune networks of (Timmis & Neal, 2000) and (de Castro & von Zuben, 2000b) described in the previous chapter. Here the author extracted metaphors such as resource competition, clonal selection, and memory cell retention to create a classification model named AIRS. However, the resultant AIRS system was not itself a network model, but a population based system. Results presented in this work are very encouraging. Benchmark data sets such as Fisher Iris data set, Ionosphere data set, and Sonar data sets were used to test the effectiveness of the algorithm. AIRS was found to perform at the same level of accuracy as some other well established techniques, such has C4.5, CART, etc. This work highlighted the need for further investigation into this model for supervised learning.

4.6.2. Unsupervised Learning

Based upon Equation 3.14 of Farmer's immune network model, the clonal selection principle and somatic hypermutation, Hunt and Cooke (1996) proposed an artificial immune network for machine-learning. Their object-oriented system was composed of a bone marrow object, a B-cell object containing antibodies, and antigens. Their network presents an evolutionary-like learning strategy and a dynamic content-addressable memory, in the sense that it is capable of forgetting previously learned information.

The authors applied their network model to two pattern recognition problems and also compared, in a theoretical basis, their AIS with other computational intelligence paradigms, such as artificial neural networks, learning classifier systems, machine-induction, and case-based reasoning. This network model also served as a step for the research that resulted in the discrete immune network model of J. Timmis and collaborators described in the framework for AIS.

Inspired in the immune network model introduced by Farmer and collaborators and by the work of Hunt, Timmis *et al.* (2000), Timmis and Neal (2001) proposed an artificial immune network for unsupervised learning. Their network is composed of a set of B-cells to be used for classification and clustering of a set of input patterns, named antigens. Each B-cell was connected to other B-cells in the network and was selected for reproduction, via the clonal selection principle, according to the degree (level) of stimulation the cell receives from the environment. The cells were represented in a Euclidean shape-space, and their stimulation level was a function of their similarity, measured via Euclidean distance, with other cells and the antigen. An immune inspired resource limited mechanism was employed to control the population of B-cells within the network, and a tool was developed to allow the visualization of the evolved network structures (Timmis, 2001).

Related Works from the Authors

Timmis, J. & Knight, T. (2001), "Artificial Immune Systems: Using the Immune System as Inspiration for Data Mining. In *Data Mining: A Heuristic Approach*, (eds.) H. A. Abbass, R. A. Sarker, and C. S. Newton, Chapter XI, Idea Group Publishing, pp. 209-230.

Timmis, J. (2000), *Artificial Immune Systems: A Novel Data Analysis Technique Inspired by the Immune Network Theory*, Ph.D. Dissertation, Department of Computer Science, University of Wales. UK.

Knight, T. & Timmis, J. (2001), "AINE: An Immunological Approach to Data Mining", *Proc. of the IEEE International Conference on Data Mining*, pp 297-304.

Timmis, J., Neal, M. & Hunt, J. (1999), "Data Analysis Using Artificial Immune Systems, Cluster Analysis and Kohonen Networks: Some Comparisons", *Proc. of the IEEE System, Man, and Cybernetics Conference*, **3**, pp. 922-927.

The work presented by de Castro and Von Zuben (2000b) used the clonal selection algorithm described in Section 3.5 to control the dynamics of an antibody repertoire when presented to a set of antigens. The antibodies corresponded to a distributed set of pattern recognizers, while the antigens were equivalent to the patterns to be recognized in a data clustering application. Both, antigens and antibodies, were represented in a normalized Euclidean shape-space, and their affinities were measured via Euclidean distance.

This system also took inspiration from the immune network theory to control the cardinality of the antibody repertoire. Thus, the antibodies were structured in an immune network fashion, and their response to the environment (antigens) followed the clonal selection principle. In a self-organized way, their network was applied to several data clustering applications and also had the goal of filtering out redundant data from a given data set.

Related Works from the Authors

de Castro, L. N. & Von Zuben, F. J. (2001), "aiNet: An Artificial Immune Network for Data Analysis", In *Data Mining: A Heuristic Approach*, H. A. Abbass, R. A. Sarker, and C. S. Newton (eds.), Idea Group Publishing, USA, Chapter XII, pp. 231-259.

de Castro, L. N. & Von Zuben, F. J., (2001), "Immune and Neural Network Models: Theoretical and Empirical Comparisons", *Int. Journal of Computational Intelligence and Applications*, 1(3), pp. 239-257.

4.6.3. Double Plasticity

Bersini (1999) argued that the immune network dynamics and metadynamics offer inspiration for the development of mechanisms of double adaptation (plasticity) for intelligent systems. Learning would be accomplished through a mechanism for parameter adaptation together with another mechanism for architectural adaptation, increasing considerably the flexibility of the machine learning paradigm.

The dynamics of a system is usually accounted for in strategies such as neural networks by weight adjustment. Learning classifier systems in contrast, inherently incorporate dynamics and metadynamics; the dynamics being played by the bucket brigade algorithm and the metadynamics by the genetic algorithm.

Bersini presented examples of the double plastic mechanisms in three problems: 1) a constructive neural network classifier, 2) the refinement and redefining of the partition of the problem space of an autonomous learning agent by reinforcement learning, and 3) the addition of linear controllers to chaotic control. Although his illustrative examples were weakly inspired by the immune network double plasticity, the author claimed they stress the importance of parametric and structural adaptation in intelligent methodologies. In addition, they show that the immune system constitutes a novel paradigm in which to search for these mechanisms.

Related Works from the Authors

Bersini, H. & Varela, F. J. (1994), "The Immune Learning Mechanisms: Reinforcement, Recruitment and Their Applications", In *Computing with Biological Metaphors*, R. Paton (ed.), Chapman & Hall, pp. 166-192.

Bersini, H. (1992), "Reinforcement and Recruitment Learning for Adaptive Process Control", *Proc. of the Int. Fuzzy Association Conference (IFAC/IFIP/IMACS) on Artificial Intelligence in Real Time Control*, pp. 331-337.

4.6.4. Concept Learning

Inspired by the self/nonself discrimination capability of the immune system, Potter and de Jong (1998) developed a co-evolutionary genetic algorithm to differentiate examples from counter-examples of a given concept. Their model was limited to the interactions of B-cells and antigens and was applied to concept learning from pre-classified positive and negative examples, equated to foreign (nonself) and self-molecules, respectively. In the case of noise free examples, the system was evolved to a point where all the foreign and none of the self-molecules were recognized.

In their model, a B-cell consisted of an antibody and a real-valued activation threshold was used to represent the binding strength required to initiate an immune response. Antigens were represented as simple binary strings, and antibodies were binary schemas (i.e., , Ab $\in$ {0,1,#}, where # is a don't care symbol) in a Hamming shape-space. A linear matching function returned the percentage of matching bits between antigens and antibodies, and this was used to compute their affinity. Besides the affinity between antibody and antigen, a B-cell also presented a fitness value proportional to the number of foreign molecules it recognizes.

4.6.5. The Baldwin Effect

The idea behind the Baldwin effect is that if learning "helps" survival, then the individuals with increased learning capabilities will have more descendants, increasing the frequency of the genes responsible for learning. Section 5.5 brings a broader discussion about the Baldwin effect.

Hightower *et al.* (1996) used a binary Hamming shape-space to model the immune system in order to study the influence of learning in the evolution of the genetic representation of antibodies. Antibodies and antigens were simply represented as bitstrings of the same length, and the match score was given by the Hamming distance taken between the two bitstrings. The binding value was a non-linear (sigmoidal) function of the match score, similar to the one illustrated in Figure 3.10(b).

By varying the learning rate (this can be equated to a somatic mutation rate) the authors showed the presence of the Baldwin effect, in the sense that learning accelerates evolution by allowing it to discover which individuals are nearest to a threshold of success. The authors claimed that the non-linear binding function was a necessary condition for the Baldwin effect to occur.

Related Works from the Authors

Perelson, A. S., Hightower, R. & Forrest, S. (1996), "Evolution and Somatic Learning in V-Region Genes", *Research in Immunology,* **147,** pp. 202-208.

4.6.6. Complexity

In order to study the generation of complexity shown in higher living organisms, such as mammals, Nagano and Yonezawa (1999) proposed a learning system based upon the thymic self/nonself discrimination capability. The authors suggested that the origin of self-organization and ordered complexity are equivalent to the establishment of a self-system and thus can be achieved by the generation of a self/nonself discrimination mechanism.

The individuals of a nonself set were composed of DNA sequences and matched against an initial self-set also composed of DNA sequences, both in a Symbolic shape-space defined over the alphabet {A,C,G,T}. These sequences were subjected to a genetic algorithm in order to observe the generation of complexity and the correlation among the DNA sequences and the self/nonself discrimination problem.

Related Works from the Authors

Nagano, S. & Yonezawa, Y., (1998), "DNA Evolutionary Process Simulated with Self-Nonself Recognition Based on Immuno-Function Mechanism", *Proc. of the IIAS, 3rd Workshop on Orders and Structures in Complex Systems*, pp. 117-130.

Nagano, S., Iwasaki, Y. & Yonezawa, Y., (1996), "Immuno Fluctuate model as Defense System Included Complexity Process", *Proc. of the 7th Int. Symposium on Micro Machine and Human Science*, pp. 257-263.

4.7   Robotics

Robotics is the research field involved in the theory, conception, design, manufacture, and operation of robots. The field is highly multidisciplinary involving computer science, electronics, mechatronics, computational intelligence, nanotechnology, bioengineering, and bioinformatics. Loosely speaking, a robot is a machine designed to execute particular tasks. It can be controlled by a human operator, a computer program, or some form of machine (computational) intelligence. An autonomous robot acts as a stand-alone system, complete with its own "controller" responsible for defining its behavior and the execution of some tasks. The last generation robots, in the research-and-development phase, might include features such as emergent behavior, self-replication, self-assembly, intelligence, and nanoscale size.

This section describes how immune principles are being applied to robotics, mainly to the autonomous navigation problem. Most of these works are based on the continuous immune network model of Farmer *et al.* (1986) described in Section 3.5. The works of Ishiguro and collaborators (Watanabe *et al.*, 1999) on the behavior arbitration of robots inspired by this network model will be fully described in Section 7.3 as one of the case studies.

4.7.1. Emergence of Collective Behavior

For a collective behavior to emerge, a set of agents must communicate with each other and with their environment. The objective of the system proposed by Lee and Sim (1997) was to enable a set of robots to undertake tasks within a given environment. The authors used a variation of the immune network model of Farmer, and the clonal selection principle to perform a cooperative control and select a group of behavior strategies for Distributed Autonomous Robotic Systems, named DARS.

In the DARS system, the robots have to individually "understand" the objective of the system, the environment, the behavior of other robots, etc., and to decide their own behavior autonomously in order to cooperate with other agents to establish and maintain the order of the whole system. No central control is supposed to exist. A clonal selection algorithm was used for transmitting high quality strategies among robots, while the immune network of antibodies controlled the interactions of individual robots. Table 4.12 summarizes the mapping between DARS and the immune system.

Table 4.12. Mapping between DARS and the immune system.

Immune System	DARS
Antigen	Environment
Antibody	Strategy of action
B-cell	Robot
T-cell	Control parameter
Stimulus	Adequate behavior
Suppression	Inadequate behavior
Plasma cell	Excellent robot
Inactivated cell	Inferior robot

Related Works from the Authors

Jun, J.-H., Lee, D.-W. & Sim, K.-B., (1999), "Realization of Cooperative and Swarm Behavior in Distributed Autonomous Robotic Systems Using Artificial Immune System", *Proc. of the IEEE System, Man, and Cybernetics Conference*, **4**, pp. 614-619.

Lee, D-W., Jun, H-B. & Sim, K-B. (1999), "Artificial Immune System for Realization of Cooperative Strategies and Group Behavior in Collective Autonomous Mobile Robots", *Proc. of the AROB'99*, pp. 232-235.

Mitsumoto *et al.* (1996) proposed a population control architecture for multiple robotic systems inspired by the immune network model of Farmer and collaborators. The authors argued that social and ecological systems have similar structures when compared to the self-organizing principles of robotic systems. Particularly, they claimed that the dynamics of the immune network is similar to a multiple robotic system and that it allows the regulation of the robotic social structure when faced with a dynamic environment. Their system was composed of robots corresponding to antibodies, and the environment was equivalent to antigens. Four types of interactions were allowed, as summarized in Table 4.13.

Table 4.13. Mapping between the immune network model of Farmer and the collective autonomous robotic problem.

	Immune Network	Multiple Robotic System
Elements	Antigen	Environment
	Antibody	Robot
Interaction 1	Antibody-Antibody stimulation	Robot-Robot stimulation
Interaction 2	Antibody-Antibody suppression	Robot-Robot suppression
Interaction 3	Antibody-Antigen stimulation	Robot-Environment stimulation
Interaction 4	Death in absence of interaction	Death in absence of interaction

Related Works from the Authors

Mitsumoto, N., Fukuda, T., Shimojima, K. & Ogawa, A. (1995), "Micro Autonomous Robotic System and Biologically Inspired Immune Swarm Strategy as a Multi Agent Robotic System", *Proc. of the IEEE Int. Conf. on Robotics and Automation*, pp. 2187-2192.

Mitsumoto, N., Fukuda, T., Shimojima, K. & Ogawa, A. (1997), "Control of the Distributed Autonomous Robotic System Based on the Biologically Inspired Immunological Architecture", *Proc. of the IEEE Int. Conf. on Robotics and Automation*, pp. 3551-3556.

4.7.2. Walking Robots

Ishiguro *et al.* (1998) applied a variation of the second-generation immune network model of Varella and collaborators (Equation 3.17) to the problem of gait acquisition of a robot with 6 legs (a hexapod). They focused on the dynamics, metadynamics, and on the high and low zone tolerances of the immune network.

For a robot to successfully walk each leg must move with an appropriate phase shift in relation to the others, so that the robot load (weight) is divided equally among the legs that are simultaneously on the floor.

No distinction was made between an antibody and a B-cell; each of them was responsible for controlling a single leg. Thus, the robot has six B-cells in total. Each B-cell had a concentration level and two thresholds, a lower and an upper threshold, responsible for determining how the legs move. When the concentration of a given B-cell (leg) exceeds the upper threshold the leg swings forward without being off the ground. In contrast, when its concentration falls below the lower threshold the leg swings backward keeping its foothold. The lower threshold was also responsible for the metadynamics: when the concentration of a given B-cell falls below it, this B-cell is replaced by a new one. The antigens correspond to the load of each leg. This way, the interaction among the B-cells allowed for the coordinate behavior of the legs, and the interaction with the environment (antigens) maintained the equilibrium of the hexapod.

Related Works from the Authors

Ishiguro, A., Kuboshiki, S., Ichikawa, S. & Uchikawa, Y. (**1996**), "Gait Control of Hexapod Walking Robots Using Mutual-Coupled Immune Networks", *Advanced Robotics*, **10**(2), pp. 179-195.

Ishiguro, A., Ichikawa, S. & Uchikawa, Y. (**1996**), "A Gait Acquisition of 6-Legged Walking Robot Using Immune Networks", *Proc. of IROS*, **2**, pp. 1034-1041.

4.8   Control

Broadly speaking, a control system can be defined as a component or series of components aimed at implementing the transformation of an input into a corresponding output response. Traditionally, control engineering was based on the foundations of feedback theory and linear system analysis, integrating several concepts. One of the present challenges to control engineers is to model and control modern, complex, and interrelated systems. This involves the development of autonomous and adaptive control systems.

The capability of the immune system to maintain the homeostasis of the organism suggests successful applications of the immune system as a novel paradigm for the improvement of modern control theory.

4.8.1. Identification, Synthesis and Adaptive Control

Bersini (1991) developed an adaptive control methodology whose basic elements were inspired by the immune recruitment mechanism, reviewed in the previous section, and the reinforcement learning approach to be discussed in Section 6.2. The other immune features addressed were viability, distribution, memory, and adaptability. The control problem was characterized by a discrete state vector in a state space $\Re^L$. His proposal relaxed the conventional control strategies, which try to drive the process under control to a precise target, in the sense that the viability corresponds to a specific zone of the state space in which the process must remain. He argued that the metadynamics of the immune system (network) is akin to a meta-control whose aim is to keep the concentration of the antibodies in a certain domain of viability so as to preserve continuously the identity of the system. He employed the immune recruitment mechanism to maintain the system within its viability domain. It was also argued that the adaptability of this model relies in its metadynamics, thus differentiating from the adaptability of neural networks based on weight adjustment.

Related Works from the Author

Bersini, H. & Varela, F. J. (**1994**), "The Immune Learning Mechanisms: Reinforcement, Recruitment and Their Applications", In *Computing with Biological Metaphors*, R. Paton (Ed.), Chapman & Hall, pp. 166-192.

Bersini, H. (**1992**), "Reinforcement and Recruitment Learning for Adaptive Process Control", *Proc. of the Int. Fuzzy Association Conference (IFAC/IFIP/IMACS) on Artificial Intelligence in Real Time Control*, pp. 331-337.

Krishnakumar and Neidhoefer (1999) introduced the concept of immunized computational systems (ICS) as those that combine a priori knowledge with the adaptability of immune systems to provide alternatives to intelligent control. They divided the intelligent control systems into several levels and pointed out the corresponding levels existing on the vertebrate immune system when it is viewed as a control system, as summarized in Table 4.14.

The proposed immunized systems were hybrids of different computational intelligence methodologies, such as fuzzy systems, artificial neural networks, and genetic algorithms. Each of these methodologies composed a building block to be used in the evolution of an immunized system. The individuals to be evolved were termed messy strings, as they combined different types of structures (neural networks and/or fuzzy systems).

Table 4.14. Intelligent control, its levels, and the immune system.

Level	Immune Response	Intelligent Control
----	Antigen	Disturbance
0	Innate immunity	Robust feedback control
1	T-cells activate B-cells	An error critic modifies the controller parameters
2	Antigen presentation by APCs, and T-cell activation	A utility function translates the disturbances into an error function and presents it to the critic, who starts the adaptation
3	Affinity maturation	The utility function adapts itself based on a planning function

Related Works from the Authors

Krishnakumar, K. & Neidhoefer, J. (1997), "Immunized Adaptive Critics for Level 2 Intelligent Control", *Proc. of the IEEE Systems, Man, and Cybernetics Conference*, 1, pp. 856-860.

Krishnakumar, K. & Neidhoefer, J. (1997), "Immunized Neurocontrol", *Expert Systems with Applications*, 13(3), pp. 201-214.

Krishnakumar, K. Satyadas, A. & Neidhoefer, J. (1995), "An Immune System Framework for Integrating Computational Intelligence Paradigms with Applications to Adaptive Control", In *Computational Intelligence A Dynamic System Perspective*, M. Palaniswami, Y. Attikiouzel, R. J. Marks II, D. Fogel and T. Fukuda (eds.), IEEE Press, pp. 32-45.

4.8.2. Sequential Control

Finding a proper execution sequence for a set of actuators such that the system achieves a desired state from a known initial state is the main goal of a sequential control approach. Ootsuki and Sekiguchi (1999) proposed a method for determining control sequences of a sequential control plant based on the immune system. They used Petri nets and the immune network theory to develop their model.

The discrete dynamic behavior of the components of a sequential control plant was modeled as state machines structured as Petri nets. Hence, the determination of control sequences became equivalent to the determination of the firing sequences for the Petri net models, which were decomposed into several sub-problems. The objective function of each sub-problem was set to satisfy constraints and minimize the objective function of a distributed immune network. The dynamics of the system were controlled by a set of differential equations responsible for describing the interactions among the network elements.

Related Works from the Authors

Ootsuki, J. S., Fujii, Y., Mizutani, H. & Sekiguchi, T. (1998), "Immune System Derived Approach for Finding Firing Sequences of a Sub-Class of Petri Nets", *Transactions of IEE-J*, **188-C**, pp. 419-427.

4.8.3. Feedback Control

Takahashi and Yamada (1997) identified two feedback mechanisms in the immune system which could provide good inspiration for the development of feedback controllers. As the first mechanism, the authors highlighted the immune regulation between activated B-cells and effector T-cells. The second relevant immune feedback mechanism was identified as being the inhibition of the adaptive immune response by suppressor T-cells.

Based on these two feedback mechanisms, the authors proposed a set of discrete equations to govern the immune feedback controller. These include equations for the concentration of antigens, helper, and effector T-cells, and antibodies. Their system used a neural network to define some parameters for the immune feedback controller. The variables of the discrete equations are real-valued vectors in an Euclidean shape-space.

Related Works from the Authors

Kawafuku, M., Sasaki, M. & Takahashi, K. (1999), "Adaptive Learning Method of Neural Network Controller Using an Immune Feedback Law", *IEEE/ASME International Conference on Advanced Intelligent Mechatronics*, pp. 641-646.

Sasaki, M., Kawafuku, M. & Takahashi, K. (1999), "An Immune Feedback Mechanism Based Adaptive Learning of Neural Network Controller", *Proc. of the 6th International Conference on Neural Information Processing*, pp.502-507.

Takahashi, K. & Yamada, T. (1998), "Application of an Immune Feedback Mechanism to Control Systems, *JSME International Journal*, **41**(2C), pp.184-191.

Takahashi, K. & Yamada, T. (1998), "Remarks on a Feedback Controller Based on an Immune Feedback Mechanism", *Japan-U.S.A Symposium on Flexible Automation*, pp.777-783.

4.9 Scheduling

A schedule might be viewed as a plan for performing work, doing an activity, or achieving an objective. It involves the specification of the order and allotted time for each element of the scheduling system. As an example, scheduling a manufacturing system corresponds to allocating machines to processes in a production sequence to fulfill objectives. A job shop scheduling problem decides a combination of sequence of jobs processed on each machine. Scheduling problems can be solved by techniques, such as mathematical programming, expert systems or simulation, and can be viewed as a particular type of optimization problem.

This section reviews those works that use immune principles for solving scheduling problems. A full case study on the work of E. Hart and collaborators (Hart *et al.*, 1999) is provided in Section 7.4.

4.9.1. Adaptive Scheduling

Mori *et al.* (1998) proposed an immune algorithm inspired by the somatic and network theories of the immune system. The former gave rise to the use of somatic recombination and hypermutation to the inducement and maintenance of diversity in an antibody repertoire. In this case, two types of antibodies were encoded in an Integer shape-space: type I was used to represent and optimize the batch sizes, and type II was used to represent the job priority. The network hypothesis was employed to address the mutual recognition among the network antibodies so as to control their proliferation.

The goal of the algorithm was to find the batch sizes and combination of sequence of orders to optimize an objective function. The authors claimed the algorithm is suitable for solving multi-modal optimization tasks, such as a scheduling problem. The affinity among antibodies was measured via the informative entropy measure (Equation 6.14), and the affinity of an antibody with the environment (antigen) corresponded to the decoded value of a given antibody, i.e., the value of the objective function evaluated for the antibody. Their algorithm to perform multi-modal optimization will be fully discussed in Section 6.5.

Related Works from the Authors

Mori, M., Tsukiyama, M. & Fukuda, T. (1994), "Immune Algorithm and its Application to Factory Load Dispatching Planning", *Proc. of the JAPAN-USA Symposium on Flexible Automation*, pp. 1343-1346.

Tsukiyama, M., Mori, M. & Fukuda, T. (1993), "Strategic Level Interactive Scheduling and Operational Level Real-Time Scheduling for Flexible Manufacturing Systems", In *Applications of Artificial Intelligence in Engineering VIII*, **2**, G. Rzevski, J. Pastor, and R. A. Adey (eds.), pp. 615-625.

Fukuda, T., Mori, M. & Tsukiyama, M. (1993), "Immune Networks Using Genetic Algorithm for Adaptive Production Scheduling", *Proc. of 15th IFAC World Congress*, **3**, pp. 57-60.

4.9.2. Scheduling in Computing Systems

King *et al.* (2001) described a biological basis for intelligent agents based upon the immune system. They stressed the primary functionalities of the immune system to be captured in intelligent agents to perform scheduling in computer systems. These are summarized in Table 4.15.

The authors also proposed two different types of agents to be developed for predictive scheduling in computer environments. One agent was named H-cell for hardware management, and another S-cell for software. The two agents were combined to reduce the overall turnaround time in responding to events. Their system also involved a hybrid with an artificial neural network model.

Table 4.15. Functionalities of the immune system to be captured by intelligent agents.

Immune System	Scheduling in Computer Systems
Antigen recognition and response	Recognition of specific hardware and/or software followed by an allocation response that will better use the computer environment's resources to perform on-going and planned tasks
Distributivity	Division of responsibility among agents for command, control, and communication
Evolutionary adaptation (self-organization)	Learning through adaptation implemented using an ART neural network
Immune memory	Embodied in the ART neural network

Related Works from the Authors

Lambert, A., King, R. L., Russ, S. H., Rajan, R. & Reese, D. S. (1999), "Adaptive Analysis for the Design of Hardware Agents Using the Artificial Immune System Model for Resource Management of Heterogeneous Systems", *Miss. State Technical Report n. MSSU-COE-ERC-98-10*, August.

King, R. L., Lambert, A. B., Russ, S. H. & Reese, D. S. (1999), "The Biological Basis of the Immune System as a Model for Intelligent Agents", *Proc. of the Int. Parallel Processing Symposium*, pp. 156-164.

4.9.3. Flow Shop Scheduling

In a classical flow shop scheduling problem, there is a number m of machines and a number j of jobs to be performed in the same order. Each job is composed of a set of stages and each stage requires a specific machine and has a fixed processing time. Cui *et al.* (2001) applied the entropy measure first studied in the context of AIS by Mori *et al.* (1993) (Section 6.5) in order to maintain the diversity of multiobjective evolutionary algorithms. The authors reported results on 2-objective flow shop scheduling problems and argued that the approach is effective in preserving the population diversity.

4.10 Fault Diagnosis

Fault diagnosis corresponds to the act or process of identifying or determining the nature and cause of a fault by detecting its symptoms promptly. This allows the avoidance of fault occurrences and the prevention of fault propagation through the identification of faulty parts.

The idea of an immune system as a special mechanism to detect anomalies and faults is quite intuitive and again, unsurprisingly, researchers have been looking into the immune system in order to develop fault diagnosis systems.

4.10.1. Sensor Network

Based upon the analogy between neural networks and distributed diagnosis models, Ishida (1990) introduced a distributed diagnosis system as an immune network model. His system was based upon a self-organizing and distributed set of units capable of testing one another. All units presented associated connection strengths over a bipolar alphabet, $\{-1,1\}$, and a reliability value. These parameters played a role in a dynamic equation used to govern the behavior of the network.

The author explored immune features, such as the recognition performed by distributed units with dynamical interactions with each other, each unit reacts based on its knowledge, and memory is realized as stable equilibrium points of a dynamical network. The diagnosis was performed by obtaining the stable equilibrium points of the network after periods of perturbation.

Related Works from the Author

Ishida, Y. (2000), "Immunity-Based Systems: A Specification and Applications", *Medical Imaging Technology*, **18**(5), pp. 703-708.

Ishida, Y. (1998), "Distributed and Autonomous Sensing Based on the Immune Network", *Artificial Life Robotics*, **2**, pp. 1-7.

Ishida, Y. (1997), "Active Diagnosis by Self-Organization: An Approach by the Immune Network Metaphor", *Proc. of the Int. Joint Conf. on Artificial Intelligence*, pp. 1084-1089.

Ishida, Y. (1996), "An Immune Network Approach to Sensor-Based Diagnosis by Self-Organization", *Complex Systems*, **10**, pp. 73-90.

Ishida, Y. & Tokimasa, Y. (1996), "Diagnosis by a Dynamic Network Inspired by Immune Network", *Proc. of the World Congress on Neural Networks*, pp. 508-511.

Ishida, Y. (1993), "An Immune Network Model and Its Applications to Process Diagnosis", *Systems and Computers in Japan*, **24**(6), pp. 646-651.

Ishida, Y. & Missezyn, F. (1992), "Learning Algorithms on Immune Network Model: Application to Sensor Diagnosis", *Proc. of the Int. Joint Conf. on Neural Networks*, **1**, pp. 33-38.

4.10.2. Prevention of Fault Propagation

Kayama *et al.* (1995) studied the problem of preventing fault propagation in industrial plants through the proper specification of faulty parts when faults occur. They proposed a hybrid system between the immune network model introduced by Ishida and discussed above, with a learning vector quantization (LVQ) strategy to detect abnormal sensor outputs in a control problem. Their system had two execution modes: training and diagnosing. In the first mode, the LVQ was responsible for extracting correlation among sensors, and in the second mode, the immune network contributed to determining faulty sensors by integrating local testing results obtained by the LVQ algorithm.

4.10.3. Hardware Fault Tolerance

Bradley and Tyrrell (2000) proposed to use the negative selection algorithm to generate a hardware fault tolerant system. Implemented with a Field Programmable Gate Array (FPGA), their approach was based upon a finite state machine, where the presence of valid states and transitions correspond to the self-behavior, and the invalid states and transitions are equivalent to antigens. Table 4.16 and Table 4.17 summarize the mapping from immunology to hardware fault tolerance in terms of entities and processes, respectively. They employed a binary Hamming shape-space to represent the states of the system and speculated that partial string matching rules must be considered in the detection of hardware faults. Another immune aspect of this work was that if a faulty state was detected a co-stimulation signal might be used to activate any number of defined responses.

Table 4.16. Hardware fault tolerance and the immune system: entity feature mapping.

Immune System	Hardware Fault Tolerance
Self	Acceptable state/state transition
Non-self (antigen)	Erroneous state/state transition
Antibody	Error tolerance conditions
Genes	Variables forming tolerance conditions
Paratope	Erroneous state/state transition tolerance conditions
Epitope	Valid state/state transition tolerance conditions
Helper T-cell	Recovery procedure activator
Memory cell	Sets of tolerance condition

Table 4.17. Hardware fault tolerance and the immune system: process feature mapping.

Immune System	Hardware Fault Tolerance
Recognition of self	Recognition of valid state/state transition
Recognition of non-self	Recognition of invalid state/state transition
Ontogenetic learning	Learning correct states and transitions
Humoral immunity	Error detection and recovery
Clonal deletion	Isolation of self-recognizing tolerance conditions
Inactivation of antigen	Return to normal operation
Life of an organism	Operation lifetime of a hardware

Related Works from the Authors

Bradley, D. W. & Tyrrell, A. M. (2001), "The Architecture for a Hardware Immune System", *Proc. of 3rd NASA/DoD Workshop on Evolvable Hardware*, pp. 193-200.

Bradley, D. W. & Tyrrell, A. M. (2000), "Hardware Fault Tolerance: An Immunological Approach", *Proc. of the IEEE System, Man, and Cybernetics Conference*, pp. 107-112.

Bradley, D. W., Sanchez, C. O-. & Tyrrell, A. M. (2000), "Embryonics + Immunotronics: A Bio-Inspired Approach to Fault Tolerance", *Proc. of the 2nd NASA/DoD Workshop on Evolvable Hardware*, pp. 215-223.

Tyrrell, A. M. (1999), "Computer Know Thy Self!: A Biological Way to Look at Fault-Tolerance", *Proc. of the 25th Euromicro Conference*, **2**, pp. 129-135.

4.10.4. Software Fault Tolerance

Software fault tolerance consists in detecting erroneous states of an algorithm and executing recovery procedures. These are usually implemented by adding formal properties to be satisfied by state variables during execution. Xanthakis *et al.* (1996) proposed an analogy between the immune system and software fault tolerance as summarized in Table 4.18, where *l-correct* corresponds to a loosely correct state. They also introduced an AIS to detect and recover erroneous states during the execution of a computer program.

Their AIS was based upon the immune network theory and was composed of antibodies (equivalent to B-cells) and T-cells. Each antibody was formed by an epitope and a paratope. The epitope consists of a simplified representation of a subset of different properties that have been verified by some state variables. The paratopes in contrast, symbolized the properties that are not verified. The AIS worked in two phases: learning and operating. In the learning phase, a population of antibodies was evolved using a GA such that the epitope of each antibody recognizes the greatest number of *l*-correct states, whereas their paratopes recognize the greatest number of erroneous states. In the second phase, a set of T-cells was created so as that, by interacting with the antibodies, the T-cells attempt to modify the defective states for the states to be tolerated.

Table 4.18. Software fault tolerance and the immune system.

Immune System	Software Fault Tolerance
Self	L-correct state
Nonself or antigen	Erroneous state
Antibody	Pair of tolerance conditions
Epitope	L-correct state tolerance condition
Paratope	Erroneous state tolerance condition
Gene used to create an antibody	Variable forming a primitive relation
Antibody proliferation	Augmentation of antibody strength
Learning during gestation	Learning l-correct states after testing
Life of the organism	Software operation

4.11   Antibody Libraries

Section 2.8 described gene libraries consisting of gene fragments that are assembled together to generate immune receptors. Throughout the lifetime of an organism, some processes can modify these receptors. For example, during an immune response the B-cell receptor genes undergo targeted mutation and selection on the basis of binding with antigens, allowing them to increase repertoire diversity and affinity with the selective antigen. Thus, an organism possesses multiple genetically encoded receptor fragments that can evolve independently of each other and may be subject to optimization, through mutation and selection, which is ultimately aimed at the survival of the organism.

This section reviews some works on theoretical immunology that study the evolution of gene libraries of antibody molecules. Although these works were not directly aimed at problem solving, they are relevant for the design of artificial immune systems for they address the problem of generating antibody repertoires.

4.11.1.   Emergent Organization

Hightower *et al.* (1995) used a genetic algorithm and a binary Hamming shape-space to study the effects of evolution on the genetic encoding of antibody molecules. A set of binary antibody molecules was evolved towards a population of binary antigens. The authors used a bone marrow model based upon gene libraries, as illustrated in Figure 3.12, to generate antibodies. Producing one antibody molecule began with a random selection of a genetic component from each of the libraries. Thus, not all genes found in the genotype (total collection of gene segments) were expressed in the phenotype (expressed antibody molecules).

The fitness of an individual was determined by its overall ability to recognize antigen molecules. It was evaluated by exposing an individual antibody to a set of antigens and testing how well it recognizes each antigen in that set. The affinity (degree of recognition) of an antibody and an antigen was measured via the Hamming distance between their attribute strings.

The authors' experimental results showed that the evolution of immune system genes could induce a high degree of genetic organization even though that organization is not explicitly required by the fitness function. The experiments also showed that the genetic algorithm could optimize complex genetic information, being able to organize the structure of the antibody libraries. The selection pressure operating on the phenotype as a whole could translate to selection pressure acting on individual genes, even though not all genes were expressed in the phenotype.

Related Works from the Authors

Perelson, A. S., Hightower, R. & Forrest, S. (1996), "Evolution and Somatic Learning in V-Region Genes", *Research in Immunology*, **147**, pp. 202-208.

Hightower, R. (1996), *Computational Aspects of Antibody Gene Families*, Ph.D. Thesis, University of New Mexico, Albuquerque, New Mexico, USA.

4.11.2. Evolution of Libraries

Oprea and Forrest (1998) argued that an intriguing feature of the immune system is its capability of building antibodies able to bind antigens previously not encountered. The authors used a similar representation as the one described above in order to study how this broad coverage of the antigenic space could be achieved, given the fact that the immune system uses a relatively small number of genes to construct its receptors. A genetic algorithm was employed to explore the strategies the antibody libraries may evolve in order to cover antigenic spaces of various sizes.

Antigens and antibodies were represented as bitstrings of the same length. The affinity between an antigen and an antibody was measured via their Hamming distance, and the fitness of an antibody was proportional to its affinity with all the antigens of a given set.

The authors argued that somatic mutation of antibody molecules already bound to antigens could improve their affinity by orders of magnitude. They derived a lower and an upper bound on the performance of the evolved libraries as a function of their size and the length of the antigen strings. They also provided insights into the strategy of antibody libraries and discussed the implications of their results for the biological evolution of antibody libraries.

Related Works from the Authors

Oprea, M. (1999), *Antibody Repertoires and Pathogen Recognition: The Role of Germline Diversity and Somatic Hypermutation*, Ph.D. Dissertation, University of New Mexico, Albuquerque, New Mexico, USA.

Oprea, M. & Forrest, S. (1999), "How the Immune System Generates Diversity: Pathogen Space Coverage with Random and Evolved Antibody Libraries", *Proc. of the Genetic and Evolutionary Computation Conference*, **2**, pp. 1651-1656.

4.12 Associative Memory

Usually, a memory is a "system" used to store and recall information. In computers, a memory usually looks like an array. An array consists of pairs where the information is stored, and an index i is assigned to it by the memory on storage. This index produces the address location of the data and the stored information can be recalled by giving the index as input to the memory. This is not a very flexible technique because the right index has to be used to recall the stored information.

A memory might be named an associative memory if it permits the recall of information based on (partial) knowledge of its contents, instead of based upon its address. The associative memories are sometimes referred to as content-addressable memories (CAM), because the stored data (the memory contents) describe their own storage location.

4.12.1. Continuous Network Model

Inspired by the large number of continuous immune network models developed in the late 1980s, Gibert and Routen (1994) proposed a dynamic associative memory. In this system, the authors explored the recognition, mutation, dynamics and metadynamics of the immune networks. They employed the dynamic equations of motion of an immune network model in order to create a content-addressable and auto-associative memory. Their algorithm is very similar to the second-generation immune network model of Varella and collaborators.

The inputs to the system corresponded to a set of antigenic patterns to be memorized and were represented in a binary Hamming shape-space. Only a set of binary antibodies composed the immune network, and the affinity between two molecules (antibody-antibody or antibody-antigen) was determined via their Hamming distances.

The concentration of antibodies was varied according to a differential equation following the general form of Equation 3.20. This differential equation was a function of the network sensitivity for each antibody type, as given by Equation 3.17. A bell-shaped function (Figure 3.21) was used as an attempt to achieve a stable state of the network.

4.12.2. Discrete Network Model

Abbattista *et al.* (1996) explored the immune recruitment mechanism (metadynamics), in order to develop a discrete associative memory. The metadynamics of this model was used to define a population of bipolar points, $\{-1,+1\}$, in an L-dimensional Hamming shape-space, representing a hypersurface. This hypersurface was likened to an associative memory whose valleys corresponded to a set of stored (memorized) patterns. The best points of the population were equivalent to attractors, i.e., local minima of the function that describes the hypersurface. The algorithm was composed of two phases: learning and recall.

In the learning phase, a population was randomly initialized, and for each individual of this population an offspring was generated by inverting a randomly chosen bit of the attribute string of its parent. Each element of the population had an assigned fitness, which was proportional to the inverse of its Hamming distance, in relation to a given input stimulus. The individuals of the population with the highest fitness values were selected as the best points. The recruitment operation then involved substituting the current individual by its offspring in cases the offspring had a better fitness than the parent; otherwise the population remained the same. This algorithm operates in a greedy (local) manner: best matching individuals are selected based upon Hamming distance, and they are then slightly mutated and reselected if this mutation promoted an increase in affinity in relation to the input pattern.

In the recall phase, a new population was presented to the population generated in the learning stage. The same steps performed for the learning phase were repeated, including the possibility of substituting a learned individual by a new one if the fitness of this new individual is larger than that of the individual determined in the learning stage.

4.13 Ecology

Ecology is a science considered being even younger than immunology. The term *ecology* was defined in 1866, seventy years after the discovery of vaccinia by Jenner (Section 2.2). Ecology might be defined as the science concerned with studying the relationships of organisms to their environment and to one another; it is a study of the interactions that determine the distribution and abundance of organisms (Brewer, 1993; Krebs, 1994).

Ecology can be examined at three levels: *individual organism level, population level*, and *community level*. While populations are groups of individuals, communities are comprised of populations of several kinds of organisms and several species that live together. The *ecosystem* is at the same level as the communities, but it takes into account its setting, or habitat, as a single interacting unit. As an example of an ecosystem, one can suggest the sea; the plants, animals and bacteria form the community; and the water, salt, dissolved gases, etc., form the rest of the system. This section reviews the works from the literature that relate the immune system and artificial immune systems with ecosystems.

4.13.1. Immune Systems and Ecosystems

Bersini and Varela (1994) suggested that their immune network model, described in Section 3.5, belongs to the same family as other biological or artificial ecosystems, such as classifier systems (Section 6.6). In this case, the immune network rather than the environment itself (antigens) would be responsible for exerting the greatest pressure in the selection of new individuals (cells and molecules) to be integrated into the system (network). This ecosystem structural metadynamics, characterized by a network-based selectivity, is based on an individual level, instead of population level. Such a view is radical for immunologists, because the external antigen input loses the main part in the development and maturation of the immune system, and it becomes an influence among others with no privileged status to direct the behavior of the immune system.

Janssen (2001) presented a new perspective for studying interactions between human activities and ecosystem management by discussing several similarities and differences between the immune system and ecosystems. The human behavior produces sustainable ecological economic systems regulated and constrained by human institutions. Researchers are trying to discover how such institutions detect problems, generate solutions, and remember successful strategies, such that the societies sustainably coevolve with ecosystems. As an illustration of the application of the immune system concept to ecological management, he suggested the response of ecological economic systems to biological invasions, as illustrated in Table 4.19. The consequences of harmful invasions of diseases, weeds, and animals to the functioning of ecosystems were directly compared to the invasion of an organism by pathogens. It was argued that one of the major differences between the two systems is in terms of their actors; while the immune systems act through cells and molecules, ecological economic systems act through human beings and institutions. An interesting aspect raised was the fact that harmful human activities sometimes continue even after they are detected, like the deforestation of tropical forests.

Table 4.19. The immune system and ecological economic systems.

Immune System	Ecological Economic Systems
Pathogen	Invaders of an ecologic economic system, such as biological invasions (pests, weeds, diseases, plants, animals, etc.), human invasions (migrants, refugees, colonists, soldiers, etc.), technological invasions (cars, computers, etc.), and cultural invasions (religion, communism, etc.)
Detection	Depend on knowledge of the system and the monitoring of particular indicators. The large uncertainty about how the system works makes the identification process difficult. For example, nuclear power plants are being closed in several countries due to the fact that their nuclear energy production is regarded as a harmful activity
Immune response	Once a harmful impact of human activities is detected, a response is organized, such as the combat of a given disease-transmitting mosquito
Memory	The memory of socioeconomic responses is embodied in the institutions through means such as laws, constitutions, rituals, religion, and so on
Maintenance	The resilience (measure of the ability of a system to persist in the presence of perturbations) of ecological economic systems is strongly influenced by how they are managed, where several management approaches can be identified, such as traditional, adaptive, and engineering management

Allen (2001) proposed to extend the comparison performed by Janssen (2001) by focusing on how resilience is maintained in complex systems under threat of invasion. He suggested that the ideas on ecological economic system management through an immune system model could be extended to ecosystems in the broad sense. It was proposed that different types of immune cells are analogous to different species in ecological systems. In immune systems, as in ecosystems, when a pathogen or perturbation exceeds the level of control inherent to one scale (e.g., the innate immune system), regulation and control at broader scales are activated (e.g., adaptive immune system). It was argued that ecological resilience is dependent upon how systems are self-organized as well as how little they are managed.

In order to discuss the validity of Janssen's immune system model for ecosystem management, Walker (2001) pointed out essential differences between the two systems. While organisms are evolved, integrated, and homeostatic, ecosystems are open and selected combinations of interacting species managed consciously by humans. In addition to the five elements of comparison suggested by Janssen (pathogen, detection, response, memory, and management), Walker proposed that the immune features of distributivity, use of stationary and dynamic components, presence of a two-signal system of activation, and compartmentalization of efforts would be other important characteristics to be used in the development of an immune system model for managing invasive species. He concluded his paper arguing that for the immune metaphor to be used as inspiration for ecosystem management, their relative costs (or the relative amounts we can afford to spend on them) should be taken into account. He also suggested that a comparison with the immune system of different organisms might provide alternative insights into ecosystems management.

Finally, Levin (2001) suggested that the weakness of the metaphor proposed by Janssen (2001) lies in the fact that ecosystems are not organisms and have not been shaped to perform particular functions. Thus, the health and integrity of an ecosystem cannot be measured.

4.14   Other Application Areas

In addition to all the domains of application of artificial immune systems discussed so far, there are several other works in the literature that do no fit into these domains. This section aims at describing these other areas or applications.

4.14.1.   Production Systems

Mori *et al.* (1997) proposed an autonomous system to control the production of semiconductors. Their approach was based upon a set of autonomous agents representing the control system. Each agent was modeled as a Petri net, and several types of agents were defined according to a component of the immune system, as summarized in Table 4.20.

Table 4.20. Agents and their immunological counterparts.

Immune System	Agents
B-cell	Detector agent
Lymphokines	Mediator agent
T-cell*	Inhibitor agent
Helper T-cell	Restoration agent

* The authors suggested that the inhibitor agent corresponded to a B-cell killing a specific antigen. This would be equivalent to an inhibitor agent inhibiting a firing transition on a Petri net. Nevertheless, we replaced their B-cell analogy by a T-cell one in order to keep the consistency of the metaphor, since the processes of killing/inhibition in the immune system are usually performed by a T-cell (killer or helper/suppressor, respectively) instead of a B-cell.

Related Works from the Authors

Fukuda, T., Mori, M., & Tsukiyama, M. (1999), "Immunity-Based Management System for a Semiconductor Production Line", In *Artificial Immune Systems and Their Applications*, D. Dasgupta (ed.), Springer-Verlag, pp. 278-288.

Mori, M., Abe, K., Tsukiyama, M. & Fukuda, T. (1998), "Artificial Immune System Based on Petri Nets and Its Application to Production Management Systems", *Proc. of the IEEE Genetic and Evolutionary Computational Conference*.

4.14.2. Intelligent Buildings

Dilger (1996) proposed an agent-based security system for intelligent home technology aiming at improving the technical facilities of a home. His security system presented two main similarities with the immune system: it was self-organized and it was capable of producing a flexible reaction according to the degree of danger. The sensors and actuators of the house were regarded as stationary agents simply defined based on states and rules.

In a later work (Dilger, 1997), the author proposed to use an evolutionary algorithm to optimize the behavior of the system, which enabled the tuning of some of its parameters. In addition, he pointed out aspects of immune-based systems that were contained in the intelligent home, such as self-definition and maintenance. He regarded the situations (presence of burglars, weather, etc.,) as antigens and the specifications of situations in a set of rules for the agents as antibodies activated by certain antigens (situations). The immune network theory was brought up by the interconnection scheme of the agents composing the security system.

4.14.3. Adaptive Noise Neutralization

Based upon the immune properties of diversity, self-tolerance, and memory, Ishida (1996b) developed an agent-based algorithm with possible applications to noise neutralization, group task achievement, model adjustment, and decision making. The author detached as one of the most striking characteristics of his algorithm its high adaptability, not only to a changing environment but also to a changing self (own system). The algorithm worked in three steps: generation of diversity; establishment of self-tolerance (recognizers corresponding to antibodies were adjusted to be insensitive to known patterns (self)); and memory of nonself (the recognizers were adjusted to be sensitive to unknown patterns (nonself)).

Related Works from the Authors

Ishida, Y. & Adachi, N. (1996), "An Immune Algorithm for Multiagent: Application to Adaptive Noise Neutralization", *Proc. of the IROS'96*, pp. 1739-1746.

Ishida, Y. & Adachi, N. (1996), "Active Noise Control by an Immune Algorithm: Adaptation in Immune System as an Evolution", *Proc. of the Int. Conf. on Evolutionary Computation*, pp. 150-153.

4.14.4. Inductive Problem Solving

Slavov and Nikolaev (1998) proposed an evolutionary search algorithm based on a discrete version of an immune network model. The algorithm was applied to solve an instance of the finite-state induction problem. Individual automata were associated with lymphocyte clones, the examples were assumed to be the antigens, and the fitness of an automaton was given by its concentration. The proliferation of an automaton (clone) was a function of two factors: the degree of recognized examples (antigens) and the automata (clones) interactions. Table 4.21 presents the mapping between their immune algorithm and the immune system.

In their model, an automaton followed a clonal selection and affinity maturation pattern of response to an example. The fitness of an automaton was governed by a discrete dynamic equation that follows the general structure of most network models given by Equation 3.20.

Table 4.21. Mapping between the immune algorithm and the immune system.

Immune System	Immune Algorithm
Lymphocyte clone	Finite-state automaton
Concentration of a clone	Fitness of the automaton
Binding capability of the clone	Recognizing capacity of the automaton
Interaction between lymphocytes	Complementarity in the automata's behavior
Antigen	Example
Antigen concentration	Power of an example
Immune network	All automata in the population

The finite-state automata employed were defined by a finite alphabet of symbols (Symbolic shape-space), a finite set of states, a transition state function, an initial state, and a set of states allowed. The affinity between two automata was proportional to the number of examples each of them recognized correctly.

4.14.5. Open WebServer Coordination

An Open WebServer corresponds to an adaptive webserver plus a framework for building a versatile server, which views various system execution policies in a web server as objects. Each object represents a policy for concurrency, an I/O event dispatching, a protocol filtering, a connection management, a caching, a logging, and a service redundancy. Suzuki and Yamamoto (2000) proposed an artificial immune network model to the design of a policy coordination facility in open webservers.

The current conditions of the system represented the antigens and each quality-of-service (QoS) policy management was regarded as an antibody. Each antibody was a symbolic string composed of a precondition, a policy, and references to stimulating antibodies and the degree of stimulation. The first two terms, precondition and policy, were equivalent to the antibody paratope, and the last term corresponded to the antibody idiotope. The dynamics of the network (concentration of antibodies) were determined by a set of differential equations based on those defined by Farmer *et al.* (1986).

Related Works from the Authors

Suzuki, J. & Yamamoto, Y. (2000), "Building an Artificial Immune Network for Decentralized Policy Negotiation in a Communication Endsystem: OpenWeb-Server/iNexus Study", *Proc. of the 4ᵗʰ World Multiconference on Systemics, Cybernetics and Informatics*, CD-ROM.

Suzuki, J. & Yamamoto, Y. (2000), "iNet: A Configurable Framework for Simulating Immune Network", *Proc. of the IEEE System, Man, and Cybernetics Conference*, pp. 119-124.

4.14.6. A Simulated Annealing Model of Diversity

In (de Castro and Von Zuben, 1999) the authors presented a simulated annealing approach aimed at generating a dedicated pool of candidate solutions that best covered a search-space. Their strategy assumed no a priori knowledge about the problem and produced a fixed-size set of potential candidates based only on the representation of the task. The algorithm induced diversity in a population by maximizing an energy function that takes into account the Hamming distance between binary strings. Its potential to machine learning applications and extension to Euclidean spaces were also discussed.

Related Works from the Authors

de Castro, L. N. & Von Zuben, F. J. (2001), "An Immunological Approach to Initialize Feedforward Neural Network Weights", *Proc. of the Int. Conf. on Artificial Neural Networks and Genetic Algorithms*, pp. 126-129.

4.14.7.   The Reflection Pattern in the Immune System

Reflection can be defined as a design principle that allows a system to have an explicit representation of itself such that it becomes easy to adapt to a changing environment. The reflection pattern generally introduces the notion of object/metaobject separation. The base units of computation in object-oriented systems are the objects (or baseobjects). A metaobject can track and control certain aspects of baseobjects. A set of metaobjects is called a metalevel, or metaspace, and a set of baseobjects are called a baselevel.

Suzuki and Yamamoto (1998) argued that the antigen processing and presentation by an antigen-presenting cell is an example of the immune reflective capability. The self/nonself discrimination problem was made equivalent to that of reflecting self in a mirror and comparing the reflected pattern with a foreign component. Under this perspective, MHC molecules would play the role of the mirror that T-cells could refer to in order to recognize intracellular pathogens. In the context of the reflection pattern, MHC molecules corresponded to metaobjects, while APCs and other lymphocytes were baseobjects because MHC controls some major immune phenomena including the recognition of intracellular pathogens by T-cells and activation of B-cells.

4.14.8.   Protein Structure Prediction

Michaud *et al*. (2001) argued that the prediction of the three-dimensional structure or conformation of a protein from its one-dimensional amino-acid sequence is an important problem to be tackled. To predict the protein structure, the authors employed the fast messy genetic algorithm (fmGA) introduced by Goldberg *et al*. (1993) and later applied it to the same type of problem in (Merkle *et al*., 1994). In their work, the authors traced a parallel between the immune system and the fmGA algorithm. This mapping will not be described here, for it would require a review of the fmGA that is outside the scope of our book.

4.15   Summary of Features and Suitability of the Framework

This chapter has attempted to make a comprehensive survey of artificial immune systems. Clearly, by the time this book reaches the bookshops, this chapter will be out of date, but it was felt that this survey needed to be done, if nothing else to provide a platform for potential researchers in the area. In order to achieve this chapter, work has been based on previous reviews of the field, coupled with vast bibliographic research. It is noted that there are other works in the field, published in conferences and journals, that were not reviewed here; no survey is completely exhaustive – so apologies to people whose work has been missed. Omissions are primarily due to not being able to locate the source documents and sometimes problems getting them translated. A list of some of these works is presented in the Further Reading section, followed by a list with the 20 papers accepted for the workshop on artificial immune systems at the Congress on Evolutionary Computation (CEC) to be held in Hawaii, May 2002.

The present review makes it clear that AIS have a vast array of application areas and are interdisciplinary in nature. For example, works on robotics, control, and optimization suggest that AIS research is attractive for engineers; papers on computational security, anomaly detection, and machine learning prove their suitability for computer scientists; works on pattern recognition and associative memories suggest they are attractive for cognitive scientists and psychologists; and so on.

Table 4.22. Most common immune principles/mechanisms used in the design of AIS and their corresponding usual roles.

Mechanism/Principle	Usual Role
Bone-marrow models	Generation of cellular and molecular repertoires
Affinity function	Quantify affinities
Somatic hypermutation	Introduction or maintenance of population diversity and/or variation
Affinity maturation	Promote learning (adaptation) through somatic hypermutation and natural selection
Clonal selection	Perform the dynamics of the system: how the immune cells and molecules are going to interact with antigens
Negative selection	Generation of a set of nonself detectors for anomaly detection
Immune network	Perform the dynamics and metadynamics of the system: how the immune cells and molecules are going to interact with each other and the antigens, and their survival

The main focuses of this review were:

1. To identify the major domains of interest and application of AIS;
2. To discuss how the problems were mapped into the AIS domain (metaphors adopted), which varies according to the application area and problem under study;
3. To stress the main immune principles used in problem solving, as summarized in Table 4.22;
4. To verify the suitability of the proposed framework for the design and formalization of artificial immune systems.

By reviewing several works on artificial immune systems, it is possible to note the importance of the first three steps of the framework introduced: 1) problem description, 2) immune principles to be employed, and 3) immune components to be used. An accurate problem description is necessary to achieve a desired solution. Choosing the immune principles that are going to govern the general behavior of the algorithm is a delicate matter; sometimes, the expected result might not be reached. The choice of "artificial" immune components is also important, but it could be noted that the metaphor has not always been accurate. It is possible to find misconceptions in the works reviewed where elements of the artificial immune system are said to have attributes or to perform functions that do not correspond to their biological counterparts. Although for the sake of problem solving the metaphor might not be a crucial issue, it is still important to keep it faithful, or the final system fails to meet the definition of what an AIS actually is.

The key aspects of the framework are the proposal of a structured approach to model immune components, the evaluation of their interactions with each other and the environment, and the review of general-purpose algorithms from the literature that have been used as "building blocks" for artificial immune systems.

The review of AIS papers allows for reflection on the generality of the framework and some conclusions can be made. As expected, not all works can be formalized using one of the four types of shape-space presented: Real-valued, Integer, Hamming, and Symbolic. In some cases, the elements representing immune cells or molecules can be as complex as a Petri net, a neural network, and a fuzzy system. Under a framework perspective, if one can identify the features of an immune receptor in relation to its ligand with an attribute string, one can also make this identification with a more complex structure, such as a neural network. Thus, it is possible to speculate on the proposal of other, more complex types of shape-spaces, such as Neural shape-spaces, Fuzzy shape-spaces or Messy shape-spaces, involving more than one of these shape-spaces. Certainly, the processes of visualization, formalization, and computing with these shape-spaces become increasingly more difficult, but this will not be pursued in this book. The argument though is very simple; anything that can be used to represent the generalized shape of a component of the immune system can be described in a particular shape-space, even if the mapping from the "artificial" to the "biological" elements cannot be made in a straightforward way.

Hopefully, the reader will now begin to appreciate the scope of AIS and its potential applications. This chapter has highlighted many areas of application where the use of AIS is very new. There still remains a great deal of work to be done to not only corroborate the results obtained by previous researchers, but also to augment and develop the ideas proposed. It is hoped that this development of AIS will help to feed into the continual refinement and augmentation of the proposed AIS framework. Additionally, there are many areas of application where AIS could be employed; that is one great excitement of this field – so much to do.

References

Abbattista, F., Di Gioia G., Di Santo G. & Farinelli A. M. (**1996**), "An Associative Memory Based on the Immune Networks", *Proc. of the Int. Conference on Neural Networks*.

Aisu, H. & Mizutani H. (**1996**), "Immunity-Based Learning – Integration of Distributed Search and Constraint Relaxation", *Proc. of the ICMAS Workshop on Immune-Based Systems*, pp. 124-135.

Allen, C. R. (**2001**), "Ecosystems and Immune Systems: Hierarchical Response Provides Resilience Against Invasions", *Conservation Ecology*, **5**(1): 15. [Online] URL: http://www.consecol.org/vol5/iss1/art15

Bersini, H. (**1999**), "The Endogenous Double Plasticity of the Immune Network and the Inspiration to tbe Drawn for Engineering Aircrafts", In *Artificial Immune Systems and Their Applications*, D. Dasgupta (ed.), Springer-Verlag, pp. 22-44.

Bersini, H. (**1991**), "Immune Network and Adaptive Control", *Proc. of the First European Conference on Artificial Life*, MIT Press, pp. 217-226.

Bersini, H. & Varela, F. J. (**1994**), "The Immune Learning Mechanisms: Reinforcement, Recruitment and Their Applications", In *Computing with Biological Metaphors*, R. Paton (ed.), Chapman & Hall.

Bersini, H. & Varela, F. J. (**1990**), "Hints for Adaptive Problem Solving Gleaned from Immune Networks", *Parallel Problem Solving from Nature*, pp. 343-354.

Bradley, D. W. & Tyrrell, A. M. (**2000**), "Immunotronics: Hardware Fault Tolerance Inspired by the Immune System", *Lecture Notes in Computer Science*, **1801**, pp. 11-20.

Brewer, R. (**1993**), *The Science of Ecology*, 2nd Ed., Saunders Environmental Library.

Carter, J. H. (**2000**), "The Immune System as a Model for Pattern Recognition and Classification", *Journal of the American Medical Informatics Association*, **7**(1), pp 28-41.

Carvalho, D. R. & Freitas, A. A. (**2001**), "An Immunological Algorithm for Discovering Small-Disjunct Rules in Data Mining", *Proc. of the Genetic and Evolutionary Computation Conference*, pp. 401-404.

Chun, J. S., Jung, H. K., Hahn, S. Y. (**1998**), "A Study on Comparison of Optimization Performances Between Immune Algorithm and Other Heuristic Algorithms", *IEEE Trans. on Magnetics*, **34**(5), pp. 2972 2975.

Chun, J. S., Kim, M. K., Jung, H. K., Hong, S. K. (**1997**), "Shape Optimization of Electromagnetic Devices Using Immune Algorithm", *IEEE Trans. on Magnetics*, **33**(2), pp. 1876 1879.

Cui, X., Li, M. & Fang, T. (**2001**), "Study of Population Diversity of Multiobjective Evolutionary Algorithm Based on Immune and Entropy Principles", *Proc. of the IEEE Congress on Evolutionary Computation*, pp. 1316-1321.

Dasgupta, D., (**1999a**), "Immunity-Based Intrusion Detection System: A General Framework", *Proc. of the 22nd NISSC*, **1**, pp. 147-160.

Dasgupta, D., (**1999b**), "An Overview of Artificial Immune Systems and Their Applications", In *Artificial Immune Systems and Their Applications*, D. Dasgupta (ed.), Springer-Verlag, pp. 3-21.

Dasgupta, D., Majumdar, N. & Niño, F. (**2001**), "Artificial Immune Systems: A Bibliography", CS Technical Report, CS-01-002 [Online] http://www.cs.memphis.edu/~dasgupta/AIS/AIS-bib.pdf

Dasgupta, D., Cao, Y. & Yang, C. (**1999**), "An Immunogenetic Approach to Spectra Recognition", *Proc. of the Genetic and Evolutionary Computation Conference*, pp. 149-155.

Dasgupta, D. & Attoh-Okine, N., (**1997**), "Immunity-Based Systems: A Survey", *Proc. of the IEEE SMC*, **1**, pp. 369-374.

Dasgupta, D. & Forrest, S. (1996), "Novelty Detection in Time Series Data Using Ideas From Immunology", *Proc. of the 5th Int. Conf. on Intelligent Systems.*

de Castro, L. N. & Von Zuben, F. J. (2000a), "Artificial Immune Systems: Part II – A Survey of Applications", *Technical Report – RT DCA 02/00*, p. 65.

de Castro, L. N. & Von Zuben, F. J. (2000b), "An Evolutionary Immune Network for Data Clustering", *Proc. of the IEEE Brazilian Symposium on Artificial Neural Networks*, pp. 84-89.

de Castro, L. N. & Von Zuben, F. J. (1999), "Artificial Immune Systems: Part I – Basic Theory and Applications", *Technical Report – RT DCA 01/99*, p. 98.

Dilger, W. (1996), "The Immune System of the Smart Home", *Proc. of the ICMAS Int. Workshop on Immunity-Based Systems*, Y. Ishida (ed.), pp. 72-81.

Dilger, W. (1997), "Decentralized Autonomous Organization of the Intelligent Home According to the Principle of the Immune System", *Proc. of the IEEE System, Mand, and Cybernetics Conference*, pp. 351-356.

Farmer, J. D., Packard, N. H. & Perelson, A. S. (1986), "The Immune System, Adaptation, and Machine Learning", *Physica 22D*, pp. 187-204.

Gibert, C. J. & Routen, T. W. (1994), "Associative Memory in an Immune-Based System", *Proc. of the 12th National Conf. on Artificial Intelligence*, pp. 852-857.

Goldberg, D. E. , Deb, K., Kargupta, H. & Harik, G. (1993), "Rapid, Accurate Optimization of Difficult Problems Using Fast Messy Genetic Algorithms", *Technical Report 93004*, University of Illinois at Urbana-Champaign, Urbana, IL., USA.

Gu, J., Lee, D., Park, S. & Sim, K. (2000), "An Immunity-Based Security Layer Model", *Proc. of the Genetic and Evolutionary Computation Conference*, Workshop on Artificial Immune Systems and Their Applications, pp 47-48.

Gaspar, A. & Collard, P. (2000), "Two Models of Immunization for Time De-pendent Optimization", *Proc. of the IEEE SMC'00*, **1**, pp. 113-118.

Hajela, P., & Yoo, J. S. (1999), "Immune Network Modeling in Design Optimization", In *New Ideas in Optimization*, D. Corne, M. Dorigo & F. Glover (eds.), McGraw Hill, London, pp. 203-215.

Hightower, R. R., Forrest S. & Perelson, A. S. (1996), "The Baldwin Effect in the Immune System: Learning by Somatic Hypermutation", In *R. K. Belew and M. Mitchell* (eds.), *Adaptive Individuals in Evolving Populations*, Addison-Wesley, Reading, MA, pp. 159-167.

Hightower R. R., Forrest, S. A & Perelson, A. S. (1995), "The Evolution of Emergent Organization in Immune System Gene Libraries", *Proc. of the 6th Int. Conf. on Genetic Algorithms*, L. J. Eshelman (ed.), Morgan Kaufmann, San Francisco, CA, pp. 344-350.

Huang, S.-J (2000), "An Immune-Based Optimization Method to Capacitor Placement in a Radial Distribution System", *IEEE Trans. on Power Delivery*, **15**(2), pp. 744-749.

Hunt, J. E. & Cooke, D. E. (1996), "Learning Using an Artificial Immune System", *Journal of Network and Computer Applications*, **19**, pp. 189-212.

Ishida, Y. (1996a), "The Immune System as a Self-Identification Process: A Survey and a Proposal", *Proc. of the ICMAS Int. Workshop on Immunity-Based Systems*, pp. 2-12.

Ishida, Y. (1996b), "Agent-Based Architecture of Selection Principe in the Immune System", *Proc. of the ICMAS Int. Workshop on Immunity-Based Systems*, pp. 92-104.

Ishida, Y. (1990), "Fully Distributed Diagnosis by PDP Learning Algorithm: Towards Immune Network PDP Model", *Proc. of the Int. Joint Conf. on Neural Networks*, pp. 777-782.

Ishiguro, A., Ichikawa, S., Shibata, T. & Uchikawa, Y. (1998), "Moderationism in the Immune System: Gait Acquisition of a Legged Robot Using the Metadynamics Function", *Proc. of the IEEE System, Man,* *and Cybernetics Conference*, pp. 3827-3832.

Janssen, M. A. (2001), "An Immune System Perspective on Ecosystem Management", *Conservation Ecology*, **5**(1): 13. [Online] URL: http://www.consecol.org/vol5/iss1/art13

Joshi, R. R. (1995), "Immune Network Memory: An Inventory Approach", *Computers Ops. Res.*, **22**(6), pp. 575-591.

Kayama, M., Sugita, Y., Morooka, Y. & Fukuoka, S. (1995), "Distributed Diagnosis System Combining the Immune Network and Learning Vector Quantization", *Proc. of the 21st IEEE Int. Conf. on Industrial Electronics, Control and Instrumentation*, pp. 1531-1536.

Kephart, J. O. (1994), "A Biologically Inspired Immune System for Computers", In R. A. Brooks & P. Maes (eds.), *Artificial Life IV Proceedings of the Fourth International Workshop on the Synthesis and Simulation of Living Systems*, MIT Press, pp. 130-139.

Kim, J. & Bentley, P. (1999a), "The Human Immune System and Network Intrusion Detection", *Proc. of the EUFIT'99*, CD ROM.

Kim, J. & Bentley, P. (1999b), "Negative Selection and Niching by an Artificial Immune System for Network Intrusion Detection", *Proc. of the Genetic and Evolutionary Computation Conference*, pp. 149-158.

King, R. L., Russ, S. H., Lambert, A. B. & Reese, D. S. (2001), "An Artificial Immune System Model for Intelligent Agents", *Future generation Computer Systems*, **17**, pp. 335-343.

Krebs, C. J. (1994), *Ecology The Experimental Analysis of Distribution and Abundance*, 4th Ed., Harper Collins College Publishers.

Krishnakumar, K. & Neidhoefer, J. (1999), "Immunized Adaptive Critic for an Autonomous Aircraft Control Application", In *Artificial Immune Systems and Their Applications*", D. Dasgupta (ed.), Springer-Verlag, pp. 221-241.

Lamont, G. B., Marmelstein, R. E. & Van Veldhuizen D. A. (1999), "A Distributed Architecture for a Self-Adaptive Computer Virus Immune System", In *New Ideas in Optimization*, D. Corne, M. Dorigo & F. Glover (eds.), McGraw Hill, London, pp. 167-183.

Lee, D-W. & Sim, K-B. (1997), "Artificial Immune Network-Based Cooperative Control in Collective Autonomous Mobile Robots", *Proc. of the IEEE Int. Workshop on Robotics and Human Communication*, pp. 58-63.

Levin, S. A. (2001), "Immune Systems and Ecosystems", *Conservation Ecology*, **5**(1): 17. [Online] URL: http://www.consecol.org/vol5/iss1/art17

McCoy, D. F. & Devarajan, V. (1997), "Artificial Immune Systems and Aerial Image Segmentation", *Proc. of the IEEE System, Man, and Cybernetics Conference*, pp. 867-872.

Merkle, L. D., Gates, G. H., Lamont, G. B. & Patcher, R. (1994), "Application of the Parallel Fast Messy Genetic Algorithm to the Protein Structure Prediction Problem", *Proc. of the Intel Supercomputer Users' Group Users Conference*, pp. 189-195.

Michaud, S. R., Zydallis, J. B., Lamont, G. B., Harmer, P. K., Patcher, R. (2001), "Protein Structure Prediction with EA Immunological Computation", *Proc. of the Genetic and Evolutionary Computation Conference*, pp. 1367-1374.

Mitsumoto, N., Fukuda, T., Shimojima, K. & Ogawa, A. (1996), "Self-Organizing Multiple Robotic System (A Population Control Through Biologically Inspired Immune Network Architecture)", *Proc. of the IEEE Int. Conf. on Robotics and Automation*, pp. 1614-1619.

Mori, M., Tsukiyama, M. & Fukuda, T. (1998), "Adaptive Scheduling System Inspired by Immune System", *Proc. of the IEEE Systems, Man, and Cybernetics Conference*, pp. 3833-3837.

Mori, M., Tsukiyama, M. & Fukuda, T. (1997), "Artificial Immunity Based Management System for a Semiconductor

Production Line", *Proc. of the IEEE Systems, Man, and Cybernetics Conference*, pp. 851-855.

Mori, M., Tsukiyama, M. & Fukuda, T. (1993), "Immune Algorithm with Searching Diversity and its Application to resource Allocation Problem", *Trans. of the Institute of Electrical Engineers of Japan*, (in Japanese), 113-C(10), pp. 872-878.

Nagano, S. & Yonezawa, Y., (1999), "Generative Mechanism of Emergent Properties Observed with the Primitive Evolutional Phenomena by Immunotic Recognition", *Proc. of the IEEE System, Man, and Cybernetics*, I, pp. 223-228.

Okamoto, T. & Ishida, Y. (1999), "Multi-agent Approach Against Computer Virus: An Immunity-Based System", *Proc. of the AROB'99*, pp. 69-72.

Ootsuki, J. T. & Sekiguchi, T. (1999), "Application of the Immune System Network Concept to Sequential Control", *Proc. of the IEEE System, Man, and Cybernetics (SMC'99)*, 3, pp. 869-874.

Oprea, M. & Forrest, S. (1998), "Simulated Evolution of Antibody Gene Libraries Under Pathogen Selection", *Proc. of the IEEE System, Man, and Cybernetics*.

Potter, M. A. & De Jong K. A. (1998), "The Coevolution of Antibodies for Concept Learning", *Proc. of the 5th Int. Conf. on Parallel Problem Solving from Nature*, pp. 530-539.

Skormin, V. A., Delgado-Frias, J. G., McGee, D. L., Giordano, J. V., Popyack, L. J., Gorodetski, V. I. & Tarakanov, A. O. (2001), "BASIS: A Biological Approach to System Information Security", *Proc. of the Int. Workshop MMM-ACNS 2001*, pp. 127-142.

Slavov, V. & Nikolaev, N. I. (1998), "Immune Network Dynamics for Inductive Problem Solving", *Proc. of the 5th Int. Conf. on Parallel Problem Solving from Nature*, pp. 712-721.

Somayaji, A., Hofmeyr, S. A. & Forrest, S. (1997), "Principles of a Computer Immune System", *Proc. of the new Security Paradigms Workshop*, pp. 75-81.

Suzuki, J. & Yamamoto, Y. (2000), "A Decentralized Policy Coordination Facility in Open WebServer", *Proc. of the SPA'00*, CD-ROM.

Suzuki, J. & Yamamoto, Y. (1998), "The Reflection Pattern in the Immune System", *Proc. of the OOPSLA'98, workshop on Non-Software Examples of Software Architecture*, CD-ROM.

Takahashi, K. & Yamada, T. (1997), "A Self-Tuning Immune Feedback Controller for Controlling Mechanical Systems", *IEEE/ASME International Conference on Advanced Intelligent Mechatronics*, CD-ROM#101.

Tarakanov A., Sokolova, S., Abramov, B. & Aikimbayev, A. (2000), "Immuno-computing of the Natural Plague Foci", *Proc. of the Genetic and Evolutionary Computation Conference*, Workshop on Artificial Immune Systems and Their Applications, pp. 38-39.

Timmis, J. (2001), "aiVIS: Artificial Immune Network Visualisation", *Proc. of EuroGraphics*, University College London, pp. 61-69.

Timmis, J., Neal, M. & Hunt, J. (2000), "An Artificial Immune System for Data Analysis", *BioSystems*, 55, pp. 143-150.

Timmis, J & Neal, M. (2001), "A Resource Limited Artificial Immune System". *Knowledge Based Systems*, 14(3-4), pp.121-130.

Toma, N., Endo, S. & Yamada, K. (1999), "Immune Algorithm with Immune Network and MHC for Adaptive Problem Solving", *Proc. of the IEEE System, Man, and Cybernetics*, IV, pp. 271-276.

Walker, B. (2001), "Ecosystems and Immune Systems: Useful Analogy or Stretching a Metaphor", *Conservation Ecology*, 5(1): 16. [Online] URL: http://www.consecol.org/vol5/iss1/art16

Watkins, A. (2001), AIRS: *A Resource Limited Artificial Immune Classifier*, M. S. Dissertation, Mississippi State University, Mississipi, USA.

Xanthakis, S., Karapoulios, S., Pajot, R. & Rozz, A. (1996), "Immune System and

Fault Tolerant Computing", In *Lecture Notes in Computer Science*, J. M. Alliot (ed.), **1063**, Springer-Verlag, pp. 181-197.

Further Reading

Chun, J. S., Cho, D. H., Kim, M. K. Lim, J. P. & Jung, H. K. (1997), "A Study on Comparison Between Immune Algorithm and the Other Algorithms", *Proc. of ISAP'97*, pp. 588-592.

Chun, J. S., Kim, M. K. & Jung, H. K. (1996), "Shape Optimization of Electromagnetic Devices Using Immune Algorithm", *Proc. of the 7th Biennial IEEE Conference on Electromagnetic Field Computation*, pp. 154.

Chun, J. S., Lim, J. P. & Jung, H. K. (1996), "Optimal Design of Permanent Magnet Type Lifter Using Immune Algorithm", *Simulation, Experiment and Design Techniques in Electrical Power Engineering*, pp. 1-4.

Chun, J. S., Lim, J. P., Jung, H. K. & Hahn, S. Y. (1997), "A Study on Comparisons of Optimization Performance Between Immune Algorithm and Other Non Deterministic Algorithms", *Proc. of COMPUMAG'97*, pp. 553-554.

Chun, J. S., Lim, J. P., Jung, H. K. & Yoon, J. S. (1997), "Optimal Design of Synchronous Motor with Parameter Correction Using Immune Algorithm", *Proc. of IEMDC'97*, pp. WB3-7.

Chun, J. S., Lim, J. P., Jung, H. K. & Yoon, J. S. (1997), "Thermal Analysis of Motor Using Immune Algorithm and Neural Network", *Proc. of ICEE'97*, pp. M05.

Jian, Z., Haifeng, D. & Sun'an, W. (2001), "The Study of Artificial Immune in Diagnosis Four-Cylinder-Air-Compressor", *Proc. of the ICTC*, pp. 89-93.

Haifeng, D. & Sun'an, W. (2001), "Data Enriching Based on ART - Artificial Immune Network", *Pattern Recognition and Artificial Intelligence* (in print).

Haifeng, D. & Sun'an, W. (2001), "Fault Diagnose of the Reciprocating Compressor Based on ART - Artificial Immune Network", *Chinese Journal of Mechanical Engineering*, (in print).

Kesheng, L., Jun, Z., Xianbin, C. & Xufa, W. (2000), "An Algorithm Based on Immune Principle Adopted in Controlling Behavior of Autonomous Mobile Robots", *Computer Engineer and Applications*, **5**, pp. 30-32.

Lei, W., Jin, P. & Li-Cheng, J. (2000), "The Immune Algorithm", *Acta Electronica Sinica*, **28**(7), pp. 74-78.

Lim, J. P., Chun, J. S. & Jung, H. K. (1997), "The Optimal Design of Permanent Magnet Motor with Parameter-Correction Using Immune Algorithm", *Proc. of SAPEC'97*, pp. 133-140.

Mori, M., Tsukiyama, M. & Fukuda, T. (1994), "Immune Algorithm and its Application to Factory Load Dispatching Planning". *Proc. of the Symposium on Flexible Automation*, pp.1343-1346.

Mori, M., Tsukiyama, M. & Fukuda, T. (1994), "Load Dispatching Planning by Immune Algorithm with Diversity and Learning". *Proc. of the 7th Int. Conf. on Systems Research, Informatics and Cybernetics*, **11**, pp.136-141.

Tazawa, I., Koakustu, S. & Hirata, H. (1997), "An Evolutionary Optimization Based on the Immune System and Its Application to the VLSI Floor Plan Design Problem", *Trans. of the Institute of Electrical Engineers of Japan*, **117-C**(7), pp. 821-828.

Williams, P. D. (2001), *Warthog: Towards an Artificial Immune System for Detecting 'Low and Slow' Information System Attacks*, M. S. Dissertation, Air Force Institute of Technology, WPAFB, OH, March. AFIT/GCE/ENG/01M-15.

Papers Accepted for the Workshop on Artificial Immune Systems – WAIS (CEC, May 2002)

Anchor, K. P., Williams, P. D., Gunsch, G. H. & Lamont, G. B., "The Computer Defense Immune System: Current and Future Research in Intrusion Detection"

Antoniou, I. & Melnikov, Y., "European Project on Immunocomputing: Objectives, Methods, Results and Perspectives"

Balthrop, J., Forrest, S. & Glickman, M. R., "Revisting LISYS: Parameters and Normal Behavior"

Bradley, D. & Tyrrell, A., "A Hardware Immune System for Benchmark State Machine Error Detection"

Cayzer, S. & Aickelin, U., "A Recommender System based on the Immune Network"

Cheh, J. J., "A Heuristic Approach to Efficient Production of Detector Sets for An Artificial Immune Algorithm-Based Bankruptcy Prediction System in Portfolio Management"

Coello Coello, C. A. & Cortes, N. C., "A parallel implementation of the Artificial Immune System to handle Constraints in Genetic Algorithms: Preliminary Results"

Costa, A. M., Vargas, P. A., Von Zuben, F. J. & Franca, P. M., "Makespan Minimization on Parallel Processors: An Immune-Based Approach"

Dasgupta, D. & Majumdar, N. S., "Anomaly Detection in Multidimensional Data using Negative Selection Algorithm"

de Castro, L. N. & Timmis, J., "An Artificial Immune Network for Multimodal Function Optimization"

Gonzalez, F., Dasgupta, D. & Kozma, R., "Combining Negative Selection and Classification Techniques for Anomaly Detection"

Janssen, M. A. & Stow, D. W., "An Application of Immunocomputing to the Evolution of Rules for Ecosystem Management"

Kim, J. & Bentley, P. J., "Toward an Artificial Immune System for Network Intrusion Detection: An Investigation of Dynamic Clonal Selection"

Michelan, R. & Von Zuben, F. J., "Decentralized Control System for Autonomous Navigation based on an Evolved Artificial Immune Network"

Nino, F. & Beltran, O., "A Change Detection Software Agent based on Immune Mixed Selection"

Qiao, Y. & Xin, X. W., "A Network IDS with Low False Positive Rate"

Singh, S. P. N. & Thayer, S. M., "A Foundation for Kilorobotic Exploration"

Tarakanov, A. & Skormin, V., "Pattern Recognition by Immunocomputing"

Watkins, A. B. & Boggess, L. C., "A Resource Limited Artificial Immune Classifier"

Wenjian, L., Xianbin, C. & Xufa, W., "An Immune Genetic Algorithm Based on Immune Regulation"

Chapter 5

The Immune System in Context with Other Biological Systems

An organism can modify the behavior of another organism in two basic ways: by interacting with it... or by orienting the behavior of the other organism...In the first case it can be said that the two organisms interact, in the second case that they communicate

– H. Maturana

5.1   Introduction

Physiology is the science that attempts to explain the physical and chemical factors responsible for the origin, development, and progression of life. Within physiology, efforts are currently being made to integrate the vast amount of the information that has been obtained from studying single cells, tissues, organs, and systems into an understanding of the way in which the whole organism responds to the environment. *Homeostasis* is the fundamental principle underlying all physiologic functions. This is the process by which an organism actively maintains a *steady state* in which all body functions can be optimally performed. It is thought that all body tissues and organs in some way exert functions that help to maintain homeostasis; however, of particular interest and importance are the nervous, endocrine, and immune systems.

Within an organism, regulation of certain functions is undertaken by two large *control systems*: 1) the *nervous system* (NS) and 2) the *endocrine system* (ES). Recent research has shown that the nervous and endocrine systems can be seen to function as a single interrelated system; this is referred to as the *neuroendocrine system* (NES). This interaction between the nervous and endocrine systems for example, can be observed in situations such as the sensation of physical discomfort common when people are subjected to anxiety, depression, or stress. Other research is attempting to relate anomalies such as cancer and other diseases with tempering and psychological conditions: a research known as *psychoneuroimmunology*. It addresses the diverse functions of the neuroendocrine and immune systems, aiming at explaining diseases known as *psychosomatic*. The central premise underlying psychoneuroimmunology is that the nervous, endocrine, and immune systems are components of a large integrated defense system. By pursuing this idea, it can be suggested that immunological strategies may offer keys to the understanding and treatment of behavioral, neural, and endocrine disorders. Indeed, behavioral, neural and/or endocrine interventions can be relevant to the treatment of immune system related diseases.

A cognitive system can be defined as the one capable of extracting information and experience from a set of input data (external environment) through the manipulation of information contained in the system itself (internal environment). By following this definition, the immune system can be regarded as cognitive, and many authors have been advocating in favor of this viewpoint. There is a great deal of debate as to the true meaning of what cognition is. There are few, however, who would deny that the central nervous system (CNS) presents cognitive capabilities. The brain has led to the development of one of the most influential computational intelligence paradigms: artificial neural networks (ANN). ANNs have been applied to a vast array of complex problems such as vision, pattern recognition, classification, and approximation, to name a few; and can be argued, display some sort of cognitive activity. By relating the IS with the CNS and by discussing relative cognitive aspects, a comparison between AIS models and ANN models can be more easily made. Based upon the cognitive argument for the IS, it may follow that artificial immune systems can also be assumed to present cognitive behaviors, given certain perspectives.

The interaction and comparison of the immune system with other systems goes far beyond the physiological (individual organism) level. Assuming a Darwinian perspective, there is strong evidence from the literature that an adaptive immune response can be regarded as a *microevolutionary* process. The immune system contributes in some way to natural selection and it is capable of maintaining stable subpopulations (species) of immune cells to fight against specific infections.

Through the study of these interactions and by making comparisons of the various systems, it is possible to develop a better understanding of the behavior of the immune system itself, leading to a deeper understanding of the proposed and reviewed artificial immune systems. For example, part of the discussion to be presented here will serve as a philosophical and conceptual explanation of why clonal selection and AIS models naturally account for the emergence of diverse, stable populations of individuals capable of covering a broad range of different antigens. This feature suggests that AIS are suitable to deal with multimodal, multiobjective, clustering, and classification problems.

The main goals of this chapter are:

- To provide an overview of the nervous and endocrine systems, from a biological perspective, with a view to being able to outline a set of similarities and differences between those systems and the immune system;
- To highlight functional and anatomical integration aspects of the nervous, endocrine, and immune systems;
- To study natural selection (evolutionary) principles in the immune system, and how these may influence the evolution of the organism;
- To discuss how the immune system and consequently artificial immune systems can be viewed as cognitive systems.

The fundamentals of the nervous system and evolutionary biology discussed in the present chapter also serve the purpose of providing the biological background for the development of some biologically motivated computing paradigms, to be discussed in the next chapter, such as artificial neural networks and evolutionary algorithms.

In an attempt to achieve the above, there clearly is a wide variety of material to be covered. In order to break this information down into manageable and related pieces of information, this chapter is organized slightly differently than the rest. Three parts have been created, each of which addresses a different (but sometimes related) topic, as follows:

Part I: contains Sections 5.2 to 5.4. The first two sections present the fundamentals of the nervous and endocrine systems from an anatomical and functional perspective, respectively. Section 5.4 discusses how and through which mechanisms these three systems (NS, ES, and IS) interact and draws out their similarities and differences.

Part II: begins with Section 5.5. This reviews the theory of evolution and natural selection, covering topics such as the Baldwin effect, niches and speciation, coevolution, and predator-prey models. Section 5.6 discusses several ideas in which the immune system can be related or contribute to natural selection.

Part III: comprises of Section 5.7. This is more discussion based and offers discourses surrounding the controversies lying behind cognition, and then, based upon several arguments from the literature, puts forward the argument of the immune system being a cognitive system.

PART I: Nervous, Endocrine and the Immune System

5.2   Fundamentals of the Nervous System

The *nervous system* (NS) plays a pivotal role for the organism. It is responsible for *informing* the organism through sensory input with regards to the environment in which it lives and moves, processing the input information, relating it to previous experience, and transformating it into appropriate actions or memories. At the early stages in the evolution of the nervous system, the processing of sensory information involves discrimination and categorization, possibly with the aid of some rudimentary learning and memory capacity (Århem & Liljenström, 1997). All multicellular animals possess some kind of nervous system, whose complexity and/or organization varies according to the animal type. Even relatively simple organisms, such as worms, slugs, and insects, have the ability to learn and store information in their nervous systems.

The main function of the nervous system is to process the incoming information such that the appropriate effector function occurs. To achieve this, the nervous system is comprised of elements that are concerned with the reception of stimuli, the transmission of *nerve impulses*, or the activation of muscle mechanisms. Functionally, the nervous system can be divided into two parts: *sensor* and *effector* (or *motor*). Sensor receptors, such as visual and taste, receive the sensorial information that may promote an immediate or late response. The effector, or motor, part of the nervous system is concerned with transmitting signals to the muscles and *glands*.

There are two main types of nerve cells: *neurons* and *neuroglia* (or simply *glia*). Neurons are responsible for the transmission and analysis of all communication signals within the brain and other parts of the nervous system, i.e., they are the functional and structural units of the nervous system. Neuroglia cells are much more numerous than neurons and account for half of the brain's weight. They provide supportive and nutritive functions for the neurons, form *myelin*, guide developing neurons, take up chemicals involved in cell-cell communication, and contribute to the maintenance of the environment around neurons. Although they have all these processes and the capability to divide throughout life, they do not conduct nerve impulses.

Neurons are grouped by function into collections of cells called *nuclei*. These nuclei are connected to form *sensory*, *motor*, and other systems. Scientists have been able to study the function of *somatosensory* (pain and touch), *motor*, *olfactory*, *visual*, *auditory*, *language*, and other systems by measuring the *physiological* (physical and chemical) changes that occur in the nervous system when these senses are activated.

Approximately 10^{11} neurons make up the human nervous system, from which half of them are located in the *brain*. Neurons have a variety of shapes and sizes, and like the nervous system, can be functionally divided into motor and sensory. Neurons can be differed from other body cells in three respects: 1) they have specialized extensions called *dendrites* and *axons*; 2) they communicate with each other through electrochemical processes; and 3) they contain specialized structures (e.g., *synapses*) and chemicals (e.g., *neurotransmitters*). Although neurons occur in a wide variety of sizes and shapes, they can be considered as consisting of three basic parts: 1) the *dendrites* and *cell body*; 2) the *axon*; and 3) the *axon terminals*. From the *cell body* (*nucleus*, or *soma*) of a typical neuron extends one or more *dendrites*. These are threadlike structures that divide and subdivide into ever-smaller branches. Another, usually longer structure called the *axon* also stretches from the cell body.

When the cell body of a neuron is stimulated, it generates an impulse that passes from the axon of one neuron to the dendrite of another. Such impulses carry information throughout the nervous system. The junction between axon and dendrite is called a *synapse*. The end branches of a *pre-synaptic neuron*'s axon make contact with the dendrites, cell body, or axon of a *post-synaptic neuron*. There is no anatomical continuity between two neurons (Ottoson, 1983). Figure 5.1 illustrates a diagrammatic representation of a neuron and the direction of signal propagation throughout the cell.

In simple animals, such as jellyfish, the nerve cells form a network capable of mediating only a relatively stereotyped response. In more complex animals, such as shellfish, insects, and spiders, the nervous system is more complicated. The cell bodies of neurons are organized in clusters called *ganglia*; these clusters are interconnected by the neuronal processes to form a ganglionated chain. Such chains are found in all vertebrates and regulate the activities of the heart, the glands, and the involuntary muscles.

While functionally the nervous system can be divided into its sensor and effector parts, anatomically it has two main divisions: *central nervous system* (CNS) and *peripheral nervous system* (PNS). The distinction between the central nervous system and the peripheral nervous system is based upon their different locations. Vertebrate animals have a *bony spine* (*vertebral column*) and a *skull* (*cranium*) in which the central parts of the nervous system are housed.

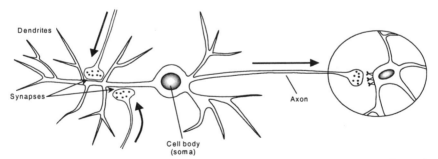

Figure 5.1. Highly diagrammatic representation of a neuron (large arrows indicate the direction of signal propagation). Signals from a pre-synaptic neuron are propagated via its axon until it reaches the synapse connecting the axon of this neuron with the dendrites of a post-synaptic neuron. After entering the post-synaptic neuron, the signal is processed in the cell body and propagated via the axon until it is propagated to another neuron.

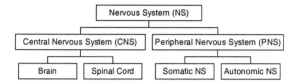

Figure 5.2.   Basic divisions of the nervous system.

The peripheral part extends throughout the remainder of the body. The part of the (central) nervous system located in the skull is referred to as the *brain*, and the one found in the spine is called the *spinal cord*. The brain and the spinal cord are continuous through an opening in the base of the skull; both are in contact with other parts of the body through the nerves. Some of the processes of the cell bodies conduct sense impressions and others conduct muscle responses, called *reflexes*, such as those caused by pain.

The peripheral nervous system can be further divided into two major parts: the *somatic nervous system* and the *autonomic nervous system*, as illustrated in Figure 5.2. The somatic nervous system consists of two elements: peripheral nerve fibers that send sensory information to the central nervous system and motor nerve fibers that project to skeletal muscle. The autonomic nervous system, again, has two main subdivisions: *sympathetic* and *parasympathetic* nervous system. This system regulates the heart muscles and smooth muscles of the *viscera* (internal organs like the stomach and intestines). It also controls the action of the glands; the functions of the respiratory, circulatory, digestive, and urogenital systems; and the involuntary muscles in these systems and in the skin. In most situations organisms are unaware of the workings of the autonomic nervous system since it functions in an involuntary, reflexive manner. Its perfect functioning is crucial in situations that cause stress and require a reflexive action like "fight or flight" situations. However, it also operates in non-emergency situations such as resting and digesting. Controlled by nerve centers in the lower part of the brain, the system also has a reciprocal effect on the internal secretions. This is controlled to some degree by the hormones of the *endocrine system* and exercising some control, in turn, on hormone production: this will be further discussed in Section 5.4.

5.2.1. Brain Structures and Functions

The brain is an extremely complex organ that has many differing functions. Among them are the processing of sensory input, serving as the originator and coordinator of motor activities, acting as the repository of experience (memory), and provide the mechanisms for intelligence which in turn lead to social and moral behaviors.

The brain is divided in two halves, a *right hemisphere* and a *left hemisphere*. The right hemisphere deals more with visual activities and organizes or groups information together. The left hemisphere tends to be the more analytical part; it analyzes information collected by the right hemisphere and also deals more with language. Research has shown that hemispheric dominance (which side of the brain does what) is related to whether a person is predominantly right-handed or left-handed. In most right-handed people (95% of people in the general population), the left hemisphere processes arithmetic, language, and speech. The right hemisphere interprets music, complex imagery, and spatial relationships and recognizes and expresses emotion. In left-handed people, the pattern of brain organization is more variable. For example, sensory input from the eyes goes to areas at the very back of the brain. Each hemisphere processes half the visual information. Visual information obtained from the left eye is processed by the right hemisphere, whereas information on the right gets processed by the left hemisphere. Alternatively, the area of the brain that controls movement is in a very narrow strip that goes from near the top of the head right down along where the ear is located.

Anatomically, the brain can be decomposed into three main structures: the *brainstem*, the *cerebellum,* and the *forebrain*, as illustrated in Figure 5.3. The *brainstem* is literally the stalk of the brain through which pass all the nerve fibers relaying input and output signals between the spinal cord and higher brain centers. It also contains the cell bodies of neurons whose axons go out to the periphery to innervate the muscles and glands of the head. The structures within the brainstem are the *midbrain, pons,* and the *medulla*. These areas contribute to functions such as breathing, heart rate and blood pressure, vision, and hearing. The cerebellum is located behind the brainstem and is chiefly involved with skeletal muscle functions and helps to maintain posture and balance and provides smooth, directed movements. The *forebrain* is the large part of the brain remaining when the brainstem and cerebellum have been excluded. It consists of a central core, the *diencephalon*, and right and left *cerebral hemispheres* (the *cerebrum*).

The outer portion of the cerebral hemispheres is called *cerebral cortex*. The cortex is involved in several important functions such as thinking, voluntary movements, language, reasoning, and perception. The *thalamus* part of the diencephalon is important for integrating all sensory input (except smell) before it is presented to the cortex. The *hypothalamus*, which lies below the thalamus, is a tiny region responsible for the integration of many basic behavioral patterns, which involve correlation of neural and endocrine functions. Indeed, the hypothalamus appears to be the most important area to regulate the internal environment (homeostasis). It is also one of the brain areas associated with emotions. Neurons of the hypothalamus are also affected by a variety of hormones and other circulating chemicals (Vander *et al.*, 1990).

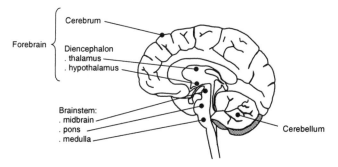

Figure 5.3.   Structural divisions of the brain as seen in a midsagittal section.

5.2.2. The Workings of the Brain

The response of the brain to direct stimulation or to stimulation of various sense organs can be measured via its electrochemical activity; this can give observers a good idea of how the brain is working. Another approach to study how the brain works is to verify brain functions after damage in some of its parts. Functions that disappear or that are no longer normal after injury to specific regions of the brain can often be associated with the damaged areas (Johnson, 1998).

Every neural response depends basically upon four processes: *reception, transmission, integration,* and *actual response* (or simply *response*). First, the organism must receive the information, a process called *reception*. The outer information (stimulus) enters the brain and is usually communicated by the spinal cord (vision and hearing do not go through the spinal cord but go directly into the brain; thus the reason why people can be completely paralyzed but still see and hear). This information is then delivered by sensory neurons to the central nervous system, the process of *transmission*, or *conduction*. In the CNS, the information provided by the sensory neurons is interpreted, and an appropriate response is determined; this process is known as *integration*. Appropriate neurons (motor) transmit the message to the selected muscles, generating the *actual response*, or *effect*. Muscles and glands are the body's chief effectors. The glands are the major constituents of the endocrine system, which will be studied separately in the next section.

The central nervous system contains millions of neurons organized into separate *neural networks*. Within each neural network, the neurons are arranged in specific pathways, or *circuits*. Neural messages travel over these circuits. Neurons are arranged so that the axon of one neuron in the circuit forms junction with the dendrites and cell bodies of the next neuron in the circuit. A junction between two neurons or between a neuron and an effector is called a *synapse*. The most familiar stimuli receptors are the organs responsible for the five senses – hearing, sight, smell, taste, and touch. However, other types of receptors, such as those of the immune and endocrine systems, located deep within the body, keep the brain apprised of changes in the internal environment. Receptors are specialized to react to specific changes in their environment; they convert various forms of inputs (e.g., sound or light) into nervous impulses. Once a neuron has been stimulated sufficiently, it transmits a nervous impulse along the entire length of its axon.

Based on how pre-synaptic and post-synaptic neurons communicate, two types of synapses have been identified: *electrical synapses* and *chemical synapses*. Most synapses in the body are thought to be chemical synapses, in which the pre- and post-synaptic cells are separated by a relatively wide space, called the *synaptic cleft*. In chemical synpases, when an impulse reaches the end of a pre-synaptic axon, it stimulates the small, bubble-like structures called *vesicles* to release chemical *neurotransmitters*, these can be *excitatory* or *inhibitory* for the synaptic cleft, as illustrated in Figure 5.4. A neurotransmitter then diffuses across the synaptic cleft and combines with specific receptors on the dendrites or cell bodies of post-synaptic neurons. When the neurotransmitter binds with the receptor on the post-synaptic neuron, it triggers a nerve impulse in this post-synaptic neuron. This way the information flows from one neuron to another along the neural circuit.

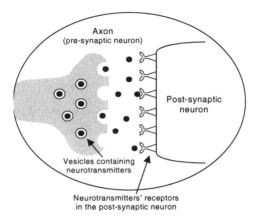

Figure 5.4. Neurotransmitter release in the synaptic cleft.

Even the simplest behavior involves the communication between thousands of neurons. It is believed that these connections and their efficiency can be modified, or altered, by experience. Only a fraction of the relevant sensory information promotes an immediate motor response. The majority of sensory information is stored for future use, with most of the storage occurring in the cerebral cortex. This information storage process is better known as *memory*. The synapses also play a role in memory. Every time a sensor signal passes through a synapse, the synapse becomes more capable of (adapted to) transmitting the same signal next time. After the sensor signals pass through the synapses a number of times, the synapses become so adapted that signals within the brain itself are capable of causing an impulse transmission through the same sequence of synapses, even when the sensor impulse is not excited. Once these *memories* are stored in the nervous system, they are part of the information processing mechanisms. *Decision making* in the central nervous system involves the comparison of new sensory information with the stored memories, where the memories assist in the selection of important sensory information.

5.3   Fundamentals of the Endocrine System

The *endocrine system* is responsible for the production, storage, and control of substances called *hormones*. A *hormone* can be defined as a chemical substance that has specific regulatory effects on the cells upon which they act. Hormone-like substances can be secreted not only by the components of the endocrine system, but also by neurons (neurotransmitters) and other types of cells, e.g., lymphokines released by T-cells. The hormones secreted by the components of the endocrine system have a great deal of influence over the body. They have many functions within the organism with the primary ones being to assist the maintenance of homeostasis, growth, reproduction, and to enable the organism to cope with stress. In terms of chemical structure, hormones generally fall into four categories: *steroids*, *amino acid derivatives*, *peptides,* and *proteins*.

The bodily organs and cells change their function in response to changes in their local environment, whilst the organism responds to alterations in both the internal and the external environment. Hormones acting on specific cells are aimed at preserving a constant physical and chemical internal environment. The secretion of a hormone is usually evoked by a change in the physiological state of the organism and results in an action that tries to restore the organism to its previous state. The return to the normal state results in the maintenance of homeostasis, where a *negative feedback* mechanism is employed to counteract the stimulus. Homeostasis operates in animals through a range of sensory receptors for change detection, in either the internal or external environment of the organism. These receptors initiate specific and appropriate responses from the immune, nervous, and endocrine system.

The organs that compose the endocrine system are sometimes called *ductless glands*, or simply *glands*, because they have no ducts connecting them to specific body parts. They are scattered throughout the body as illustrated in Figure 5.5. As examples, the *pituitary* is in the brain, the *thyroid* is in the neck, the *adrenal glands* are just along the kidneys, and the *sexual glands* (*ovaries* or *testes*) are located in the sexual organs.

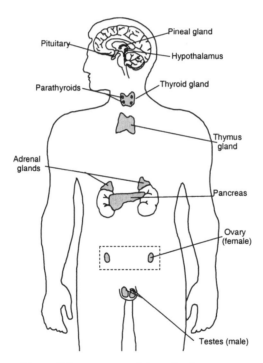

Figure 5.5. Anatomy of the endocrine system.

Table 5.1 summarizes the major endocrine glands and the main functions of the hormones they secrete. In order not to overload this section, a list of endocrine hormones will not be presented, rather the focus will be on their physiological functions according to their secretory gland. For references on the hormone types and names, see Vander *et al.* (1990), McClintic (1985), Campbell (1990), Salomon *et al.* (1990), and Guyton (1991).

The hormones secreted by the endocrine glands are released directly into the bloodstream or lymph. They are differentiated from the *exocrine glands*, such as the *sweat glands* or the *salivary glands*, that release their secretions through ducts directly to target areas, e.g., the skin or the inside of the mouth. Some of the body's glands are described as *endo-exocrine* glands because they secrete hormones as well as other types of substances. As hormones can travel in the blood and lymph, they are able to reach virtually all bodily tissues. Yet, the body's response to hormones is highly specific, in some cases involving only a single organ or group of cells. In other words, despite the ubiquitous distribution of a hormone mainly via the blood, only certain cells are capable of responding to the hormone. In addition, at any one time there may be several different types of hormones present in the blood.

Table 5.1.   Major endocrine glands and the roles of their secreted hormones.

Gland	Hormone Function
Ovary	To develop and maintain female sex organs and characteristics
Testis	To develop and maintain male sex organs and characteristics
Pancreas	To lower blood sugar, increase glycogen storage, stimulate protein synthesis, and suppress release of insulin and glucagon
Adrenal glands	To constrict blood vessels, increase heart rate and blood pressure, stimulate muscle contraction, raise blood glucose levels, increase metabolic rates, regulate sodium, water and potassium excretion by the kidney, and contribute to secondary sex characteristics
Thymus	To stimulate T-cell development in thymus and maintenance in other lymph tissue, involved in some B-cells developing into plasma cells
Parathyroid gland	To increase blood calcium concentration, decrease blood phosphate level
Thyroid	To increase oxygen consumption and heat production; stimulate, increase and maintain metabolic processes; and inhibit calcium release
Pituitary gland	To increase water absorption, raise blood pressure, stimulate contraction of pregnant uterus, and release breast milk after childbirth, stimulate bone and muscle growth, promote protein synthesis and fat mobilization, and stimulate production and secretion of thyroid hormones
Hypothalamus	To respond to signals from the nervous system and release hormones that act on the pituitary gland; it acts as a liaison between the brain and the pituitary gland
Pineal gland	To regulate the wake-sleep cycle

When a hormone reaches a target cell, an initial interaction occurs between the hormone and the cell receptor, i.e., molecules of the target cell that have a specific capacity to bind with the hormone. Often hormones have *synergistic* effects; that is, the presence of one enhances the effect of the other. As with the immune system, the recognition of a hormone by a cell receptor is made possible by the configuration of portions of the receptor molecules such that a match (binding) exists between them and the specific hormone. It is the presence of the hormone-receptor combination that initiates the chain of intracellular biochemical events leading ultimately to the cell's overall response.

The receptors in the target cell are usually located in one of two sites: within the cell nucleus (mainly steroid hormone receptors) or in the plasma membrane (nonsteroid hormone receptors, e.g., proteins, amines, and peptides). When a peptide hormone binds with a receptor on the cell membrane, it makes use of a *second messenger* to relay a hormonal message to the appropriate sites within the cell. This second messenger is responsible for altering the cell activity.

Conversely, steroid and thyroid hormones are relatively small, lipid-soluble molecules that pass easily through the plasma membrane of a target cell, through the cytoplasm, and into the nucleus. Specific protein receptors into the nucleus bind with the hormone to form a hormone-receptor complex. This complex interacts with specific sites on the DNA, activating appropriate genes and leading to the synthesis of the needed proteins. These proteins may stimulate changes in cell activities. Figure 5.6 illustrates the processes of recognition and cell activation when stimulated by a steroid hormone.

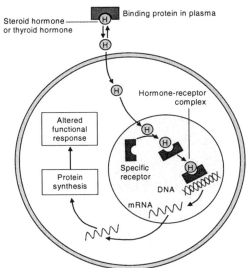

Figure 5.6.   Steroid hormones are secreted by an endocrine gland and enter the target cell, binding to a specific receptor in the cell nucleus. The hormone-receptor complex binds with a protein associated with the DNA molecule, and activates transcription of new RNA and synthesis of specific proteins. The proteins mediate the response characteristic of the hormone's action (reproduced with permission from [Vander *et al.*, 1990]. © *The McGraw-Hill Companies, 1990*).

When an endocrine gland is stimulated by appropriate inputs, the bursts of hormone release occur more frequently, so that the average plasma concentration of the hormone increases. In contrast, in the absence of stimulation or in the presence of active inhibitory inputs, the bursts decrease in frequency or stop altogether, and the plasma concentration of the hormone decreases. The final result of a hormone stimulation of its target cell is an alteration in the rate at which the target cell performs a specific activity. Muscle cells increase or decrease contraction, epithelial cells and other cell types alter their rates of water or solute transport, and gland cells secrete more or less of their secretory products. The direct outcome of many of these observed changes is a hormone-induced change in the activity of an enzyme in the cell. Certain hormones induce both the synthesis of new enzyme molecules and an altered activity of the enzyme molecules already present in the cell. The advantages of this dual effect are considerable. Induction of new enzyme synthesis requires hours to days, whereas the activation of molecules already present can occur within minutes. Thus, the hormone simultaneously exerts a rapid effect and sets into motion a long-term adaptation.

The *pituitary gland*, also named *hypophysis cerebri*, is found at the base of the brain and is connected to the hypothalamus by the hypophysical stalk. It is considered the master gland because its hormones, either directly or indirectly, affect the functioning of the entire endocrine system. Due to the fact that the pituitary is located in the brain and has both neural and humoral (blood) connections to the hypothalamus, it is also the endocrine gland traditionally associated with cognitive control.

It is now known that a number of endocrine glands receive direct neural input via the autonomic nervous system and respond to that neural input in concert with the hormonal secretions of the pituitary. The pituitary, through a series of hormonal feedback loops, acts as the principal regulator of these responses, but this regulation can be overridden via input from the nervous system.

5.3.1. The Workings of the Endocrine System

The endocrine system responds to stimuli as follows.

1. Glands and nerve cells signal endocrine glands in response to stimuli such as temperature changes, hunger, fear, and growth needs.
2. In response, endocrine glands release hormones that carry instructions to specific cells. These hormones travel all around the body or just to neighbor cells looking for special binding proteins, the receptors, which are located in and on the target cells.
3. Once bound, the receptor interprets the hormone's message and carries out its instructions by starting one of two distinct cellular processes. The receptor can:
   a. Turn on genes to make new proteins, which causes long-term effects such as growth or sexual and reproductive maturity;
   b. Alter the activity of existing cellular proteins, which produce rapid responses such as a faster heart beat and varied blood sugar levels.

Too much or too little hormone can be harmful to the body; therefore hormone levels are regulated by a feedback mechanism that is essential for an ideal body function. Growth hormones control height and bone structure, too little causes *dwarfism*, too much causes *gigantism (acromegaly)*. Sex steroid hormones (*oestrogens, progestins, androgens*) help develop, regulate, and maintain male and female sex characteristics (breast size, bone density, muscle development, sperm production), cycles (uterine growth, pregnancy), and behavior. Several mechanisms influence the feedback relationships like the change that a hormone produces also serves to regulate that hormone's secretion (negative feedback).

5.4   Immune-Neuro-Endocrine Interactions

All vertebrate animals, from fish to mammals, have an immune, a nervous, and an endocrine system. Although each system has its specific functions, they are all interconnected and dependent on one another in order to:

- Maintain the body's internal state (homeostasis);
- Coordinate functions of highly differentiated cells, tissues and organs;
- React to stimuli from inside and outside the organism;
- Regulate growth, development, and reproduction; and
- Produce, use, and store energy.

As discussed in Section 2.2, at the beginning of the second half of the 20th century, the majority of research efforts were directed at understanding the molecular and cellular basis of the immune response, immune diversity and tolerance mechanisms. As a result of this research, the following is now known: the structures of the main antigenic receptors (antibodies and TCRs); the types and subtypes of cells that participate in an immune response; the molecular and genetic basis of the differentiation and diversification of immune cells; the biochemical and molecular basis of immune cell activation and how their interaction with and reception of information from APCs. In contrast, much less is known about how immunological cells and their products interact with other bodily systems and about the consequences of such interactions for the functioning of the immune system. Thus, the comprehension of the immune system organization raised essential questions concerning its physiological functioning within the whole organism.

The interactions of the immune, endocrine, and nervous systems are very complex, since each of these systems is intrinsically complex. Furthermore, the amount of information coming from the research literature is by now enormous and in some cases, contradictory or difficult to interpret. However, there is anatomical, biochemical, and pharmacological evidence suggesting that functional immune-neuro-endocrine interactions can occur at certain levels.

Table 5.2 presents a functional view of the three systems (immune, nervous, and endocrine) and discusses some evidence that the immune and neuroendocrine mechanisms can affect each other. In summary, neuroendocrine agents can influence immune selection, homing, recirculation, trafficking, cytokine production, cellular interactions, antigenic presentation, effector functions, and auto-regulatory processes. In contrast, lymphokines and other immune cell derived products can affect hormonal production, cellular metabolism, food intake, neuronal activity and growth, thermoregulation, sleep and behavior, to name a few.

Table 5.2.　Immune, nervous and endocrine systems: functions, components and interactions.

System	Function	Components	Interactions
Immune	Defend the body against foreign invaders and malfunctioning cells that may cause infection	Bone marrow Adenoids Tonsils Thymus Lymph nodes Spleen Lymphatic vessels Peyer's patches Appendix	Different immune cell populations have receptor profiles for modulators like neurotransmitters and endocrine hormones The thymus synthesize different thymus hormones Immune products coexist in neuroendocrine tissue
Nervous	Reception of stimuli, transmission of nerve impulses, and activation of muscle mechanisms	Peripheral nervous system (autonomic and somatic) Central nervous system (brain and spinal cord)	Neural cells express receptors for cytokines, hormones, and neurotransmitters The brain can stimulate defense mechanisms against infection The hypothalamus control the pituitary and other endocrine glands Neural products coexist in immune and endocrine tissue
Endocrine	Secrete hormones into blood and other body fluids aiming at regulating metabolism, growth, water and mineral balance, response to stress and reproduction	Pineal gland Adrenal gland Pituitary gland Hypothalamus Thyroid Parathyroid Pancreas Thymus Ovaries Testes	Endocrine cells express receptors for cytokines, hormones, and neurotransmitters Hormones provide feedback to the brain that affect neural processing Reproductive hormones affect the development of the nervous system Endocrine products coexist in immune and nervous tissue

The hypothalamus is an excellent example of the interactions between these three major physiologic systems of the human body. Anatomically, the hypothalamus is part of the brain; it is located beneath the thalamus in the diencephalon (Figure 5.3). Signals from the limbic system are the primary neural trigger for the hypothalamus. Electrochemical signals from the hypothalamus trigger the autonomic nervous system as well as the pituitary. Nevertheless, the hypothalamus also produces a variety of hormones that are conveyed through a group of blood vessels to the pituitary, triggering the release or inhibition of the corresponding pituitary hormones. Furthermore the hypothalamus is an integral part of a series of feedback loops which not only regulate many systemic physiologic processes, but also adjust those processes to deal with environmental or internal changes and/or threats to the organism. As part of this feedback system, the hypothalamus senses the amount of certain hormones in the blood, the amount of neural stimulation in the limbic system, and the amount of certain thymic hormones. This information is then processed by the hypothalamus and adjustments in both neural and hormonal secretions are accomplished. The adjustment can be either to restore homeostasis or to move in either direction from it, depending upon the result of the combined information processed by the hypothalamus (Ripka & Ripka, 1995).

In a broad sense, the reciprocal effects between the neuroendocrine and immune systems can be classified as follows (Besendovsky & del Rey, 1996):

1. *Immune, endocrine, or neural cells can express receptors for cytokines, hormones, neurotransmitters, and neuropeptides*

Reciprocal expression of receptors for products of the nervous, endocrine, and immune systems constitutes the basis of the immune-neuro-endocrine interactions or communication. The presence of receptors for hormones, neurotransmitters, and peptides on immune cells has already been established. Several observations like the alteration of patterns of hormonal and neural activities following the antigenic inoculation in health individuals allowed the introduction of molecular bidirectional communication models between the neuroendocrine and immune systems, as depicted in Figure 5.7. It is important to stress that the same molecular signals and corresponding receptors are used to regulate the system itself and the communication between them.

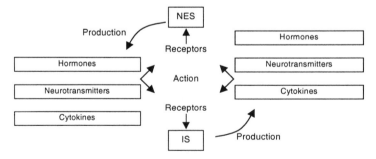

Figure 5.7. A molecular mechanism of communication between the immune and neuroendocrine systems through the sharing of signaling molecules and their receptors (reproduced with permission from [Blalock, 1994]. © *Hogrefe & Huber Publishers, 1994*). NES/IS: Neuroendocrine/Immune system.

2. *Immune and neuroendocrine products coexist in lymphoid, endocrine, and neural tissue*

For exerting reciprocal immune-neuro-endocrine effects, hormones, neurotransmitters, and neuropeptides must reach immune cells and conversely, neuroendocrine structures need to become exposed to products of activated immune cells. In addition to being exposed to hormones, immune organs are innervated. Evidence from several fields of investigation indicates a bi-directional link between the nervous and the immune system. Both primary and secondary lymphoid organs are innervated by nerves derived from ganglia of the sympathetic nervous system. This innervation shows similarities in the patterns of fiber distribution and in principles of general organization on these organs. Additionally, there is experimental evidence that cytokines influence endocrine structures as humoral signals and are also present in the brain.

3. *Endocrine and neural mediators can affect the immune system*

Hormones, neurotransmitters, and cytokines contribute to immunoregulation. Hormone administration can lead to a depressed or stimulated immune response, depending on the kind and dose of hormones and the timing of their administration. There is abundant evidence showing that direct manipulation of the brain, e.g., by stimulating different parts of it, can affect the immune response. The effects on the immune response caused by stress and circadian rhythms and the complex phenomena of conditioning of the immune response also show that processes integrated at the level of the central nervous system can affect immune functions. The influence of hormones and neurotransmitters in the immune system go beyond this and can affect the negative and positive selection of thymocytes, the specificity of the immune responses, the production of cytokines and their receptors, and the lymphocyte recirculation and trafficking.

4. *Immune mediators can affect endocrine and neural structures*

Certain cytokines, antibodies and thymic hormones can serve as mediators in the bi-directional communication between the immune and neuroendocrine systems. Furthermore, stimulated lymphoid cells can produce pituitary-like hormones. Cytokines can strongly affect the nervous behavior, including neuronal growth and differentiation, nerve repair, food intake, sleep, and thermoregulation. They can also affect the general host homeostasis through metabolic derangements.

The information exchange among the nervous, endocrine, and immune systems through hormones, neurotransmitters, and cytokines is summarized in Figure 5.8. When the exchange of signals occurs between immune and neuroendocrine structures that are distant from each other, a long loop circuit is established. When immune-neuro-endocrine communication is based on signal exchange, at either peripheral or central levels, local interactions are established. Long loop circuits and local interactions are also interconnected. The degree of activity of the immune-neuro-endocrine network can be affected at the level of the immune system after antigenic stimuli or at the level of the central nervous system sensorial and psychological stimuli. The branching out arrows indicate the consequences of interactions between immune, nervous, and endocrine systems for the whole organism.

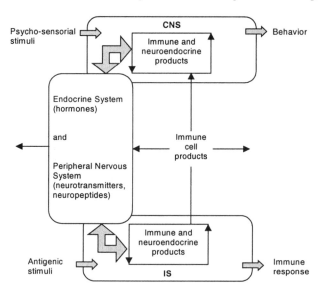

Figure 5.8. Information exchange among the nervous, endocrine, and immune systems (reproduced with permission from [Besendovsky & del Rey, 1996]. © *The Endocrine Society, 1996*). CNS: central nervous system; IS: immune system.

5.4.1. Similarities and Differences

As discussed, the nervous, endocrine, and immune systems are functionally interrelated. It is now possible to contrast properties of each of these systems:

- *Anatomy*: while neurons have fixed positions in the central and peripheral nervous systems, the immune cells are mobile and circulate throughout the body. The nervous system has its central part located in the brain and spinal cord and has several branches throughout the body. Although the components of the immune and endocrine systems are not anatomically interconnected as in the nervous system, their components are spread along the organism and are functionally interconnected;

- *Structure*: the nervous system present hierarchies, while the immune and endocrine systems are decentralized;

- *Interconnectivity*: in the nervous system, the connections among cells are mediated by axons, synapses, and dendrites and can be visualized in a microscope. Under the immune network perspective, the nervous and immune systems have their components functionally interconnected as a network, presenting excitatory (stimulatory) or inhibitory (suppressive) effects on neighboring cells. In the immune network theory, the cells and molecules are capable of recognizing and being recognized, sustaining a communication network with less obvious characteristics than the neural networks. The idea of a communication network can also be suggested for the endocrine system in the form of hormone secretion and reception by many cells and organs through their molecular interactions;

- *Cellular population*: the immune and nervous systems consist of a large number of diverse cells. In humans, the nervous system consists of approximately 10^{11} neurons and the immune system contains approximately 10^{12} lymphocytes. In both cases, individual cells are highly specific. The endocrine system is basically composed of glands, which secrete chemicals that affect the behavior of cells in the immune and nervous systems;

- *Functional division*: the central nervous system can be functionally divided into a sensorial and a motor part. Analogously, the immune system can be functionally divided into two parts: a recognition and an effector part. The same division, as the one for the immune system, can be made for the endocrine system. The recognition part of both systems is responsible for recognizing specific molecules (antigens or hormones) and responding by producing and releasing other specific molecules (lymphokines and antibodies or hormones) that will alter the function of other cells;

- *Input signals (stimuli)*: the great diversity of components in these system ensures that the appropriate response is made to a great variety of stimuli. The nervous system recognizes and responds to physiologic stimuli received from our five senses: hearing, sight, smell, taste, and touch. The immune system recognizes and responds to the shape of diverse molecules (antigens) that cannot be perceived by the nervous or endocrine systems. The glands of the endocrine system are capable of recognizing and responding to several types of hormone-like stimuli: the hormones themselves, some neurotransmitters, and lymphokines. As the immune system can recognize non-physiologic stimuli, Blalock (1994) suggested that it can be viewed as our "sixth sense";

- *Multidirectional communication*: as discussed in Section 5.4, the components of each of these three systems are capable of communicating with elements of the systems themselves and with the other systems as well;

- *Types of communication signals (stimuli)*: while the nervous system uses electrochemical communication signals among neurons, the immune and endocrine systems employ primarily chemical signals. In fact, as illustrated in Figure 5.7, a single communication network can be derived for all systems;

- *Response to stimuli*: the nervous system responds to input stimuli by generating several types of signals that promote actions like moving and breathing. The immune system usually responds to the input stimuli by reproducing immune cells, secreting antibody molecules, and promoting the elimination of foreign substances either alone or combined with immune molecules. The endocrine system usually responds by promoting or inhibiting the secretion of specific hormones;

- *Maturation of the system*: in humans, the neuroendocrine as well as the immune system are still immature at birth. Fetal and newborn brains present a paucity of synaptic connections as compared to the adult brain. Myelination and motor control are incomplete, and much programming by sensory input is required. The brain suffers biochemical and physiological changes. The immaturity of the immune system is reflected by an inability to respond to certain antigens as well as by a reduced capacity of macrophages to present antigens or to produce cytokines. In the endocrine system, some hormones are present in low levels in neonates;

- *Adaptation*: in the nervous system, the learning and memory acquisition processes are thought to be consequences of the alteration of connection strengths and patterns of connections among neurons, and not of the alteration of the neurons themselves. Additionally, the brain can be thought of as constituting a type of content-addressable memory, such that frequent death of individual neurons does not drastically affect the brain behavior as a whole. With respect to the immune system, the knowledge is stored in the cells themselves (in their receptors), or in specific clones; the learning happens through the variation in clone sizes and receptor structures. A hormone may induce an increase in the number or affinity of receptors for a second hormone, thus being capable of adapting itself to the current state of the internal environment;

- *Parallel processing*: all systems use parallel processing where the stimuli are simultaneously processed in many different parts;

- *Memory*: the capability of presenting memory distinguishes the nervous and immune systems from all others. The memory of an event might last for many years. Early life experience in the immune and nervous system has lifelong effects on behavior and immunity;

- *Knowledge inheritance*: the knowledge stored by the immune and nervous systems during the lifetime of an individual is not automatically passed to subsequent generations, even if this inheritance supplies the individual with an apparent selective advantage over the others. Section 5.6 discusses how the immune evolution influences species evolution. However, processes like feeding a neonate with a maternal milk are able to transfer some types of information (antibody molecules) to the progeny;

- *Self-identification*: the neural and immune systems have a deep notion of themselves, i.e., of the self. One of the most important roles of the immune system is to distinguish between self and nonself. From a philosophical perspective, the immune self/nonself discrimination can be compared to one of the most primitive functions of the nervous system: the consciousness;

- *Individuality*: each human being has its own set of systems, from nervous to endocrine. These systems might resemble each other only to the extent that they are organized according to the same general pattern. It is the organization defining a type of organism that determines the mode of functioning of any given kind of system, not any particular pattern of connectivity or specificities. As the immune and nervous systems are capable of learning from experience, at the end of life these two systems reflect the environment in which the individual subject was inserted;

- *Presence of cell receptors*: the cells of all the three systems display receptors that allow the communication among them and with external elements. Some neurons are only capable of recognizing very specific stimuli, while others present more general receptors. The immune and endocrine systems have receptors highly specific to their ligand or hormone, respectively;

- *Contextual recognition*: some immune cells learn to recognize and respond to certain antigenic patterns in specific contexts, e.g., in the context of an infection. This phenomena is similar to the context dependent recognition of signals received by the nervous system;

- *Approximate recognition*: all systems share the property that a perfect recognition is not necessary for the triggering of a response; a "fuzzy" or a partial stimulus might suffice. A memory can be retrieved by the immune and nervous systems given a similar stimulus, not necessarily identical, to a previously recognized one. Although the endocrine system is not known to show memory type behavior, it can also respond to molecular patterns that are not exactly the complement of their receptors;

- *Robustness*: the ideal functioning of the immune and nervous systems is apparently insensitive to small damages to its components and structure. It is known however that relatively small doses of hormones and neurotransmitters can significantly alter the behavior of the organism. The feedback mechanisms of the endocrine system are quite effective;

- *Feedback mechanisms*: all three systems are regulated by feedback mechanisms. Examples of negative feedback mechanisms are present in the nervous system. When it is too cold for example, the brain sends signals to the muscles so that they constrain and start shivering in order to reduce the loss of heat by the skin. Negative feedback mechanisms can also be found in the immune and endocrine systems. The information regarding the status of an immune response is fed back into the immune system. When the antibody production is sufficient to counteract the given invading antigen, some immune cells (particularly suppressor T-cells) start producing and releasing cytokines that inhibit antibody synthesis, thus leading to the end of the adaptive immune response. In the endocrine system, the information regarding the hormone level or its effect is fed back into the gland, which then responds in a homeostatic manner.

- *Delayed response*: like the immune system, the endocrine system also presents a fast response (such as the innate immunity) by stimulating already present molecules on a given cell and a slower response (such as the adaptive immunity) by inducing the synthesis of new enzymes, which might take days to start exerting their functions. The responses of the nervous system may also present temporal delays, e.g., the understanding of a methematical theorem sometime after reading the proof.

- *Environmental description*: the immune and nervous systems are designed such that, independently of the pattern of connections or cellular (and molecular) interactions, a repertoire (population) of elements might exist and be diverse enough to describe the environment;

- *Corollary of environmental description*: the corollary of the previous statement suggests that both systems are highly fault tolerant due, mainly, to redundancy and diversity.

5.4.2. Summary

In an attempt to place the immune system in some context with other biological systems, this part has discussed two complex systems within an organism: the nervous and the endocrine system. The nervous system is responsible for the processing of sensory inputs and the appropriation of reactions. The endocrine system is responsible for the production, release, and control of hormones within an organism body in response to stimuli. By examining these systems it is possible to observe the immune system as part of a complex process within an organism that does not operate in isolation, but rather as one part in a complex structure. Numerous interactions between the immune, nervous, and endocrine systems were discussed, with similarities and differences being drawn. By studying these interactions, it may be possible to create new *artificial* systems that combine these three systems.

Having discussed the immune system in context with other bodily systems, it is now possible to take a higher level view and see if the immune system has any relationship with the (macro-)process of evolution, and if so, what can be learnt from that.

PART II: The Evolution of Species and the Immune System

5.5   Evolutionary Biology

Work by J. B. Lamarck in the 19th century proposed the initial hypotheses regarding the theory of evolution. This work proposed that the adaptation of the individuals to the environment as the core of evolution. According to Lamarck, the organs that develop intense activity grow and become more efficient, and those that are little used become weary and degenerate (use and disuse law). It was thought that these alterations could be passed to the descendants through inheritance, thus the descendants acquired characteristics of the parents. Then, after several generations the accumulation of these variations could lead to the emergence of new species. In the eyes of Lamarck, different species of animals developed exactly what they needed to survive; with inheritance of acquired characteristics during the lifetime of an individual being the driving force behind evolution.

When C. Darwin began his research, the Lamarckian evolutionary theory was already known. However, Darwin was primarily concerned with how evolution occurs and how individuals became adapted to their environment. Darwin pointed out two determining factors of an evolutionary process: *natural selection* and *genetic variation*; and presented the following hypotheses to explain the origin of species (Darwin, 1859):

1. The number of offspring tends to be larger than the number of parents;
2. The number of individuals in a species remains approximately constant;
3. From (1) and (2) one can conclude that there will be competition to survive;
4. There are genetic variations within the same species of individuals.

This *natural selection principle* indicates that those individuals whose variations are better adapted to the environment will have a greater probability of surviving and reproducing. As a complement to these ideas, three additional hypotheses were added leading to the so-called *neo-darwinism*:

5. Any sort of continual variation must be responsible for the introduction of novel information in the genetic material of the organisms;
6. There is no limit for the variations to occur; and
7. Natural selection allows the preservation of the new information corresponding to a better adaptation.

After a few *generations*, the most adapted (or the most *fit*) individuals dominate the species. *Selection* (competition and exclusion) exists to eliminate those (or reduce the number of) individuals whose behavior is not appropriate, thus avoiding a population explosion. It is important to note that evolution optimizes the behavior, not the genetic information (Atmar, 1994).

The basic difference between Darwinian and Lamarckian ideas can be summarized as follows. For Lamarck there was a mapping from environmental conditions and expressed characteristics (*phenotype*) to the genetic information (*genotype*). In contrast, for Darwin the environmental conditions and genetic information (*genotype*) determines the expressed characteristics (*phenotype*).

The beginning of the 20th century was marked by the debate between neo-lamarckists and neo-darwinists. Neo-lamarckists denied natural selection and proposed that inherited effects of environmental direct action over the organisms was the basis of evolution. However, neo-darwinists rejected all about Darwin's theory of evolution with the exception of natural selection, which was assumed to be the core of evolution.

Later, research from *genetics* explained that genes determine individual characteristics and that it was these genes, and not the expressed characteristics, which are the elements transmitted through generations. This discovery rocked the foundations of Lamarckism as acquired characteristics were shown not to be inherited. Genetics also demonstrated that the genetic code of a population could change depending on three factors: *migration*, *genetic recombination,* and *mutation*.

Migration introduces new genes in a population, as far as the migrants carry their genetic code and reproduce with individuals from another population. Genetic recombination is a consequence of sexual reproduction. Although it does not introduce new genes in a population, it guarantees new genetic combinations in the individuals of the population. The mutations, most important factors of alteration in the genetic code, produce variations in the genes that can be transmitted to the next generation, i.e., mutations are capable of altering the inheritable characteristics of an organism. Mutations are somewhat random but are strongly constrained by the ability to survive as well as by what genes it has to work with.

Evolution through natural selection is a consequence of adaptation, and under appropriate conditions produces new species, a process termed speciation (Krebs, 1994). Three distinct forms of adaptation can be identified in natural selection:

- *Phylogenetic adaptation*: accumulation of acquired behaviors in the germ cells of a species;
- *Sociogenetic adaptation*: adaptive behaviors are accumulated during the life in a group (society); and
- *Ontogenetic adaptation*: appropriate behaviors are acquired by trial and error during the lifetime of an individual.

5.5.1. The Baldwin Effect

Learning can be broadly defined as any lasting change in behavior resulting from previous experience (Cotman & Lynch, 1990). During the lifetime of an organism, learning does not directly affect the genetic code of an individual. As a consequence, sociogenetic and ontogenetic adaptations cannot be directly transmitted to descendants. However, some evolutionary biologists have been discussing an indirect effect of learning in evolution, inspired by the evolutionary ideas of J. M. Baldwin (Baldwin, 1896). These ideas, known as the *Baldwin effect*, were proposed as a "new factor in evolution".

The idea behind the Baldwin effect is that if learning contributes to the survival of an organism, then the individuals with increased learning capabilities will have higher survival probabilities and thus an increased capability of generating a large number of descendants. If the behavior of an individual is stable, so that the best things to learn remain constant, then this can indirectly lead to a genetic encoding of a characteristic that originally had to be learnt. In summary, the capability to acquire a certain desired characteristic allows the organism to survive and supplies it, together with genetic variation, with the possibility of independently discovering the desired characteristic. Without this learning, the survival probability (and the opportunity of a genetic discovery) decreases. In this indirect pathway, learning can affect evolution even if the subject learnt cannot be directly transmitted.

The Baldwin effect works in two steps. First, the ability of an individual to adapt to its environment during its lifetime (known as phenotypic plasticity) allows it to adapt to a partially successful mutation, which might otherwise be useless to the individual. Secondly, given sufficient time, evolution may find a rigid mechanism that can replace the plastic mechanism. Thus, a behavior that was once learned (first step) may eventually become instinctive (second step).

5.5.2. Species and Niches

The concept of *species* is an important but difficult one to define in biology. There is little agreement on a definition for species. The idea for species came about as the result of observing the effects of several processes: reproduction, mutation, gene flow, and genetic drift. New *traits* in the population result from these processes and are selected through natural selection, which favors different characteristics in different situations. The accumulation of differences eventually yields different species.

Mayr (1942) introduced the most widespread and accepted concept of biological species, as follows: "Species are groups of actually or potentially interbreeding natural populations, which are reproductively isolated from other such groups." Populations are not assigned to different species if they are merely isolated by topographic barriers such as bodies of water; if they resemble one another closely, they are presumed to be potentially capable of interbreeding.

Conceptually, individuals are members of the same species if their genes can be traced through the generations to unite in a parent individual under natural conditions. In practice, biological species are not recognized by genetic criteria, but by phenotypic differences that are taken as evidence of genetic distinctness. It is possible to have overlapping characteristics between two species, yet distinct differences in one or more characteristics are taken to imply genetic isolation.

Even if external or physical (phenotypic) similarity is taken as the common basis for identifying individuals as being members of the same species, the possibility of interbreeding is the species' most remarkable property. Individuals of a species are able to interbreed with one another but not with members of other species. The ability to interbreed is of great evolutionary importance, as it determines that species are independent evolutionary units. Different species have independently evolved different gene pools because they are reproductively isolated. Therefore, genetic changes can only originate in single individuals, and they can only spread to members of their own species, not to individuals of other species.

The concept of a *niche* is proposed at an ecological level in two ways. A niche is defined as the region consisting of the set of possible environments in which the species can persist; members of one species occupy the same ecological niche. In natural ecosystems, there are many different ways in which animals may survive (grazing, hunting, on water, etc.), and each survival strategy is called an ecological niche. However, it is generally recognized that the niche of a single species may vary widely over its geographical range. The other fundamental concept of niche was proposed by Elton (1927) "The niche of an animal means its place in the biotic environment, its relations to food and enemies;" where the term *biotic* refers to life, living organisms. Thus, niche in this case was used to describe the role of an animal in its community Krebs (1994).

5.5.3. Coevolution

Coevolution can be simply defined as a change in the genetic composition of one species (or group of individuals) in response to a genetic change in another. It embodies the idea of some reciprocal evolutionary change in interacting species, where there must be reasonable evidence that the traits in each species were a result of, or evolved from, the interactions of the two species. The term is usually attributed to Ehrlich and Raven (1964) by their study of butterflies on plants. However, the notion was very present in the book *On the Origin of Species* by Darwin (1859). Ehrlich and Raven (1964) documented the association between species of butterflies and their host plants noting that noxious compounds produced by some plants determined the usage of certain plants by butterflies. The implication was that the diversity of plants and their poisonous compounds contributed to the generation of diversity of butterfly species.

In discussing coevolution, it is convenient to distinguish three cases, according to the nature of the ecological relations between the interacting species:

- *Competition*: the presence of each species inhibits the population growth of the other;
- *Exploitation*: the presence of species A stimulates the growth of species B, while species B inhibits the growth of A. Examples are predator-prey and host-parasite interactions;
- *Mutualism*: the presence of each species stimulates the growth of the other.

Species that occupy different niches can coexist side by side without competition. However, if two species occupying the same niche are brought into the same area, there will be competition for a single resource. This will lead to the eventual weakening of one of the species and its ultimate extinction. However, if the species compete for a range of resources, it is possible that they will partition the resources between them and that both survive. Hence, diversity of species is partially dependent on them occupying a diverse set of niches, competing for a range of resources, being geographicaly separate.

5.5.4. **Predator-Prey and Host-Parasite Interactions**

There are a number of enemies for a species; these include its natural predators and organisms that cause diseases and parasites (parasitism). *Predation, parasitism*, and *disease* are overwhelmingly important aspects to life for all species. Many features of organisms are adaptations that have evolved to escape predators, resist pathogens, and capture as food species that have evolved elaborate capabilities of escape and defense.

In many cases these *predator-prey* interactions are unstable and result in the extinction of one species. In contrast, there is support for the view that host-parasite interactions are an important cause both of genetic *polymorphism* (occurrence of different forms, stages, or types in individual organisms or in organisms of the same species, independent of sexual variations) and of continuing evolutionary change. In this case, one species is not extinct due to predation or parasitism by the other, but they coevolve leading to the appearance of novel forms of individuals within the species.

Although no species is entirely free of predation, all have escaped some of their potential predators and parasites by evolving mechanisms of defense. A clear example is found in the case of the immune defense mechanisms against pathogens. Consider the vertebrate immune system: it has developed an efficient and effective multilayered system of defense against pathogens. In the case of less complex mechanisms of defense, several examples can be taken from nature. Many plants and animal species possess spines, stinging hairs, protective armor, or noxious chemicals that render them unpalatable to some predators.

In Sections 2.9 and 3.2, it was argued that the clonal expansion of the immune cells to overcome the rapid proliferation of pathogens might be viewed as a typical predator-prey situation. As a matter of fact, there are several authors supporting the hypothesis that parasites play a role analogous, or at least complementary, to that of predators, herbivores, or resource limitation in influencing the population biology of plants and animals, including humans (e.g., Anderson & May, 1979; May & Anderson, 1979; Hassell & Anderson, 1989). Consider the case of viruses and bacteria (*microparasites*): they are characterized by having a small size relative to the host, short generation times, extremely high rates of reproduction within the host, and a tendency to induce a degree of immunity to re-infection in those hosts that survive the initial exposure. The duration of infection is normally short when compared to the expected lifespan of the host. Due to these characteristics, the infected host serves as the basic unit of ecological study.

Most of the predator-prey models stem either from the original model of Lotka (1925) and Volterra (1926) or some variation of it. This model (Lotka-Volterra) assumes that the system is closed involving coupled interactions, involves predation a function of prey density, and is framed in continuous time. In a simple form, the model assumes that the number of predator depends on the size of the prey population, acting on the predators birth rate. The basic Lotka-Volterra equations can be described as follows:

$$\frac{dx}{dt} = k_1 xy - k_2 x \quad,$$

$$\frac{dy}{dt} = k_3 y - k_4 yx$$

(5.1)

where x is the density of predators, y is the density of prey, k_1 is the reproduction rate of predators per prey eaten, k_2 is the predator mortality rate, k_3 is the intrinsic rate of prey population increase, and k_4 is the predation rate coefficient.

These equations lead to the behavior that the predator population declines due to lack of prey, but increases due to an abundance of food. In contrast, the prey population declines because few escape predation, and it increases because many escape predation.

The following tries to construct a similar model looking at the clonal expansion principle, for example. If an antigen (prey) invades our body and starts reproducing, the immune cells will have to have their specific clones (predators) expanded in order to produce a sufficient number of antibodies and other effector cells to combat this antigenic proliferation. If the population of antigens is of size zero, the immune cells will not reproduce (proliferate) at all. The number of antigens depends on the number of immune cells and molecules acting on the antigenic death rate. In other words, if the number of immune cells and molecules is low, most antigens will survive and reproduce. Thus, immune cells and molecules limit antigens, and immune cells and molecules are limited by antigens.

If we substitute antigens by mice, and immune cells and molecules by foxes, for example, we come to realize that the immune example given above clearly fits a predator-prey model of Lotka-Volterra. In fact, if we contrast the continuous immune network models (equations) discussed in Section 3.5 (and other similar models), it is possible to realize that they also follow the principles of the Lotka-Volterra predator-prey model (equations).

5.6   Evolution and the Immune System

The process of natural selection can be seen to act on the immune system at two levels. First, recall that lymphocytes multiply based on their affinity with a pathogen. The higher affinity lymphocytes are selected to reproduce, a process usually named *immune microevolution*. Secondly, there is an *immune contribution to natural selection,* which acts by allowing the multiplication of those people carrying genes that are most able to provide maximal defense against infectious diseases coupled with minimal risk of autoimmune diseases. In the latter case, there are indications that immune-neuro-endocrine interactions may also contribute to natural selection. In addition to natural selection, the formation of biological *niches and species of immune cells and molecules* can be studied.

5.6.1. Immune Microevolution

Individual organisms suffer ontogenetic adaptation in several ways: the muscles become stronger the more they are used, the behavior varies along time, and so on.

It is suggested that ontogenetic adaptation occurs within the vertebrate immune system as well.

To understand the *immune microevolution*, or the evolution within the immune system, a brief summary of the clonal selection principle and affinity maturation of B-cells is appropriate (Section 2.9). The clonal selection principle presupposes that a large number of B-cells containing antigenic receptors is constantly circulating throughout the organism. The great diversity of this repertoire is a result of the random genetic recombination of gene fragments from different libraries plus the random insertion of gene sequences during cell development. This huge repertoire diversity virtually guarantees that at least one cell will produce an antibody capable of recognizing, thus binding with, any antigen that invades the organism: an immune feature named repertoire completeness. The antigen-antibody binding stimulates the production of clones of the selected cells, where successive generations result in the exponential growth of the selected antibody type. Some of these antibodies remain in circulation even after the immune response ceases, constituting a sort of immune memory. Other cells differentiate into plasma cells, producing antibodies in high rates. Finally, during reproduction, some clones suffer an affinity maturation process, where somatic mutations are inserted with high rates (hypermutation) and, combined with a strong selective mechanism, improve the capability (Ag-Ab affinity and clone size) of these antibodies to recognize and respond to the selective antigens.

The functioning of an adaptive immune response, based upon the clonal selection principle, reveals it to be a remarkable 'microcosm' of Charles Darwin's theory of evolution, with the three major principles of *reproduction with inheritance, genetic variation,* and *natural selection*, each playing an essential role. During the cell proliferation (reproduction) there is no crossover; the progenies of a single cell are copies (clones) of the parent cell and are subjected to a somatic mutation process. Natural variation is provided by the variable gene regions responsible for the production of highly diverse population of antibodies. Selection then occurs such that only antibodies able to successfully bind with an antigen will reproduce and be maintained as memory cells.

The similarity between adaptive biological evolution and the production of antibodies is even more striking when one considers that the two central processes involved in the production of antibodies – genetic recombination and mutation – are the same ones responsible for the biological evolution of sexually reproducing species. The recombination and editing of immunoglobulin genes underlies the large diversity of the antibody population, and the mutation of these genes followed by the selection of the high affinity variants serves as a fine-tuning mechanism. In sexually reproducing species, the same two processes are involved in providing the variations on which natural selection can work to fit the organism to the environment. Thus, cumulative blind variation and natural selection, which over many millions of years resulted in the emergence of mammalian species, remain crucial in the day-by-day ceaseless battle for survival of this species. It should also be noted that recombination of immunoglobulin genes involved in the production of antibodies differs somewhat from the recombination of parental genes in sexual reproduction. In the former, nucleotides can be inserted and deleted at random from recombined immunoglobulin gene segments (Section 2.8), and the latter involves the crossing-over of parental genetic material, generating an offspring that is a genetic mixture of the chromosomes of its parents.

Whereas adaptive biological evolution proceeds by cumulative natural selection *among* organisms (or among organisms and selfish genes (Dawkins, 1989)), research on the immune system has now provided the first clear evidence that ontogenetic adaptive change can be achieved by cumulative blind variation and selection *within* organisms.

Another similarity between the immune function and biological evolution can be observed in our own knowledge of how each one of these mechanisms operates. Our comprehension of the adaptability of an organism and its environment evolved from an instructionist explanation, of the same kind as proposed by Lamarck, to a purely selective model, similar to neo-darwinism. These stages appeared in the development of evolutionary theory, as discussed in the previous section, as well as in the history of immunology, as discussed in Section 2.2.

Finally, note that selectionist principles play different roles in the evolution of species and in the immune microevolution. In evolutionary theory, selectionist principles explain how species become more and more adapted to their environment, thus explaining the evolution of species. However, evolutionary theory says nothing about the mechanisms behind this adaptive behavior. Selectionist principles can explain the functioning of the immune system. These principles clarify the mechanisms responsible for the adaptability of the immune system. This way, the immune system can be considered to be more important than natural evolution as a metaphor in understanding adaptation in an unknown environment (Manderick, 1994).

5.6.2. Immune Contribution to Natural Selection

The immune system contributes to homeostasis by recognizing and eliminating foreign antigens and altered self-antigens. However, homeostasis as a product of natural selection contributes to evolution as long as the survival of one individual would not threaten the survival of other members of the species. In this sense, when referring to homeostasis mediated by the immune system, it is necessary to consider that an individual infected by a pathogenic microorganism may not only have his own life compromised, but might also be a medium capable of transmitting this agent to other healthy individuals. Therefore, there are situations in which immune mediated homeostasis enters into conflict with evolution. This would be the case for example, when individuals who, although having a fully operative immune system cannot deal, or deal ineffectively, with an infective agent. The longer those individuals survive, the greater the threat to the species. This conflict between immune homeostasis and natural selection may be overcome by mechanisms referred to as *anti-homeostatic* functions of the immune system.

Some immune processes may have been acquired in evolution to limit homeostasis. This would have occurred when the survival of an individual compromised the survival of other members of the species. For example, it was demonstrated that some cytokines, rather than the products of the infectious agents that cause the disease, are responsible for the promotion of a series of deleterious neuroendocrine and metabolic derangements that will lead to the death of the individual (Besendovsky & del Rey, 1996).

An alternative way in which the immune system can contribute to evolution is through the association of immune and reproductive functions. The inhibitory effects of certain cytokines on reproductive functions may serve to avoid the transmission of microorganisms to the progeny via the placenta or the milk. Cases where the development of the immune system is deficient, e.g., animals lacking a thymus and therefore T-cells, are usually associated with sexual insufficiency (Besendovsky & Sorkin, 1974). A phenotypical association seems to exist between the function of the primary lymphoid organs that control the development of the immune system and the reproductive capability. It appears to reflect a selective force to impede the reproduction of immunodeficient animals, while favoring the reproduction of individuals capable of developing an efficient immune system.

5.6.3. Niches and Species within the Immune System

The definition of a species given previously applies only to individuals that perform sexual reproduction. Individuals with asexual reproduction, such as lymphocytes and bacteria, are classified into different species according to criteria such as external morphology, chemical and physiological properties, and genetic constitution. However, under a philosophical perspective, one can ask if species are 'single individuals' or 'classes of individuals'. For example, individuals with asexual reproduction do not exchange genetic material (do not reproduce) with other species, so would every individual be a species? The two different hierarchical levels of biological systems discussed in Chapter 1 seem to be appropriate to tackle this situation. In the following discussion, the focus will be on the study of species and niches of cells within an organism, i.e., in the physiologic level instead of in the ecological level in which the concept of a species as interbreeding individuals is the most accepted one.

By the tracing of ancestry, organisms have been found to resemble each other in descending degrees, so that they can be classified into groups and sub-groups. Classifications are often plainly influenced by chains of similarities, geographical distribution, and reproductive patterns. C. Darwin wrote: "On the principle of the multiplication and gradual divergence in character of the species descended from a common progenitor, together with their retention by inheritance of some characters in common, we can understand the excessively complex and radiating affinities by which all the members of the same family or higher group are connected together. For the common progenitor of a whole family, now broken up by extinction into distinct groups and subgroups, will have transmitted some of its characters, modified in various ways and degrees, to all the species; and they will consequently be related to each other by circuitous lines of affinity of various lengths ... " (Darwin, 1859, Chapter 14).

Thus, under Darwin's viewpoint, a species can be conceptually understood as a set of individuals descended from a common progenitor. The attempt with this argument is to view individual lymphocyte clones as different species of cells within the immune system. The concept of niches, species, and population diversity in computational intelligence is relevant for the development of clustering algorithms and search methods capable of performing multimodal and multiobjective function optimization, in a way to be elucidated in the next chapter.

The diversity issue addressing lymphocyte repertoire has also already been discussed in Chapter 2. Furthermore, it was argued that clonal selection is worthy as a revalidation of Darwinian models of natural selection, in which reproductive, mutational and selective events occur. Every time an adaptive immune response is mounted against a bacterium, for example, a multitude of antibody clones with high antigenic affinity is elicited in detriment of the cells with the smallest antigenic affinity. The formation of any single one of these antibody clones is not itself sufficient to confer immunity. Thus, in the case of introduction of bacteria into the body, there has to be a production of different types of antibodies, each of which is directed only against one definite quality or metabolic product of the bacteria. There must be enough "species of antibodies" to combat the bacteria. Each individual lymphocyte clone can be viewed as a "species of immune cells" capable of protecting our organism against a specific type of antigenic stimulus. This way, the amount of cell species in the immune system has to be diverse enough to account for any type of invasion by a pathogenic microorganism.

As a matter of fact, no new term is being coined here, nor is there an attempt to explore any new branch in biology, examples can be found in the literature where authors refer to "species of antibodies", e.g., J. Lederberg (1988). By bringing up this discussion, it is our intention to state that the immune system is not only diverse but it is capable of maintaining different types (species) of antibodies each one capable of covering a 'niche' specific to an antigenic type or species. In the next chapter the concepts of niches and species, under a computational perspective, will be explored and examples from the literature in which a great number of AIS were shown to naturally account for the formation of stable diverse populations capable of maintaining multiple solutions (niches or species) to complex problems will be described.

5.6.4. Summary

This part has discussed a number of issues relating to the comparison of the immune system with other biological mechanisms, such as evolution, species and niches, coevolution, and predator-prey interactions. By broadening the view of the immune system to incorporate these ideas, it is possible to see the immune system in context with the larger scale biological processes. These perspectives help to explain how the immune system can act as part of a larger system (such as evolution) and the strategies it employs to achieve this (niching and species). Perhaps most pertinent to this book, is the fresh perspectives these viewpoints can give to artificial immune systems. Indeed, some of these ideas will be explored in Chapter 6, but the ideas do represent a significant challenge to researchers in AIS for them to take on board and help to drive forward research on AIS.

PART III: Cognition and the Immune System

5.7 Cognition

A symposium named "Cerebral Mechanisms in Behavior" held in September 1948 on the campus of the California Institute of Technology, U.S.A., laid the foundation for *cognitive science*. However, it is a nearly unanimous agreement that the field started officially around 1956 (Gardner, 1985). The concepts involved in such a wide and interdisciplinary subject vary among authors and fields of research. For example, with a very broad and sometimes controversial viewpoint, the biologist H. Maturana defined *cognition* as a biological phenomenon that can only be studied as such. According to him, a cognitive system has an organization that defines a domain of interactions in which it can act with relevance to the maintenance of the system itself, and the process of *cognition* is the actual (inductive) acting (or behaving) in this domain. Thus, living systems are cognitive systems, and living, as a process, is a process of cognition; a property valued for all organisms, with and without a nervous system (Maturana, 1970). Under this standpoint, a single cell or even a plant can be defined as a cognitive system. Nevertheless, most authors take as the subject matter of cognitive science human cognition and intelligence, functions usually reserved for the brain. But if the major subject of cognitive science is to study cognition, and its definition varies among authors and fields, it remains for this book to define a standpoint in relation to what cognition means from an immune perspective. Thus, the intent in this section is to provide the reader with some philosophical and scientific discussions on an issue termed *immune cognition*. To do so, arguments will be drawn from the literature suggesting that the immune system presents the required features to be characterized as a cognitive system, as far as some specific viewpoints of cognition are taken into account.

In a more restrictive sense than the one proposed by Maturana (1970), *cognitive science* might be viewed as an interdisciplinary field whose efforts draw on the resources of a number of disciplines such as psychology, computer science and artificial intelligence, neurobiology, linguistics, and philosophy (Edelman, 1992; von Eckardt, 1996). It thus relies on the concept of "mental" representations and on a set of assumptions collectively called the *functionalist position*. From this perspective, human beings behave according to knowledge made up of symbolic mental representations. *Cognition*, then, consists of the manipulation of these symbols. Psychological phenomena are described in terms of functional processes. The efficacy of such processes resides in the possibility of interpreting items as symbols in an abstract and well-defined way, according to a set of rules. Such set of rules constitutes what is known as a *syntax*. The exercise of the syntactical rules is a form of *computation*, in the broad sense of the manipulation of information according to a definite procedure. Such well-defined processes constitute *semantic* representations, by which it is meant that they unequivocally specify what their information represents in the world.

Under this computational (or artificial intelligence) assumption, particularly suitable for our purposes, the central intuition behind cognitivism is that intelligence, including human intelligence, can actually be defined as computations performed on information representations (Varela *et al.*, 1991). The key notions, in this case, are those of *representation* and *intentionality*. The cognitivist argument is that intelligent behavior presupposes the ability to represent the world as being certain ways (Dennett, 1978).

5.7.1. Immune Cognition

The expression *cognitive* was imported into immunology from psychology. In Psychology, it refers to the superior functions of the brain, such as object recognition, identification of the organism, and intentionality (Mitchison, 1994). The initial goal was to emphasize that the immune system in some way *knows* what it is looking for when it encounters an antigen, i.e., its internal organization endows it with certain intentionality. Some immunologists like I. Cohen, F. Varela, A. Coutinho, and N. Jerne deal with *immune cognition* as based upon the self/nonself discrimination paradigm and/or the immune network theory. Other more conservative authors, adopt a *recognition* point of view for the immune system, or see the immune system as a *sensorial*, instead of cognitive, system. T. Tada (1997) presented a different paradigm proposing that systems like the immune and central nervous system can be denominated *supersystems*.

The idea of recognition as a kind of selective adaptive matching has been around in immunology for some time. The identification of foreign elements to the organism implicitly requires that some immune component is performing this identification, or recognition. Recognition is a *perceptive* event (registration of sensory stimuli) and, thus, has to be sustained in some sort of cognitive apparatus (Tauber, 1997). This standpoint reflects the richness hidden in terms like recognition, learning, and memory, properties pertinent to the immune system.

N. Jerne with his network theory is considered to be the true author of the cognitive model of the immune system (Tauber, 1997). The cognitive view of the immune network theory, presented in Section 2.11, is rooted in two premises:

- The immune system is composed of a universe of internal images that are only recognized because they are expressed in a language known to the system; and
- The immune system is self-defined, i.e., it is designed to know itself.

In this way, the self-elements promote a certain pattern of response, while the nonself induces another type of response. This is based not in the intrinsic nature of the nonself, but in the fact that the immune system perceives the foreign antigen in the *context* of invasion or degeneracy. The key elements are the antibodies that act as antigens through their idiotypic domains, thus existing an internal image of the universe of antigens. The mutual recognition among the immune components (B-cells and antibodies) form a large interconnected network, the immune or idiotypic network, of elements that communicate with each other.

When the immune system is viewed as a cognitive entity, it may represent a complement to the nervous system. For the immune system to act, it first has to perceive, recognize, and decide what mechanisms to put into action in order to operate. It can thus be inferred that it performs a sort of cognitive function, where the immune and nervous systems are viewed analogously. Both systems have perceptive properties: the capability of distinguishing between the internal and external universes. Information processing is central for their functioning and the respective perceptive properties are linked to effector mechanisms. Besides the functional analogies, the increasing evidence of their interdependence, through messenger molecules, neurotransmitters, and hormones was discussed previously. With the adoption of the immune network paradigm proposed by Jerne (1974), the similarities between these systems are even more striking.

Following this same contextualist approach to the immune cognition, I. Cohen (1992a,b) defined a cognitive system as one capable of extracting information and fashioning experience out of raw input data by deploying information already contained in the system. Thus, a cognitive system acts through a sense of direction with intentionality, it is not a passive information processor, or a memory of information; it is designed to manipulate particular information from the domain in which it operates (Cohen, 1992a). I. Cohen (1992b) also proposed the concept of an *immunological homunculus* as an internal image of the self, acquired by early recognition of self-antigens both in the thymus and in the periphery. The self-image being, in fact, composed of the repertoires of T- and B-cells that deal with the self-antigens.

In general terms, a *homunculus* might be defined as the little man that "sits at the top of the mind", acting as an interpreter of signals and symbols in any instructive theory of mind. This interpreter must have a variety of psychological or intentional traits: it must be capable of comprehension and must have beliefs and goals. It can use its internal representation to inform itself and assist it in achieving its goals.

Although this general concept of a homunculus has been criticized by several researchers (e.g., Skinner, 1971; Dennett, 1978; Edelman, 1992), there is a strict relationship between the immunological homunculus proposed by Cohen (1992b) and the most general definition of a homunculus described above. Both are rooted in the idea that the system will be capable of performing its task more efficiently through the gathering and processing of information if it is endowed with an internal representation of the environment in which it is placed. This way it can define the niche in which it must operate. Antigens are recognized as nonself because they are presented in a context that indicates their pathology – they are causing damage to the host organism. Autoimmunity is viewed as a normal characteristic of the immune system that constantly tries to identify and monitor the elements of the host. If these self-antigens are altered in a contextual form, their meanings change, and an immune response might be triggered. Hence, self is no longer an entity, rather it emerges dynamically in a self-identification process that changes continuously along the lifetime of an individual.

Similarly, a theory based on the definition of self and the immune network hypothesis was developed by A. Coutinho and his collaborators (Coutinho *et al.*, 1984; Varela *et al.*, 1988; Coutinho, 1989; Bersini & Varela, 1994; Varela & Coutinho, 1991). They suggested that the global properties of the immune system like self/nonself discrimination and self-tolerance cannot be understood through the analysis of individual components. It was proposed that the essential properties of the immune networks such as structure, dynamics, and metadynamics, together with clonal selection, constitute powerful approaches for the study of specific cognitive aspects of the immune system, such as recognition, learning, and memory. Immune memory was assumed to be a clonal characteristic, at least in the context of secondary responses, and antigenic recognition (directly related to memory) is probably the most appealing cognitive immune property. They classified the immune system as belonging to a class of biological systems whose adaptability relies on a continuous generation of novel elements (cells and molecules) to handle an unpredictable and varying set of situations (antigens).

Based upon the immune network models proposed by Farmer *et al.* (1986) and Varela *et al.* (1988) and the study of selective theories, Manderick (1994) discussed how selectionism could be applied to an understanding of autonomous cognitive systems. He argued that the adaptability principles incorporated by evolutionary systems, such as ecosystems and the immune and nervous systems (under the theory of neuronal group selection, TNGS, proposed by Edelman in 1987), are crucial for the understanding of cognitive behaviors. As pointed out by Varela and his collaborators (Varela *et al.*, 1988), he stressed as the main cognitive properties of the immune system its pattern recognition, learning, and memory capabilities.

Still sustaining the immune network paradigm, Vaz and de Faria (1988) argued that immune processing is explicitly symbolic. There is a correspondence between an exterior world of antigens (epitopes) and an interior world of receptors (paratopes) manufactured by lymphocytes. A great number and diversity of epitopes would be in balance with a great and diverse number of paratopes. The immune and nervous systems are defined as cognitive systems formed by large networks of interconnected elements presenting several degrees of world perception. The network idea was approached, and cognition was viewed as a function of the pattern of connectivity among the elements of the immune network. Both systems, neural and immune, were said to operate in a parallel and distributed fashion, with a great degree of redundancy, using multiple elements that are equivalent in the performance of some tasks.

Up to the third edition of their book, A. Abbas, A. Lichtman and J. Pober (1998) divided an adaptive immune response into three distinct phases: 1) cognitive phase, 2) activation phase, and 3) effector phase. The cognitive phase consists of the recognition and binding of foreign antigens to the specific receptors on lymphocytes, prior to the antigenic stimulation. Under this viewpoint, cognition was equated to recognition followed by binding, in accordance with most of the viewpoints discussed so far. In the fourth and last edition of their book, released in the year 2000, the authors changed from a *cognitive* to a *recognitive* view of the immune principles of recognition and ligation. The adaptive immune response is now divided into recognition, activation, and effector phases.

Based upon a conceptually different point of view, Blalock (1994) approached the immune system as a sensorial system, such as the nervous system, but he attributed cognition only as a process resulting from stimuli like physiological, emotional, etc. He proposed that the immune system is capable of recognizing and responding to stimuli that cannot be perceived by the nervous system like bacteria, viruses, tumors, and so on. These stimuli would go unnoticed if not for the immune system. A virus cannot be seen by a naked eye, it cannot be smelt or tasted, it makes no noise, but it can be perceived by the symptoms it causes. This occurs through the recognition of this stimulus by immune cells, which convert it into chemical information such as hormones, neurotransmitters, and cytokines. These signals are received by the neuroendocrine system resulting in psychological and physiological changes. Apparently, the sensorial operation of the immune system imitates the neuroendocrine system in the sense that a specific stimulus promotes a particular response that results ultimately in a physiologic response.

Besendovsky and del Rey (1996) followed the same approach as Blalock. They argued that the intercommunication between the immune and the neuroendocrine systems (Section 5.4) implies that the immune system is a receptor sensorial system. However, the sensory function of the immune system does not imply that the central nervous system will always react to signals derived from immune cells. A neuroendocrine response to immune signals occurs in a threshold-dependent manner, and only seldom do such responses become cognitive. A cognitive sensation is expected to be more often than not related to stimuli that occur as a consequence of the disease rather than to the elicited immune response itself. The authors also suggested another interesting phenomenon that might reflect the reception of signals from immune cells at the central nervous system level: the behavior condition of certain immune responses. This implies that the immune system is capable of informing the brain about the effect of the stimuli, and the brain, in turn, would mediate the conditioned stimulation or inhibition of the immune response.

Finally, Tada (1997) introduced the term "supersystem" to designate highly integrated vital systems, like the nervous and immune systems. The many elements of a supersystem are interrelated through mutual adaptation and co-adaptation, producing a self-regulated and self-organized dynamic system. The system is also self-contained but open to environmental stimuli that can be translated into internal messages for the self-regulation and expansion processes. A supersystem is characterized by its self-regulation generation of its many components through stochastic processes following selection and adaptation (consequences of self-organization), individuality, and decision making as a response to stimuli.

As a conclusion of the several approaches to the immune cognition discussed above, it is important to remark that cognition in the immune system also implies consciousness: the properties of intentionality and personality. Both are unique and depend on the history and individual experiences of each organism (Tauber, 1994). Cognitive principles embodying the ideas of intentionality and symbolic manipulation (or computation) can be generically applied to the immune and nervous systems; both deal with:

- *The search for a context*: when to act;
- *Signal extraction from noise*: how to focus recognition; and
- *The response problem*: what decision to take.

Based upon these arguments, we defend cognition as a property intrinsic to the immune system: *immune cognition*. Furthermore, we can highlight the immune system's capability of complementing and/or regulating the neural recognition capabilities, thus cognition through the perception of stimuli that cannot be directly detected by our five senses (hearing, sight, smell, taste, and touch).

5.8   Chapter Summary

The overall goal of this chapter was to introduce the reader to the wider context of biological systems and processes and determine where the immune system fits in this broader perspective. This chapter introduced to the reader to the nervous and endocrine systems. Through exploring these systems at a high level, it was possible to draw out some similarities and differences between these biological systems. It could also be seen that these systems (immune, nervous, and endocrine) all interact in various ways within an organism, targeting different stimuli and anomalies, but working towards the same goal, the one of homeostasis. The idea of the immune system being, in some small part, an aspect of the evolutionary process and, indeed, the immune system itself being an evolutionary process was discussed. It was argued, for example, that clonal selection can be considered as an evolutionary-like process. The final section outlined ideas (some controversial) that the immune system can be considered to be a cognitive system, much like the nervous system.

Another intent of this chapter was to raise many questions as to where the immune system fits in the biological world and what could be learnt from that. By discussing the fundamentals of some biological systems (e.g., the nervous system) and evolutionary biology, this chapter will help prepare the reader to understand some of the biologically motivated paradigms which are discussed in the following chapter, in particular artificial neural networks and evolutionary algorithms. It is hoped that this chapter has stimulated the reader to explore new avenues of research and to look more carefully into biology as a great source of inspiration for the development of computational systems. It is also expected that the relationship between the immune system (AIS) with other biological systems is explored, thus leading to a better understanding of the behavior of AIS and how they can be put in context (hybridized) with other already well-established techniques.

References

Abbas, A. K., Lichtman, A. H. & Pober, J. S. (1998), *Cellular and Molecular Immunology*, W, B, Saunders Company.

Anderson, R. M. & May, R. M. (1979), "Population Biology of Infectious Diseases", Part I, *Nature*, **280**, pp. 361-367.

Århem, P. & Liljenström, H. (1997), "On the Coevolution of Cognition and Consciousness", *J. theor. Biol.*, **187**, pp. 601-612.

Atmar, W (1994), "Notes on the Simulation of Evolution", *IEEE Trans. Neural Networks*, **5**(1), pp. 130-148.

Baldwin, J. M. (1896), "A New Factor in Evolution", *American Naturalist*, **30**, pp. 441-451.

Bersini, H. & Varela, F. J. (1994), "The Immune Learning Mechanisms: Reinforcement, Recruitment and Their Applications", In *Computing with Biological Metaphors*, R. Paton (ed.), Chapman & Hall, pp. 166-192.

Besendovsky, H. O. & del Rey, A. (1996), "Immune-Neuro-Endocrine Interactions: Facts and Hypotheses", *Endocrine Reviews*, **17**(1), pp. 64-102.

Besendovsky, H. O. & Sorkin, E. (1974), "Involvement of the Thymus in Female Sexual Maturation", *Nature*, **249**, pp. 356-358.

Blalock, E. J. (1994), "The Immunec System Our Sixth Sense", *The Immunologist*, **2**/1, pp. 8-15.

Campbell, N. A. (1990), *Biology*, 2nd Ed., Redwood City, CA: Benjamin/Cummings Publishing Company, Inc.

Cohen, I. R. (1992a), "The Cognitive Principle Challenges Clonal Selection", *Imm. Today*, 13(11), pp. 441-444.

Cohen, I. R. (1992b), "The Cognitive Paradigm and the Immunological Homunculus", *Imm. Today*, 13(12), pp. 490-494.

Cotman, C. W. & Lynch, G. S. (1990), "The Neurobiology of Learning and Memory", In P.D. Eimas & A. M. Galaburda (eds.), *Neurobiology of Cognition*, MIT Press.

Coutinho, A. (1989), "Beyond Clonal Selection and Network", *Imm. Rev.*, 110, pp. 63-87.

Coutinho, A., Forni, L., Holmberg, D., Ivars, F. & Vaz, N. (1984), "From an Antigen-Centered, Clonal Perspective of Immune Responses to an Organism-Centered, Network Perspective of Autonomous Activity in a Self-Referential Immune System", *Imm. Rev.*, 79, pp. 152-168.

Darwin, C. (1859), *On the Origin of Species by Means of Natural Selection*, 6th Edition, [Online Book] www.literature.org/authors/darwin.

Dawkins, R. (1989), *The Selfish Genes*, Oxford University Press.

Dennett, D. C. (1978), Brainstorms: Philosophical Essays on Mind of Psychology, Brighton Harvester.

Edelman, G. M. (1992), Bright Air, Brilliant Fire, On the Matter of the Mind, Basic Books.

Edelman, G. M. (1987), Neural Darwinism The Theory of Neuronal Group Selection, Basic Books.

Ehrlich, P. R. & Raven, P. H. (1964), "Butterflies and Plants: A Study in Coevolution", *Evolution*, 18, pp. 586-608.

Elton, C. (1927), *Animal Ecology*, Sidgwick and Jackson, London.

Farmer, J. D., Packard, N. H. & Perelson, A. S. (1986), "The Immune System, Adaptation, and Machine Learning", *Physica 22D*, pp. 187-204.

Gardner, H. (1985), The Mind's New Science: A History of the Cognitive Revolution, Basic Books, New York.

Guyton, A. C. (1991), *Textbook of Medical Physiology*, 8th Ed., W. B. Saunders Company.

Hassel, M. P. & Anderson, R. M. (1989), "Predator-Prey and Host-Pathogen Interactions", In Cherret, J. M. (ed.), *Ecological Concepts The Contribution of Ecology to an Understanding of the Natural World*, Blackwell Scientific Publications.

Jerne, N. K. (1974), "Towards a Network Theory of the Immune System", *Ann. Immunol.* (Inst. Pasteur) 125C, pp. 373-389.

Johnson, G. (1998), *Traumatic Brain Injury Survival Guide*, Online Book, [Online] www.tbguide.com.

Krebs, C. J. (1994), *Ecology The Experimental Analysis of Distribution and Abundance*, 4th Ed., Harper Collins College Publishers.

Lederberg, J. (1988), "Ontogeny of the Clonal Selection Theory of Antibody Formation", *Annals of the New York Ac. of Sc.*, 546, pp. 175-182.

Lotka, A. J. (1925), *Elements of Physical Biology*, Williams and Wilkins, Baltimore (Reissued as *Elements of Mathematical Biology* by Dover, 1956).

Manderick, B. (1994), "The Importance of Selectionist Systems for Cognition", In: *Computing with Biological Metaphors*, R. Paton (ed.), Chapman & Hall.

Maturana, H. (1970), "Neurophisiology of Cognition", In P. L. Garvin (ed.), *Cognition: A Multiple View*, Spartan Books, pp. 3-24.

May, R. M. & Anderson, R. M. (1979), "Population Biology of Infectious Diseases", Part II, *Nature*, 280, pp. 455-461.

Mayr, E. (1942), *Systematics and the Origins of Species*, Columbia University Press.

McClintic, J. R. (1985), *Physiology of the Human Body*, 3rd Ed., John Wiley & Sons.

Mitchison, N. A. (1994), "Cognitive Immunology", *The Immunologist*, 2/4, pp. 140-141.

Ottoson, S. D. (1983), *Physiology of the Nervous System*, New York: Oxford University Press.

Ripka, J. F. & Ripka, F. T. (1995), *The Body Immortal*.

Solomon, E. P., Schmidt, R. R. & Adragna, P. J. (1990), *Human Anatomy & Physiology*, Saunders College Publishing.

Skinner, B. F. (1971), *Beyond Freedom and Dignity*, Alfred A. Knopf: New York.

Tada, T. (1997), "The Immune System as a Supersystem", *Ann. Rev. Imm.*, 15, pp. 1-13.

Tauber, A. I. (1997), "Historical and Philosophical Perspectives on Immune Cognition", *Journal of the History of Biology*, 30, pp. 419-440.

Tauber, A. I. (1994), "The Immune Self: Theory or Metaphor", *Imm. Today*, 15(3), pp. 134-136.

Vander, A. J., Sherman, J. H. & Luciano, D. S. (1990), *Human Physiology The Mechanisms of Body Function*, 5th Ed., McGraw-Hill Book Company.

Varela, F. J. & Coutinho, A. (1991), "Second Generation Immune Networks", *Imm. Today*, 12(5), pp. 159-166.

Varela, F. J., Anderson, A., Dietrich, G., Sundblad, A., Holmberg, D., Kazatchkine, M. & Coutinho, A. (1991), "Population Dynamics of Antibodies in Normal and Autoimmune Individuals", *Proc. Natl. Acad. Sc. USA*, 88, pp. 5917-5921.

Varela, F. J., Coutinho, A. Dupire, E. & Vaz, N. N. (1988), "Cognitive Networks: Immune, Neural and Otherwise", *Theoretical Immunology*, Parte Dois, A. S. Perelson (ed.), pp. 359-375.

Vaz, N. M. & de Faria, A. M. (1988), "Cognitive Aspects of the Immune Activity", *Ciência e Cultura* (in Portuguese), 40(10), pp. 981-986.

Volterra, V. (1926), "Variazioni e Fluttuazioni Del Numero D'individui in Specie Animali Conviventi", *Memorie della R. Accaddemia Nazionale dei Lincei*, 2, pp. 31-113 [Translation in Chapman, R. N. (1931) *Animal Ecology*, McGraw Hill, New York, pp. 409-448].

Von Eckardt, B. (1996), *What is Cognitive Science?*, MIT Press.

Further Reading

Physiology

Bullock, J., Boyle, J. & Wang, M. B. (1984), *Physiology*, New York: J. Wiley, Pennsylvania: Harwal Pub.

Campbell, N. A. (1990), *Biology*, 2nd Ed., Redwood City: Benjamin/Cummings Publishing Company, Inc.

Guyton, A. C. (1991), *Textbook of Medical Physiology*, 8th Ed., W. B. Saunders Company.

Mackenna, B. R. & Callander, R. (1998), *Illustrated Physiology*, Churchill Livingstone.

McClintic, J. R. (1985), *Physiology of the Human Body*, 3rd Ed., John Wiley & Sons.

Ottoson, S. D. (1983), *Physiology of the Nervous System*, New York: Oxford University Press.

Solomon, E. P., Schmidt, R. R. & Adragna, P. J. (1990), *Human Anatomy & Physiology*, Saunders College Publishing.

Vander, A. J., Sherman, J. H. & Luciano, D. S. (1990), *Human Physiology The Mechanisms of Body Function*, 5th Ed., McGraw-Hill Book Company.

Neuro-Immune-Endocrine Interactions (Psychoneuroimmunology)

Ader, R. (2000), "On the Development of Psychoneuroimmunology", *Eur. J. of Pharmacology*, **405**, pp. 167-176.

Ader, R., Felten, D. L. & Cohen, N. (Eds.) (1991), *Psychoneuroimmunology*, 2nd Ed., Sand Diego, Academic Press.

Altman, F. (1997), "Where is the 'Neuro' in Psychoneuroimmunology?" *Brain, Behavior, and Immunity*, **11**, pp. 1-8.

Berczi, I., Chow, D. A. & Sabbadini, E. R. (1998), "Neuroimmunoregulation and Natural Immunity", *Domestic Animal Endocrinology*, **15**(5), pp. 273-281.

Besendovsky, H. O. & del Rey, A. (1996), "Immune-Neuro-Endocrine Interactions: Facts and Hypotheses", *Endocrine Reviews*, **17**(1), pp. 64-102.

Blalock, E. J. (1994), "The Immune System Our Sixth Sense", *The Immunologist*, **2**/1, pp. 8-15.

Blalock, E. J. (1992), *Neuroimmunoendocrinology*, 2nd Ed., Chemical Immunology, 43.

Bonamin, L. V. (1994), "O Estresse e as Doenças", *Ciência Hoje*, **17**(99), pp. 25-30.

Carlson, S. L. (1997), "Lymphocyte Trafficking in the CNS and Periphery: Relationship to Neural-Immune Interactions", *Brain, Behavior and Immunity*, **11**, pp. 243-244.

Felten, D. L., Felten, S. Y., Ackerman, K. D., Bellinger, D. L., Madden, K. S., Carlson, S. L. & Livnat, S. (1990), "Peripheral Innervation of Lymphoid Tissue", In *The Neuroendocrine-Immune Network*, S. Freier (ed.), CRC Press, pp. 9-18.

García, A., Martí, O., Vallès, A., Dal-Zotto, S. & Armario, A. (2000), "Recovery of the Hypothalamic-Pituitary-Adrenal Response to Stress", *Neuroendocrinology*, **72**, pp. 114-125.

Heijnen, C. J. (2000), "Who Believes in 'Communication'?", *Brain, Behavior, and Immunity*, **14**, pp. 2-9.

Heijnen, C. J. & Kavelaars, A. (1999), "The Importance of Being Receptive", *J. of Neuroimmunology*, **100**, pp. 197-202.

Mašek, K., Petrovický, P., Ševčík, J., Zídek, Z. & Franková, D. (2000), "Past, Present and Future of Psychoneuroimmunology", *Toxicology*, **142**, pp. 179-188.

Olff, M. (1999), "Stress, Depression and Immunity: The Role of Defense and Coping Styles", *Psychiatric Research*, **85**, pp. 7-15.

Roszman, T. L. & Brooks, W. H. (1990), "Signalling Pathways of the Neurotransmitter-Immune Network", In *The Neuroendocrine-Immune Network*, S. Freier (ed.), CRC Press, pp. 53-67.

Shavit, Y., Yirmiya, R. & Beilin, B. (1990), "Stress Neuropeptides, Immunity, and Neoplasia", In *The Neuroendocrine-Immune Network*, S. Freier (ed.), CRC Press, pp. 163-175.

Solomon, G. F. (1993), "Whither Psychoneuroimmunology? A New Era of Immunology, of Psychosomatic Medicine, and of Neuroscience", *Brain, Behavior, and Immunity*, **7**, pp. 352-366.

Sternberg, E. M. & Gold, P. W. (1997), "The Mind-Body Interaction in Disease", *Scientific American – Special Issue "Mysteries of the Mind"*, pp. 8-15.

Weigent, D. A. & Blalock, J. E. (1987), "Interactions Between the Neuroendocrine and Immune Systems: Common Hormones and Receptors", *Immun. Reviews*, **100**, pp. 79-108.

Evolution of Species

Baldwin, J. M. (1896), "A New Factor in Evolution", *American Naturalist*, **30**, pp. 441-451.

Belew, R. K. & Mitchell, M. (Eds.) (1996), *Adaptive Individuals in Evolving Populations: Models and Algorithms*, Massachusetts: Addison-Wesley.

Escobar, W. (1999), "Defining Species", *Critical Thinking*, Brooks/Cole Biology Research Center.

Futuyma, D. J., (1979), *Evolutionary Biology*, Sinauer Associates, Inc.

Hassel, M. P. & Anderson, R. M. (1989), "Predator-Prey and Host-Pathogen Interactions", In: Cherret, J. M. (ed.), *Ecological Concepts The Contribution of Ecology to an Understanding of the Natural World*, Blackwell Scientific Publications.

Morgan, C. L. (1896), "On Modification and Variation", *Science*, **4**, pp. 733-744.

Osborne, H. F. (1896), "Ontogenic and Phylogenic Variation", *Science*, **4**, pp. 786-789.

Roughgarden, J. (1976), "Resource Partitioning Among Competing Species – A Coevolutionary Approach", *Theor. Population Biol.*, **9**, pp. 388-424.

Smith, J. M. (2000), *Evolutionary Genetics*, 2nd Ed., Oxford University Press.

Smith, J. M. (1987), "When Learning Guides Evolution", *Nature*, **329**, pp. 761-762.

Turney, P., Whitley, D. & Anderson, R. (eds.) (1996), "Evolution, Learning and Instinct: 100 Years of the Baldwin Effect", *Evolutionary Computation*, Special Issue on the Baldwin Effect, **4**(3).

Williams, G. C. (1992), *Natural Selection: Domains, Levels, and Challenges*, Oxford University Press.

Chapter 6

AIS in Context with Other Computational Intelligence Paradigms

Scientific progress may result from the application of ideas in one domain to another one

– B. Manderick

6.1 Introduction

In order to propose a framework to design artificial immune systems introduced in Chapter 3, inspiration was taken from the two most influential biologically motivated computing paradigms: artificial neural networks (ANNs) and evolutionary algorithms (EAs). It was argued that to design an ANN it is necessary to define a representation for an artificial neuron, a network structure to interconnect the neurons, and a learning algorithm to adjust the network weights. In the case of evolutionary algorithms, it was suggested that a given encoding scheme (representation) plus procedures for selection, reproduction, and genetic variation were necessary to design an EA. Similarly, the framework to engineer artificial immune systems was proposed as being comprised of a representation scheme, a set of functions to evaluate interactions between the elements of the system and the environment, and a set of immune algorithms.

For a reader familiar with ANNs and EAs, several similarities and differences between AIS and these approaches have probably come to mind, in particular when comparing bone marrow and thymus models with EAs and when comparing immune networks with artificial neural networks. In addition, these three paradigms have been broadly hybridized to create more powerful computational tools that overcome particular limitations of a given strategy, thus increasing their practical applications. In light of this, the present chapter starts by presenting the fundamentals of artificial neural networks and evolutionary algorithms and raising a brief discussion about their practical applications. It is not the goal of this chapter to provide a deep review of any of these paradigms, but to provide a novice reader to these fields with the minimum concepts necessary to grasp how AIS can be seen in context with ANNs and EAs. Additionally, specific topics on evolutionary algorithms, such as niches and species (Section 5.5) and genetic programming will be emphasized so as to prepare the reader for a discussion about the hybrids between AIS and EAs, benefits and their outcomes.

After contrasting the three approaches, a survey of the literature concerning the hybrids of AIS with ANNs and AIS with EAs is presented. The survey follows the standard adopted in Chapter 4, in which the metaphors employed were stressed and how the works fit into the proposed framework for designing AIS was empasized.

Two of the hybrid algorithms surveyed in this chapter, namely Forrest's (Forrest *et al.*, 1993) and Mori's (Mori *et al.*, 1993) immune algorithms, have been broadly used by other researchers on AIS; this is one reason why they are described in more detail in this chapter (because of this, it may appear a little disparate from the other hybrids reviewed, but it was felt a worthwhile exercise to undertake).

This chapter also considers artificial immune systems in context with other computing paradigms. For instance, hybrids of AIS with case-based reasoning (CBR) and fuzzy systems (FS) can be found in the literature. Additionally, AIS have been compared with learning classifier systems (CS) and have even been implemented using DNA computing. To make the text more comprehensive, a very brief introduction to all these fields (CBR, FS, CS, and DNA computing) will be provided before the hybrids or comparisons are reviewed. A tentative list of future research on the direction of creating hybrids and contrasting these many paradigms will also be proposed.

This chapter is organized as follows. Section 6.2 describes the fundamentals of artificial neural networks, and Section 6.3 presents an introduction to evolutionary computation. Section 6.4 contrasts AIS with ANN and EA regarding aspects such as components, interaction with the environment, generalization capability, and so on. Section 6.5 surveys the works from the literature that integrate these different methodologies and summarizes the benefits of creating these hybrid systems. Section 6.6 place AIS in context with other approaches, such as case-based reasoning, fuzzy systems, classifier systems, and DNA Computing. Finally, hints on how to integrate artificial immune systems with some of the other paradigms are given, so that the reader may have new lines of research and application to follow.

6.2   Fundamentals of Artificial Neural Networks

In order to develop artificial or computational models of the brain, its functions (e.g., vision), or some of its parts (e.g., the cerebral cortex), research on *artificial neural networks* (ANN) has to be multidisciplinary, involving areas such as neurophysiology, psychology, physics, computation and engineering.

Neurophysiologists study the potential of individual neurons to respond to stimuli, while psychologists study brain functions dealing with its cognitive aspects. Psychologists also use techniques derived from artificial neural networks to create models of different brain behaviors and functions. In contrast, engineers and computer scientists are trying to design artificial systems capable of performing similar tasks as their biological counterparts. Abilities such as generalization and the processing of incomplete or imprecise information and massive parallelism are desirable in artificial systems and organisms; these are properties that can be observed in the brain. As with the paradigm of artificial immune systems introduced in this book, ANNs are mostly concerned with the development of techniques for problem solving.

An artificial neural network can be defined as a massively parallel distributed processor, made up of simple processing units, which has a natural propensity for storing experiential knowledge and making it available for use (Haykin, 1999).

ANNs are inspired by the human nervous system (Section 5.2) and present a number of resemblances with it:

- It is composed primarily of a set of information processing cells known as *neurons*;
- Ensembles of interconnected neurons form structures known as *neural networks*;
- Knowledge is acquired by the neural network from the environment through a *learning* or *training* process; and
- Interneuron *connection strengths*, known as *synaptic weights* (or simply *weights*), are used to store the acquired knowledge.

6.2.1. Biological and Computational Terminology

Figure 5.1 illustrates a diagrammatic representation of a biological neuron with the directions of signal propagation throughout the cell. Highly abstract models of biological neurons were proposed in order to design artificial neural networks; these *artificial neurons* are also referred to as *nodes*, or *units*. McCulloch and Pitts (1943) designed the first neural network. They proposed an artificial model for a neuron (Figure 6.1), as a binary processing unit and proved this unit was capable of performing several logical operations (e.g., OR, AND).

Mathematically, the neuron of Figure 6.1 can be expressed as

$$y = f(u) = f(x_1 w_1 + x_2 w_2 + ... + x_L w_L) = f(\mathbf{w}^T \mathbf{x}), \tag{6.1}$$

where y is the output of the neuron, u its activation, $f(\cdot)$ its activation function, x_i ($i = 1,...,L$) is the i-th component of the input vector $\mathbf{x}$, and w_i ($i = 1,...,L$) is the i-th component of the weight vector $\mathbf{w}$.

Artificial neural networks have been developed as generalizations of mathematical models of human cognition or neural biology assuming that:

- *Physiologic stimuli* are received from the environment by a set of input or sensory units;
- Information processing occurs in several elements named *neurons*;
- Signals are propagated from a neuron to another through a set of *connections*;
- Each connection has an associated *strength* that, in a typical neural network *weights* the transmitted signal; and
- Each neuron applies an *activation function* (usually non-linear) to its network input (weighted sum of the input signals) to determine its output.

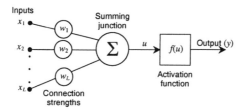

Figure 6.1.   Functional representation of an artificial neuron.

Three main aspects usually characterize an artificial neural network: 1) the pattern of connectivity among units (*network architecture* or *structure*); 2) the method of determining connection strengths (*learning* or *training algorithm*); and 3) the *activation function* of the network neurons. In order to place these ideas in context, it is useful to map the terminology from the biological nervous system discussed in the previous chapter into the computational domain, as summarized in Table 6.1.

Table 6.1.   Mapping the biological to the computational terminology for neural networks.

Biology		Computation
	Soma	Summing junction
Neuron	Synapse	Connection strength
	Activation	Given by an activation function
Neural network		Network of artificial neurons
Network structure		Pattern of connectivity among neurons
Environmental stimuli		Input data (patterns)
Learning		Alteration of network "free parameters"
Generalization		Response to unknown input patterns

6.2.2. Neural Network Architectures

The way in which neurons are structured (interconnected) in an artificial neural network is intimately related to the learning algorithm that is used for the network training. In addition, this interconnectivity affects the network storage and learning capabilities. In general, it is possible to distinguish three main types of network architectures: *single-layer feedforward networks*, *multi-layer feedforward networks*, and *recurrent networks*.

Single-Layer Feedforward Networks

The simplest case of layered networks consists of an *input layer* of nodes whose output feeds the *output layer*. Usually, the input nodes are linear, i.e., they simply propagate the input signals to the output layer of the network. In contrast, the output units are usually processing elements, such as the neuron depicted in Figure 6.1. The signal propagation in this network is purely positive (*feedforward*): signals are propagated from the network input to its outputs and never the opposite way (*backward*). This architecture is illustrated in Figure 6.2(a) and the direction of signal propagation in Figure 6.2(b).

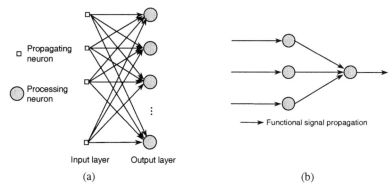

Figure 6.2. *Single-layer feedforward* neural network. (a) Network architecture. (b) Direction of propagation of the functional signal.

Multi-Layer Feedforward Networks

The second class of feedforward neural networks is known as multi-layered networks. These are distinguished from the single-layered by the presence of one or more *intermediate* or *hidden* layers. By adding one or more hidden layers, the non-linear computational processing and storage capability of the network is increased. The output of each network layer is used as input to the following layer. The learning algorithm used to train this type of network requires the backpropagation of an error signal calculated between the network output and a desired output. This architecture is illustrated in Figure 6.3(a) and the direction of signal propagation is depicted in Figure 6.3(b).

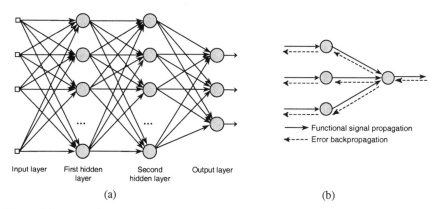

Figure 6.3. *Multi-layer feedforward* neural network. (a) Network architecture (legend as depicted in Figure 6.2). (b) Direction of propagation of the functional and error signals.

Recurrent Networks

The third class of networks is known as recurrent networks, distinguished from feedforward networks for they have at least one *recurrent* (or *feedback*) loop. For example, a recurrent network may consist of a single layer of neurons with each neuron feeding its output signal back to the input of other neurons, as illustrated in Figure 6.4. The recurrent loop has an impact on the network learning capability and performance because it involves the use of particular branches composed of retard units (Z^{-1}) resulting in a non-linear dynamic behavior (assuming that the network has non-linear units).

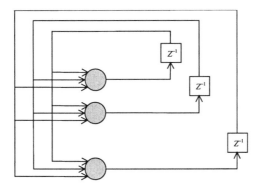

Figure 6.4.   Recurrent neural network architecture with no hidden layer.

6.2.3. Learning Paradigms

In the context of artificial neural networks, *learning* (or *training*) corresponds to the process by which the network's "free parameters" are adapted (adjusted) through a mechanism of presentation of environmental (or input) stimuli. In the standard neural network learning algorithms, the free parameters correspond to the connection strengths (weights) of individual neurons. However, more recent learning algorithms are capable of dynamically adjusting several other parameters, such as the network architecture and the activation function of individual neurons. The environmental or input stimuli correspond to a set of input data (or patterns) that is used to train the network (see Table 6.1).

Neural network learning, thus implies in the following sequence of events:

- Presentation of the input patterns to the network;
- Adaptation of the network free parameters; and
- Altered pattern of response for the input patterns.

With standard learning algorithms a neural network learns through an iterative process of weight adjustment. The type of learning is defined by the way in which the weights are modified. The three main learning paradigms are: 1) supervised learning, 2) unsupervised learning, and 3) reinforcement learning.

Supervised Learning

This learning strategy has the concept of a *supervisor* or *teacher*, who has the knowledge about the environment in which the network is operating. This knowledge is represented in the form of a set of *input-output samples* or *patterns*. Supervised learning is typically used when the class of data is known *a-priori* and this can be used as the supervisory mechanism, as illustrated in Figure 6.5. The network free parameters are adjusted through the combination of the input and error signals, where the error signal is the difference between the desired output and the current network output. Once the supervised learning process is complete, it is then possible to present an *unseen* item to the network, which will then classify that item, with a certain degree of accuracy, into one of the classes used in the training process.

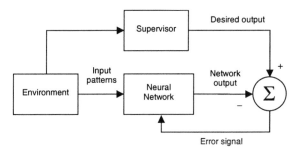

Figure 6.5.   In supervised learning, the environment provides input patterns to train the network and a supervisor has the knowledge about the environment in which the network is operating.

Consider a simple example, let neuron k be the only output unit of a feedforward neural network, as illustrated in Figure 6.6. Neuron k is stimulated by a signal vector $\mathbf{x}(t)$ produced by one or more hidden layers, that are also stimulated by an input vector. Index t is the discrete time index or, more precisely, the time interval of an iterative process that will be responsible for adjusting the weights of neuron k. The only output signal $y_k(t)$, from neuron k, is compared with a *desired output*, $d_k(t)$. An error signal $e_k(t)$ is produced:

$$e_k(t) = d_k(t) - y_k(t). \tag{6.2}$$

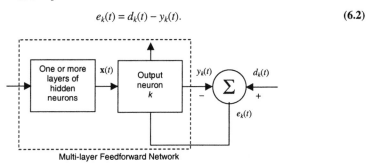

Figure 6.6.   Error-correction learning. At each time step, the network output is compared with the desired output and the error is calculated.

The error signal acts as a control mechanism responsible for the application of corrective adjustments in the weights of neuron k. The goal of supervised learning is to make the network output more similar to the desired output at each time step, i.e., to *correct the error* between the network output and the desired output. This objective can be achieved by minimizing a *cost function* (also called *performance index, error function*, or *objective function*), $\Im(t)$, which represents the instant value of the error measure:

$$\Im(t) = \frac{1}{2}e_k^2(t) \cdot \qquad\qquad (6.3)$$

Unsupervised Learning

In the *unsupervised* or *self-organized* learning paradigm, there is no supervisor to evaluate the network performance in relation to the input data set, as illustrated in Figure 6.7. Note that in this figure there is no error information being fed back into the network, the classes of the data are *unknown* or *unlabelled* and the presence of the supervisor no longer exists. The network adapts itself to statistical regularities in the input data, developing an ability to create internal representations that encode the features of the input data and thus, generate new classes automatically. Usually, self-organizing algorithms employ a *competitive learning* scheme.

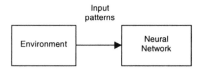

Figure 6.7.   Self-organizing learning.

In *competitive learning*, the network output neurons compete with each other to become activated, with a single output neuron being activated at each iteration. This property makes the algorithm appropriate to discover salient statistical characteristics within the data that can then be used to classify a set of input patterns.

There are three basic elements in a competitive learning strategy for neural networks:

- A set of neurons with the same characteristics, except for their associated weights;
- A limit imposed in the weight of each neuron; and
- A competition mechanism among neurons. The neuron that 'wins' the competition is called *winner*.

Individual neurons learn to specialize on ensembles (*clusters*) of similar patterns; in effect they become *feature extractors* for different classes of input patterns. In its simplest form, a *competitive neural network*, i.e., a neural network trained using a competitive learning scheme, has a single layer of output neurons that is fully connected. There are also lateral connections among neurons, as illustrated in Figure 6.8, capable of inhibiting neighbor neurons.

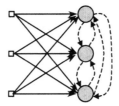

Figure 6.8. Simple competitive network architecture with direct excitatory (feedforward) connections (solid arrows) from the network inputs to the network outputs and inhibitory lateral connections among the output neurons (dashed arrows).

For a neuron k to be the winner, the distance between its corresponding weight vector $\mathbf{w}_k$ and a certain input pattern $\mathbf{x}$ must be the smallest measure (among all the network output units), given a certain metric $\| \cdot \|$ usually taken to be the Euclidean distance. Therefore, the idea is to find the output neuron whose weight vector is most similar (has the shortest distance) to the input pattern presented.

$$k = \arg \min_k \|\mathbf{x} - \mathbf{w}_k\|, \quad \forall k. \tag{6.4}$$

If a neuron does not respond (i.e is not the winner) to a determined input pattern, no learning takes place for this neuron. However, if a neuron k wins the competition, then an adjustment $\Delta \mathbf{w}_k$ is applied to the weight vector $\mathbf{w}_k$ associated with the winning neuron k

$$\Delta \mathbf{w}_k = \begin{cases} \alpha(\mathbf{x} - \mathbf{w}_k) & \text{if } k \text{ wins the competition} \\ 0 & \text{if } k \text{ loses the competition} \end{cases}, \tag{6.5}$$

where α is a *learning rate* that controls the step size given by $\mathbf{w}_k$ in the direction of the input vector $\mathbf{x}$.

Reinforcement Learning

Reinforcement learning is distinguished from the other approaches as it relies on learning from direct interaction with the environment but does not rely on explicit supervision or complete models of the environment. Often, the only information is a scalar evaluation that indicates how well the neural network is performing. This is based on a framework that defines the interaction between the neural network and its environment in terms of the current values of the network's free parameters (network state), network response (actions), and rewards. Situations are mapped into actions so as to maximize a numerical reward signal (Sutton & Barto, 1998).

Reinforcement learning is also distinguishable by the use of trial and error search and delayed reward; there is a trade-off between *exploration* and *exploitation*. To obtain more reward, a reinforcement learning network must prefer actions that it has tried in the past and found to be effective in producing reward. In contrast, to discover such actions it has to try actions that it has not selected previously. Thus, the network has to exploit what it already knows in order to obtain reward, but it also has to explore in order to make better action selections in the future. Figure 6.9 illustrates the network-environment interaction in a reinforcement learning system, highlighting that the network output is fed into the environment that provides it with a reward signal according to how well the network is performing.

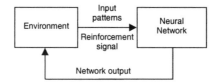

Figure 6.9. In reinforcement learning, the network output provides the environment with information about how well the neural network is performing.

6.2.4. Activation Functions

The *activation function* determines how the current state of a neuron and its internal activation is going to be modified in order to produce the neuron output. When dynamic properties are involved in the definition of the neuron activation, differential (continuous case) or difference (discrete case) equations are used. In order to keep the desired simplicity for the artificial neurons, the activation is usually defined as an algebraic function of their current internal input, which is independent of previous activation values. The activation functions are usually monotonically nondecreasing and present non-linearities associated with saturation. The most common activation functions employed in feedforward networks are the *linear*, *logistic* or *sigmoid*, and *Gaussian* or *radial basis* functions, depicted in Figure 6.10.

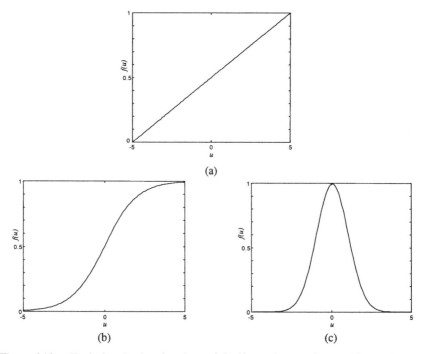

Figure 6.10. Typical activation functions of feedforward networks. (a) Linear: $f(u) = u$. (b) Logistic or sigmoid: $f(u) = (1 + exp^{-u})^{-1}$. (c) Gaussian: $f(u) = exp(-u^2/2)$.

6.2.5. Practical Aspects of Artificial Neural Network Training

In order to apply ANNs to any problem, several considerations have to be made:

- *Model selection*: a suitable network architecture, which might include several hidden layers, connections, and units, has to be chosen. The number of network inputs is usually dependent upon the input data set;
- *Initialization of the weight vectors*: most network models, mainly feedforward networks, are sensitive to the initial values chosen for the network weights. This sensitivity can be expressed in several ways, such as guarantee of convergence, convergence speed, and convergence to local optima solutions;
- *Convergence speed and analysis*: if one considers practical applications of ANN to real-world problems, then a guarantee of convergence is usually required. In general, a network is said to have converged when its response is satisfactory, according to a certain performance measure. The convergence can be affected by the size and complexity of the input data set, and the convergence speed may be a strong limitation to the practical application of ANNs;
- *Parameter setting*: most neural network models require a priori definition of a set of training parameters, such as a learning rate and a stopping criterion.

The problem to be solved greatly influences the choice of the network structure (feedforward or recurrent) and the learning paradigm (supervised, unsupervised, or reinforcement learning). Once the type of network structure and learning algorithm have been selected, the next step in designing a neural network is the model selection, i.e., what network architecture would be suitable to solve the problem at hand. Model selection can be dealt with several approaches, among which *constructive*, *pruning,* and *evolutionary* methods are the most common. Basically, constructive algorithms define the network architecture by adding one unit, layer, or connection at a time during the network learning, until a satisfactory network response is attained. In contrast to the constructive algorithms, pruning strategies start with a large network of cells and iteratively remove 'useless' connections, units, or layers from the network, until a satisfactory pattern of response is reached. Most constructive algorithms incorporate pruning phases in their processes of network model construction. Evolutionary algorithms have also been largely used to search for an appropriate neural network structure.

The strategies used to initialize the network weights vary according to the type of network. For example, discrete Hopfield networks (Hopfield, 1982) usually set weight vectors according to the input data set; there is no iterative network training. The adaptation process of this class of network is performed after a storage phase by presenting a novel input pattern and iterating the network until it reaches a stable state. In the case of feedforward neural networks trained with a backpropagation learning algorithm, the initial set of weights for each layer can be initialized either by taking into account the information contained in the input data set or not. These methods tend to position the initial weight vectors in regions of the space that favor the convergence speed and generalization capabilities of the networks.

There are a number of stochastic processes usually involved in neural network training, making it difficult to present formal proofs of network convergence. As an example, for a class of self-organizing networks, proposed by T. Kohonen (1982) and termed self-organizing maps, convergence can only be guaranteed for some particular cases. Also, convergence is guaranteed because these networks use decaying parameters, which make that the network reaches a stationary state after a certain number of iteration steps. In the case of multi-layer feedforward networks however, convergence speed can be increased in several orders of magnitude by using enhanced learning algorithms, such as second-order gradient-based methods or other alternative approaches. Convergence criteria are usually based upon a minimal value for a given error function or cross-validation strategy.

Finally, the adoption of self-adaptation during training constitutes an interesting approach to reduce the number or alleviate the importance of user-defined parameters. This can help to automate the network learning process and increase its computational capabilities. In the case of feedforward networks for example, line search procedures can be used to automatically determine the learning rate at each iteration. Also, gain and slope of (sigmoid) activation functions can be automatically adjusted. This can be achieved through calculating their derivatives and minimizing an error function associated with the derivatives.

6.2.6. Summary

This section has introduced the reader to some of the basic aspects concerned with the design of artificial neural networks. The brain has some remarkable characteristics, and although its full workings are unknown, interesting metaphors have been extracted to create useful computational intelligence tools. The basic component of any artificial neural network is an artificial neuron with a set of connections that allow it to receive and process input stimuli. The artificial neuron performs an inner product between an input vector and its weight vector (connection strengths), resulting in the neuron activation. Finally, the neuron output is determined after its activation is passed through an activation function. Neurons can be structured in a number of different architectures, such as single-layer feedforward, multi-layer feedforward, and recurrent networks, depending on the desired functionality and problem area. The three main learning paradigms were reviewed: supervised, unsupervised, and reinforcement learning. Practical aspects of using ANNs were then outlined, such as model and parameter selection and network initialization. These aspects were discussed because they are important for the reader to better understand the usefulness of hybridizing AIS with ANNs (Section 6.5), and also to give insights into how to develop new hybrid algorithms (Section 6.7).

6.3   Fundamentals of Evolutionary Computation

Evolutionary algorithm (EA) is the general term encompassing a number of search and optimization procedures that have their origin and inspiration in the biological processes of evolution (Section 5.5). *Evolutionary computation* (EC) is the name used to describe the field of investigation that concerns evolutionary algorithms. An EA maintains a population of individuals, each of which represents a search point in the space of potential solutions to a given problem. The algorithm evolves this population through processes of reproduction, genetic variation, and selection. Evolutionary algorithms can be divided into three major groups:

- *Evolutionary Programming* (EP), originally developed by Fogel, Owens, and Walsh (Fogel *et al.*, 1966) in the United States and recently refined by Fogel (1991);
- *Evolution Strategies* (ES), initially proposed in Germany by Rechenberg (1973) and Schwefel (1965); and
- *Genetic Algorithms* (GA), developed by Holland (1975) in the United States.

Using genetic algorithms as a basis, other evolutionary algorithms were subsequently developed. One significant approach are *classifier systems* (Section 6.6) as proposed by Holland (1975) and another being the evolution of computer programs, known as *genetic programming* (Koza, 1992). This section reviews the basics of evolutionary computation, emphasizing algorithms that account for the formation of niches and species in a population of candidate solutions to a problem and emphasizing genetic programming. The goal is to provide the reader with the minimum knowledge necessary to place AIS in context with EAs.

6.3.1. Biological and Computational Terminology

The biological terminology that is employed in evolutionary algorithms represents a high-level abstraction (metaphor) from the real biological entities. The computational systems invariably correspond to a much simpler structure than their biological counterparts. Section 5.5 discussed the natural evolutionary processes from the biological viewpoint. The remainder of this section maps the biological terminology into the computational domain.

Evolutionary algorithms usually operate with populations of individuals, of single or multiple species, which evolve within a pre-defined environment. As illustrated in Figure 1.1, reproduced here for convenience as Figure 6.11, all living organisms are composed of cells, and each germ cell contains the same set of one or more *chromosomes* – DNA strings – that serve as identifiers for the organism. A chromosome can be conceptually divided into *genes* (functional blocks of DNA), each one encoding a particular protein. Simply put, a gene can be seen as a code for a particular *trait* such as skin color. The different settings of a trait are called *alleles*. Each gene is located in a particular position (*locus*) in the chromosome (Mitchell, 1998).

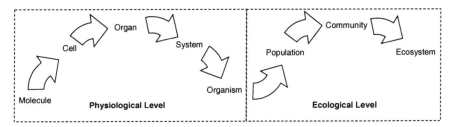

Figure 6.11.   A hierarchical division of biological systems.

Many organisms have multiple chromosomes in each cell, with the full collection of genetic material of an organism being termed the *genome*. The expression *genotype* refers to the particular set of genes contained in a genome. Two individuals with the same genome have the same genotype. The genotype of an organism leads to its *phenotype*, i.e., its mental and physical characteristics, such as eye and skin color.

Organisms whose chromosomes are arranged in pairs are called *diploids*, while organisms with individual chromosomes are said *haploids*. Usually, species with *sexual reproduction* (between two individuals) are diploids, while species with *asexual reproduction* (of a single individual, such as lymphocyte reproduction) are haploids. During sexual reproduction, a *genetic recombination* or *crossover* occurs: in each one of the parents, genes are exchanged between each pair of chromosomes to form a *gamete* (single chromosome), and the gamete of both parents form pairs constituting a complete set of diploid chromosomes. In haploid reproduction, genes are exchanged between the chromosomes of each one of the parents. The *offspring* are subjected to *mutation*, in which *nucleotides* (elementary bits of DNA) are mutated from parent to offspring. The *fitness* of an organism is typically defined as the probability that the organism will live to reproduce (*viability*) or as a function of the number of offspring the organism has (*fertility*).

Restricting our discussion to the genetic algorithms, Table 6.2 presents a mapping between the biological terminology presented and its computational counterpart. It can be noted that the majority of applications of genetic algorithms employ haploid encoding based upon a single chromosome.

Table 6.2.　　Mapping the biological into the computational terminology for GAs.

Biology	Computation
Haploid chromosome	Bitstring that represents a candidate solution
Gene	A single bit or a block of bits
Allele	Values that can be assigned to each position of the chromosome
Crossover	Exchange of genetic material between chromosomes
Mutation	Random exchange of a certain bit in a chromosome
Genotype	Bit configuration in the chromosome of an individual
Phenotype	Decoding of one or more chromosomes

6.3.2. Standard Evolutionary Algorithm and its Process

Evolutionary algorithms were inspired by the neo-Darwinian theory of evolution, briefly reviewed in Section 5.5. As such, the main processes that compose an evolutionary algorithm include reproduction with inheritance, genetic variation, and (natural) selection. Most evolutionary algorithms follow the same standard sequence of steps:

1. *Initialization*: generate an initial population of individuals (parents). This is often accomplished by randomly sampling from the space of possible solutions;
2. *Evaluation*: evaluate the quality of the behavior of the system for all individuals of the population. A performance index is assigned to each individual describing its fitness in relation to the environment;
3. *Selection*: apply selective operators to determine which individuals will be selected for reproduction, and with what frequency;
4. *Reproduction and genetic variation*: generate a novel population of individuals (offspring) by reproducing the selected ones and randomly varying the offspring. This random variation is usually performed by genetic operators, such as crossover and mutation;
5. *Cycle*: the individuals selected in Step 3 compose the new population of parents and are subjected to reproduction and genetic variation in Step 4. Convergence is assumed when a pre-defined solution is met or a fixed number of generations have been performed.

Each time Steps 2 to 4 are completed, a *generation* is said to have occurred. This process of 'simulated evolution' is thus a result of the successive application of a (natural) selection mechanism, which increases the probability of highly fit individuals to survive over the generations, followed by the application of "artificial" reproduction and genetic variation of the selected fittest individuals.

An evolutionary algorithm searches for a solution using a set of candidate solutions, or 'artificial chromosomes'; the space where the possible solutions are held is termed *a search space*. A *fitness landscape* is a representation of a mapping from the space of all possible genotypes to their respective fitnesses.

6.3.3. Genetic Algorithms

A *genetic algorithm* (GA) can be defined as a stochastic algorithm whose search method tries to model the biological phenomena of genetic inheritance and natural selection (Michalewicz, 1996). Simple genetic algorithms constitute abstract models of natural evolution and operate with a fixed size population and individuals represented by "genetic strings" of fixed length. New populations evolve through a probabilistic fitness proportionate selection of individuals, producing, via crossover and mutation, offspring similar to the parents. The main characteristics of a GA can be summarized as follows:

- Population-based search;
- The use of cost (fitness, objective, or adaptability) functions instead of derivatives or other type of auxiliary knowledge; and
- The use of probabilistic transition rules (selection and reproduction mechanisms) instead of deterministic.

Given a problem, how do we know if a GA can solve it effectively? There is no rigorous answer to this question, though several intuitive aspects can be raised (Mitchell, 1998):

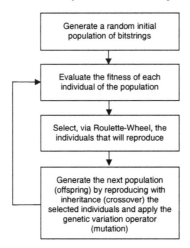

Figure 6.12.   Standard genetic algorithm.

- If the search space is large, neither perfectly smooth nor unimodal, is unknown, or if the fitness function is noisy, then the GA will have a good chance of being a competitive approach;
- If the search space is smooth or unimodal, then *gradient* or *hill climbing* methods are much superior to the GA; and
- If the search space is well understood (such as in the *travelling salesman problem* – TSP), heuristics can be introduced in specific methods, including the GA, such that they present good performances.

After defining an appropriate genetic representation to the problem, a *standard genetic algorithm* can be described by the block diagram of Figure 6.12. This algorithm has the following properties (de Jong, 1994): 1) binary encoding; 2) reproduction and selection via *Roulette Wheel*; 3) single-point crossover; and 4) single-point mutation. Note that it is composed of the three basic steps of all evolutionary algorithms: evaluation, selection, and reproduction with inheritance.

In the *Roulette Wheel* (RW) selection method, the probability of selecting a chromosome (individual of the population) is directly proportional to its fitness value. Figure 6.13 depicts the RW applied to a population composed of four individuals. To play the roulette means to obtain a value from a random number generator with uniform distribution in the interval [0,1]. The value obtained is going to define the chromosome to be chosen as depicted in Figure 6.13(b).

Single-point crossover is realized as follows. Given two parent chromosomes, a random position (locus) is chosen and the genetic material of the strings is exchanged. Each individual has a crossover probability p_c. In the *mutation process*, a position in the chromosome is randomly chosen and its bit is switched from $0 \rightarrow 1$ or from $1 \rightarrow 0$. The mutation probability p_m defines the rate at which each locus can be mutated. Figure 6.14 illustrates the single-point crossover and mutation processes for binary strings of length $L = 8$.

Ind.	Chromosome	Fitness	Degrees
1	0001100101010	16	240
2	0101001010101	4	60
3	1011110100101	2	30
4	1010010101001	2	30

(a)

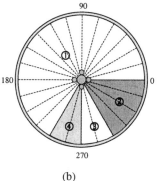

(b)

Figure 6.13. Example of Roulette Wheel for a population with 4 individuals.

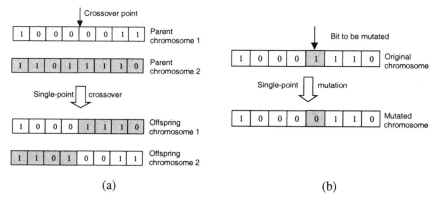

(a)   (b)

Figure 6.14. Basic operators of genetic variation. (a) Single-point crossover. (b) Single-point mutation.

6.3.4. Niches and Species in Evolutionary Algorithms

As discussed in the previous chapter, the specialization permitted by sexual differentiation is carried further in nature through speciation and niche exploitation. The inducement of niches and species in evolutionary algorithms can help the evolutionary search for solutions by providing the capability of locating *multiple optima* (*multimodal search*) and also by generating populations capable of maintaining *increased diversity levels* (*diverse populations*). In this case, each peak of a multimodal fitness function is considered to be analogous to a niche. In contrast, the definition of a species in an evolutionary algorithm is not very clear if one considers the biologically accepted concept of a species (Section 5.5) as a group whose individuals are capable of breeding together. It is safer to use this terminology in the context of evolutionary algorithms that explicitly employ *speciation* mechanisms.

It is possible to identify two different types of evolutionary algorithms that account for the formation of stable diverse populations occupying different regions of the search space: *niching* and *speciation* methods. Nevertheless, if one considers the general case of algorithms with this capability of locating multiple solutions to a given problem, strategies such as the *sequential location of niches, ecological GAs* and *immune system models* can be added to these methods. Indeed, one of the arguments we have been discussing (Section 5.6) is that artificial immune systems are good at maintaining diverse repertoires of cells and molecules and also at locating a large number of optima solutions to a problem. This section reviews niche and species methods from the perspective of evolutionary algorithms, and Section 6.5 surveys work from the literature in which AIS have been hybridized with EAs to improve population diversity and the search for multiple solutions.

Niching Methods

Niching methods extend evolutionary algorithms to domains that require the location and maintenance of multiple solutions (e.g., multimodal and multiobjective optimization). These methods can be divided into categories based upon structure and behavior. To date, two of the most successful categories of niching methods are *fitness sharing* and *crowding*. Both categories contain methods that are capable of locating and maintaining multiple solutions within a population, whether these solutions have identical or distinct fitness values. A sharing or a crowding evolutionary algorithm distinguishes its niches by determining similarities between individuals through the application of a *genotypic* or a *phenotypic* distance measure. This means that the similarity between two individuals can be measured by comparing their chromosomes or by comparing their fitness values.

Fitness sharing, first introduced by Goldberg and Richardson (1987), is a fitness scaling mechanism that alters only the fitness assignment stage of a GA. From a multimodal function optimization perspective, if similar individuals are required to share fitness, then the number of individuals that can reside in any portion of the fitness landscape is limited by the fitness of that portion of the landscape. This sharing results in individuals being allocated to optima regions of the fitness landscape. The number of individuals residing near any peak will theoretically be proportional to the height of that peak. Sharing works by reducing the fitness of each individual of the population by an amount related to the number of similar individuals in the population. Specifically an individual shared fitness f_s is given by:

$$f_s(x_i) = \frac{f(x_i)}{\sum_{j=1}^{N} sh(d(x_i, x_j))},$$
(6.6)

where $sh(\cdot)$ is the sharing function given by Equation (6.7), and $d(\cdot, \cdot)$ is a distance measure used to evaluate the similarity between pairs of individuals in the population:

$$sh(d) = \begin{cases} 1 - \left(\dfrac{d}{\sigma_{share}}\right)^{\alpha}, & \text{if } d < \sigma_{share}, \\ 0, & \text{otherwise} \end{cases}$$
(6.7)

where α is a constant that regulates the shape of the sharing function (usually set to 1), and σ_{share} represents a threshold of dissimilarity.

Crowding techniques work basically by inserting new individuals into the population to replace similar ones. These methods tend to spread individuals among the most prominent peaks of the search space and do not allocate individuals of the population proportionally to fitness (de Jong, 1975). The *sequential niching algorithm*, for instance, runs a standard GA multiple times and maintains the best solution of each run off-line. At the end of each run, the algorithm derates the fitness function at all points within a certain radius of the best solution. This change to the fitness function discourages future runs from revisiting the same area (Beasley *et al.*, 1993).

Speciation Methods

Speciation methods for evolutionary algorithms were developed based upon the biological concept of a species: a set of interbreeding organisms. These methods work basically through the use of *mating restriction* schemes. Deb (1989) proposed mating restriction algorithms in order to solve multimodal function optimization problems using genetic algorithms. Mating restriction is performed by determining the distances between individuals such that appropriate mates are chosen. If the distance between two individuals is less than a pre-defined threshold they are allowed to mate (crossover), otherwise other individuals are sampled from the population until all members are exhausted or a suitable mate is found. As in the case of niching methods, mating restriction is performed according to a phenotypic or a genotypic distance between individuals.

To account for the formation of niches and species in evolutionary algorithms, the three main methods can be summarised as follows:

- *Fitness sharing*: reduce individual fitnesses according to their similarity;
- *Crowding*: maintain diversity by replacing similar individuals with new ones; and
- *Speciation*: restrict mating according to the similarity among individuals.

6.3.5. Genetic Programming

Genetic programming (GP) constitutes a type of evolutionary algorithm developed as an extension of genetic algorithms. In GP, the data structures that suffer adaptation are representations of computer programs; the fitness evaluation involves the execution of the programs. Thus, GP involves a search based upon the evolution of the space of possible computer programs such that, when run, they will produce the best fitness.

The main question responsible for the appearance of genetic programming was "How can computers learn to solve problems without being explicitly programmed to do so?" The major barrier is in the deterministic characteristic of most computational intelligence approaches.

In its original form, a computer program is basically the application of a sequence of function arguments: *functional paradigm*. Implementing GP is conceptually straightforward when it is associated with programming languages that allow the manipulation of a computer program in the form of data structures. Originally, GP was undertaken in the programming language LISP (Koza, 1992).

In GP, a problem is defined by a *representation* and a *fitness function*. The representation consists of *functions* and *terminals* that define a language. The computer programs in the defined language are the individuals of the population that can be represented in the form of *trees*. These individuals (programs) must be run so that one can obtain the corresponding candidate solution (Kinnear Jr., 1994). Figure 6.15 illustrates a tree structure representing the function $f = (x - y) - (a + b)$ in GP. The evolutionary process is performed basically by exchanging sub-trees among individual trees, possibly introducing variations in some nodes or branches of a given tree, and selecting the fittest trees within a population.

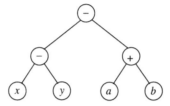

Figure 6.15.   Tree representing the program (or function) $f = (x - y) - (a + b)$ in GP.

6.3.6. Practical Aspects of Evolutionary Algorithms

In the same vein as the discussion proposed for the practical aspects of neural networks, it is possible to identify the following aspects to be accounted for when applying an evolutionary algorithm to a given task:

- *Model selection*: the representation for the individuals of the population, the number of individuals in the population, the evaluation function(s), and the selection operators, all influence the performance of an EA;
- *Initialization of the population*: due to the type of exploratory search performed by evolutionary algorithms, the initialization of the population is in most cases, not of crucial importance for the final performance of the algorithm. However, a priori knowledge of a given task can be used to bias the initial population of individuals towards the solution;
- *Convergence speed and analysis*: as with neural networks, guarantee of convergence in a reasonable amount of time might be a limiting factor while applying an evolutionary algorithm to real-world problems. In addition, formal proofs of convergence are very hard to derive;
- *Parameter setting*: several parameters influence the performance of an evolutionary algorithm, such as the variation operators and their probabilities.

Theoretical results regarding the convergence rate of evolutionary algorithms, more specifically genetic algorithms, have been difficult to obtain due to the fact that these algorithms incorporate complex nonlinear stochastic processes. This problem is usually attacked by theoretical methods, such as Markov chain analysis, that have to make numerous assumptions to make the problem computationally tractable. As a result, the true algorithm is not studied, but a simplified version of it. Thus, one may question the degree to which what can be proven for the simplified procedure still holds for the original procedure (Fogel, 1994). This is the reason why the majority of the work done up to now consist of efforts to quantify the performance by empirical studies, which suggest that GA performance is problem dependent.

Most methods used to tackle the problems of model selection and parameter adjustment in an evolutionary algorithm fall into the category of adaptive evolutionary algorithms. Eiben *et al.* (1999) proposed a taxonomy for the problem of parameter setting in EAs, as illustrated in Figure 6.16. They proposed two major strategies: *parameter tuning* and *parameter control*. The difference between parameter tuning and parameter control is that the former is performed prior to running the algorithm, while the latter occurs during the run. According to this taxonomy, methods for changing the value of a parameter can be classified into one of three categories:

- *Deterministic*: the value of a strategy parameter is altered through a deterministic rule;
- *Adaptive*: some form of feedback from the search is used to determine the direction and/or magnitude of the change to the parameter; and
- *Self-adaptive*: this strategy embodies the idea of evolution of evolution, in which the parameters to be adapted are encoded into the chromosomes and undergo genetic variation.

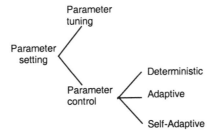

Figure 6.16.   Taxonomy for parameter setting in evolutionary algorithms.

6.3.7. Summary

This section briefly introduced the field of evolutionary computation. The main focuses were on genetic algorithms, mechanisms to induce and maintain population diversity, niches, and species in EAs, and genetic programming. Based upon a population of individuals, an evolutionary algorithm is implemented by the repetitive application of evaluation, selection, reproduction, and genetic variation operators. The importance of population diversity and the formation and maintenance of niches and species in EAs is mainly for applications that require a broad exploration of the search space and the determination of multiple solutions, such as clustering, multimodal, and multiobjective problems. EAs have similar practical aspects as neural networks: however, as a good search strategy, they have been used as tools to search for suitable architectures and parameters in ANNs, as will be discussed in Section 6.5.

6.4   Contrasting the Approaches

In the previous chapter, the neuroendocrine system and the theory of evolution were reviewed. Together with the fundamentals of the immune system provided in Chapter 2, it was possible to outline several similarities and differences between these biological systems and processes.

Through the use of biological systems as inspiration, artificial neural networks (ANN) and evolutionary algorithms (EA) have been developed. As with the biological systems, it is possible to draw out several similarities and differences among their computational counterparts. There have been a few early attempts at comparing AIS with ANN models (e.g., Dasgupta, 1997, 1999; de Castro and Von Zuben, 2001a). Dasgupta (1997, 1999) compared the two systems focusing on their biological equivalents, while in (de Castro & Von Zuben, 2001a) the authors compared their artificial immune network model (aiNet) with self-organizing neural networks.

This section is aimed at identifying the main characteristics of AIS according to the framework proposed in Chapter 3 and contrasting them with the ANNs and EAs, which have just been reviewed. The focus will be on shape-spaces with an attribute string representation (more sophisticated shape-spaces are outside the scope of this volume). The comparison of approaches to be presented is thus of a higher level than the works existing in the literature; it is neither focused on the biological system, nor it is biased to particular models.

In Section 3.5, it is possible to identify two main types of immune algorithms: 1) population-based (bone marrow and thymus models), and 2) network-based (continuous and discrete immune network models). In the population-based immune algorithms, the components of the AIS are usually assumed to be discrete sets of cells and/or molecules that interact only with the external environment (antigens). In contrast, in the immune network algorithms, the components of the AIS interact with each other and the external environment under a network structure. To outline the main similarities and differences among AIS, ANN, and EA, both population-based and network-based models will explicitly be taken into account. The comparison will be made by identifying several features of each paradigm, from the basic components and how they are structured to possible characterizations of the approaches.

6.4.1. Basic Components (Units)

The shape-space formalism was proposed as an approach to create abstract models of immune cells and molecules. In the simplest population-based artificial immune systems, these basic components are represented by attribute strings in a given shape-space. In some applications however, the basic components of the system can be more complex structures, such as a neural or a Petri network. When considering immune network models, the immune cells also include a set of connections that allow them to be linked to other network cells. An immune network cell can also perform some form of computation (e.g., to calculate its stimulation level) and it can carry additional information (e.g., its cross-reactivity threshold and an attribute string representing an antibody molecule). Therefore, immune network cells can be information storage and processing elements.

In neural networks, the basic unit is an artificial neuron composed of a set of connection strengths, a summing junction, and an activation function, as illustrated in Figure 6.1. Like an artificial immune cell, the artificial neuron is also an information-processing and storage element, which receives a set of stimuli from the environment and performs some form of computation with it in order to determine the neuron output. Nevertheless, immune and neural cells have different constituent parts and perform completely different forms of computation. Immune cells store information in individual connection strengths and in the attribute strings representing antibody molecules, while the information stored in an artificial neuron is basically contained in its connection strengths; the body of the neuron is an information processing element. The primary computation performed by an artificial neuron is the inner product of its weight vector (connection strengths) with an input vector. In contrast, each connection of an artificial immune cell corresponds to a link with another cell in the network, and its strength corresponds to the degree of interaction between these two cells. Thus, the information contained in the connections of artificial neurons and immune cells perform different roles in each paradigm.

In the case of evolutionary algorithms the individuals of the population (chromosomes) are usually represented by strings. These can be real-valued, integer, binary, etc., and these are dependent on the problem under evaluation, which is also the case for shape-spaces. The type of EA (ES, EP, and GA) also influences the representation to be used for the components of the algorithm. In the case of genetic programming for instance, the individuals of the population correspond to computer programs generated from a set of terminals represented in the form of (parse) trees. For the simplest population-based AIS using attribute strings, the encoding schemes of an EA and an AIS are in essence the same, the difference lying in aspects such as the algorithms used to govern the behavior of the system over time and their sources of inspiration (metaphor).

6.4.2. Structure (Architecture)

In population-based AIS and evolutionary algorithms, the components of the systems are structured around matrices, which represent repertoires of cells/molecules or populations of individuals (chromosomes). These matrices can have fixed or variable sizes. These components are discrete in the sense that they are not linked to any other element through a connection. They interact with each other indirectly, via an affinity or fitness function, and genetic variation operators in the case of crossover in EAs (see section on "interaction with other components").

In artificial immune networks and artificial neural networks the members of the population are organized in a network-like structure. In most cases, immune networks have an architecture that follows or represents the spatial distribution of the antigenic patterns, while neural networks have pre-defined architectures. Even in the case of dynamically adjusting neural network architectures (see section on "metadynamics"), the pattern of connectivity, number of neurons, layers, and/or connections vary in a deterministic fashion, with the exception of neural networks constructed using evolutionary algorithms.

6.4.3. Knowledge Storage (Memory)

In this context, knowledge can be thought of as the information contained in the system that is a result of its interaction with the environment and the interaction among elements of the system itself. Those parameters that are pre-defined are not considered knowledge of the system, though they are necessary to run the system and reproduce results.

The attribute strings representing the repertoire(s) of immune cells and molecules, and their respective numbers, constitute most of the knowledge contained in a population-based artificial immune system. If one assumes an AIS with adaptive parameters, such as the cross-reactivity threshold, then these parameters are also part of the memory of the system, and their final values are direct results of the interaction with the environment. With artificial immune network models, in addition to the attribute strings, the connection strengths among units also carry information. They quantify the interactions among the components of the AIS themselves. In most cases, memory is content-addressable and distributed.

In the standard (earliest) neural network models, knowledge was stored only in the connection strengths of individual neurons. In more sophisticated strategies such as constructive and pruning algorithms and networks with adaptive parameters, the final number of network layers, neurons, connections, and the shapes of their respective activation functions are results of the network interaction with the environment and, thus, part of the network knowledge. The memory is usually self-associative or content-addressable and distributed.

Each individual chromosome represents the knowledge contained in an evolutionary algorithm. Again, in the case of EAs with adaptive parameters, these can be considered part of the knowledge acquired by the algorithm as a result of its interaction with the environment. Memory is content-addressable and distributed.

6.4.4. Adaptation (Dynamics)

Adaptation is the term used here to express the alteration or adjustment in the structure and free parameters of a system in response to stimulation by other components of the system and the interaction with the environment. The adaptation of free parameters has been termed dynamics in the context of artificial immune systems. Structural adaptation in contrast, has been termed metadynamics. Although both evolutionary and learning processes involve adaptation, there is an important conceptual difference between them (Section 5.5). Evolution can be seen as a change in the genetic composition of a population of individuals during successive generations, resultant from natural selection acting on the genetic variation among individuals. In contrast, learning can be seen as a long lasting change in behavior as a result of previous experience. Whilst AIS may present both types of adaptation, learning and evolution, ANNs adapt through learning procedures and EAs through evolutionary procedures.

Adaptation and learning in an artificial immune system involve basically two aspects: 1) varying the number of cells and molecules in the system, and 2) altering the shapes (attributes) of attribute strings. Those elements that best perform their task (e.g., recognizing an antigen or optimizing a function) are selected to proliferate on a clonal expansion basis; a procedure that increases the number of elements which have proven to be useful. During clonal expansion, immune cells are subject to affinity maturation, in which their antigenic affinity is altered through mutation followed by a selective process. In the case of immune networks, learning can also involve the other two aspects: 3) the modification, addition, and removal of connection strengths among different network elements, and 4) the recruitment of novel elements and death of useless ones (metadynamics).

Artificial neural networks adapt to the environment based upon a learning algorithm that alters the network's free parameters, which are primarily the connection strengths between neurons, but can also include the number of connections, neurons, layers, activation functions, and their shapes.

Adaptation in evolutionary algorithms involves basically the variation in the genetic information contained in populations of individuals, i.e., the alteration of attributes in the chromosomes.

In all cases, the use of parameters that vary with time also correspond to part of the system's adaptation procedure.

6.4.5. Plasticity and Diversity (Metadynamics)

Metadynamics refers basically to two processes: 1) the recruitment of new components into the system, and 2) the elimination of useless elements from the system. This term is often known as plasticity and endows the system with the capability of adapting its structure according to the environment. As a consequence of metadynamics, the architecture of the system can be more appropriately adapted to the environment, and its search capability (diversity) can be increased by the recruitment of novel components. In addition, metadynamics can reduce redundancy within the system by eliminating surplus components.

Population-based AIS usually have a fixed repertoire size. Some attribute strings are clonally expanded (or positively or negatively selected), but the final population size is defined a priori. In the case of immune networks however, metadynamics is one of its most intrinsic features. Individual cells and/or connections are constantly being added to or removed from the network, a reason why immune networks are sometimes called double plastic structures: they can adapt their basic components and their structures as well.

In the standard artificial neural network models, adaptation is only a result of altering the network connection strengths. In more sophisticated neural network learning algorithms, however, metadynamics are already incorporated. For instance, constructive algorithms allow the insertion and/or pruning of individual neurons, connections, and even layers in the network. Thus constructive networks can be classified as double plastic systems as well.

Metadynamics in evolutionary algorithms corresponds to the insertion and elimination of individual chromosomes into and from the population, resulting in a population with varying size; a property not usually accounted for in EAs. Only some of the EAs with parameter control strategies allow for population with varying sizes.

6.4.6. Interaction with Other Components

Population-based AIS are mainly composed of discrete sets of elements represented by attribute strings that exert no direct influence on other elements of the system; they only interact with the environment. In immune network models however, the network cells are usually connected to other cells in the network through a connection that quantifies the degree of interaction between the network cells. The connection strengths between two cells can be stimulatory or suppressive, contributing to the probability of survival and clonal expansion of the cell.

Artificial neural networks are composed of a set (or sets) of interconnected neurons whose connection strengths assume any positive or negative values indicating an excitatory or inhibitory influence to the neuron. The interaction with other neurons in the network occurs explicitly through these connection strengths, where a single neuron receives and processes inputs from the environment or other network neurons, including itself.

Although in evolutionary algorithms, the individuals of the population are not directly connected to other elements of the population, they interact with each other through their reproduction operators and/or fitness function. The simplest type of interaction among individuals in an EA is via a crossover operator responsible for the exchange of genetic material between two chromosomes. If we take into account EAs with explicit niching and species formation for example, the interaction among individuals occurs in other levels as well. Niching GAs involve fitness sharing, where similar individuals are required to share fitness, and crowding methods, where similar individuals are replaced by new ones. In these approaches, the interaction between individuals is performed through the evaluation of a similarity (distance) between them. Speciation methods for GAs are mainly based upon mating restrictions, where sexual reproduction occurs among elements within the same species. Like niching GAs, speciation methods also require that individuals interact with each other through a similarity measure, but in this case, the exchange of genetic material is restricted to the species. In a more complex framework, co-evolutionary algorithms refer to the simultaneous evolution of two or more species with coupled fitness (Potter & de Jong, 1998), thus the interaction with other elements occurs at two levels, within and between species.

6.4.7. Interaction with the Environment

In all biologically inspired computing methods discussed so far (AIS, ANN, and EA) the environment is usually represented by a set of input patterns to be learnt, recognized and/or classified, or a function to be optimized (either minimized or maximized).

In artificial immune systems, an attribute string is compared with the information received from the environment. If there is an explicit antigenic population to be recognized, all or some antigens can be presented to the whole or parts of the AIS. At the end of the learning or recognition phase, each component of the AIS might represent an internal image of a portion of the environment in which it is inserted. When a function is to be optimized, the attribute strings might represent the encoded values of input variables for the function. In this case, these strings will have to be decoded and the function evaluated for each of the decoded strings.

Artificial neurons have connections that receive input signals (data patterns) from the environment or other neurons in the network. These signals are propagated through the connections until they reach the body of the neuron where they are processed and an output is generated. A neural network is usually used to approximate, classify, or optimize the information received from the environment.

An evolutionary algorithm interacts with the environment similarly to an artificial immune system. Most evolutionary algorithms are used to perform a form of search procedure, thus individual chromosomes represent encoded values of a given cost function that evaluate the direction and quality of the search. The algorithm is usually employed to evolve a population of potential candidate solutions, where a single member is going to specify the best solution and represent the environment. In approaches like the Michigan (Holland, 1975), the whole population represents the solution and hence the environment. Niching and species methods usually maintain subpopulations of individuals that interact with separate parts of the environment, though migration (the process by which individuals move along different niches) allows individuals to perform a better exploration of the search space.

6.4.8. Threshold

Antigenic recognition in the immune system is not perfect; a close match between the shapes of an antigen and its receptor is sufficient to elicit an immune response. This is modeled in artificial immune systems through the use of a cross-reactivity or affinity threshold ε that defines a small surrounding region around the shape of an attribute string representing an immune cell or an antigen.

The majority of neuron models include a bias (or threshold) b that corresponds to an external parameter of the artificial neuron, as depicted in Figure 6.17. The presence of this bias in the neuron model can be added to the mathematical expression of the neuron described in Equation (6.1), resulting in Equation (6.8):

$$y = f(u) = f(x_1 w_1 + x_2 w_2 + ... + x_L w_L + b) = f(\mathbf{w}^T \mathbf{x} + b), \tag{6.8}$$

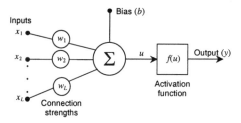

Figure 6.17. Artificial neuron with a bias.

where y is the neuron output, u its activation, $f(\cdot)$ its activation function, x_i ($i = 1,...,L$) the i-th component of the input vector $\mathbf{x}$, and w_i ($i = 1,...,L$) the i-th component of the weight vector $\mathbf{w}$. This threshold determines the neuron output, i.e., it indicates how sensitive the neuron output is in relation to its activation u.

In an evolutionary algorithm there is no explicit threshold. Nevertheless, one can understand the probabilities of the genetic variation operators, such as mutation and crossover probabilities, as thresholds for the promotion of genetic variations in individual chromosomes. If this view is taken, then parameters like the hypermutation rate can also be seen as other thresholds of AIS.

6.4.9. Robustness

As knowledge is distributed over the many components of the system, damage or failure to individual elements does not significantly deteriorate the performance of the whole system or network. All the three paradigms discussed (AIS, ANN, and EA) are highly robust due mainly to the presence of populations or networks of components. The attribute strings, neurons, and chromosomes, can act collectively, cooperatively, and competitively to accomplish their particular tasks.

6.4.10. Generalization Capability

In a broad sense, generalization can be defined as the process of formulating general concepts by abstracting common properties of instances. Under a computational intelligence perspective, generalization corresponds to the capability of a system to respond appropriately to a set of input data unknown to the system. It means that the system is adapted based upon a given set of input data and another data set, different from (or a modification of) the other one, is used to evaluate the system's generalization capability.

In artificial immune systems, a given attribute string m can match not only strings that are its exact complement, but also strings that are "reasonably" complementary to it. The universe of attribute strings that can be matched by m is modelled using the cross-reactivity threshold ε. Any string lying in a volume V_ε resulting from the definition of the cross-reactivity threshold is said to match m. Therefore, if the AIS was adapted to a given antigen that defined the current attributes of m, the definition of ε will allow m to match any string contained in V_ε, thus generalizing the information carried by m. In addition to cross-reactivity, some immunologists (e.g., Inman, 1978; Perelson & Weisbuch, 1997), speculate that antibodies can also be multispecific, in the sense that they can bind with antigens of relatively different structures, as far as enough interactions are established between the antigen and the selected antibody. Multispecificity, then, contributes to the generalization capability of AIS.

ANNs are known to be efficient in generalizing the input patterns, provided that appropriate learning is performed. There are basically two ways in which an ANN can attain a satisfactory generalization performance (Prechelt, 1998): 1) by reducing the number of dimensions of the parameter space, or 2) by reducing the effective size of each dimension, i.e., by model selection or by regularization/cross-validation. Model selection techniques include constructive and pruning methods, while regularization and cross-validation methods act basically on the cost function to be minimized and convergence criterion, respectively.

When EAs are applied to tasks like pattern recognition (e.g., Jones *et al.*, 1993) and classification (e.g., Holland, 1987), the generalization issue is of great importance. However, as most evolutionary algorithms are used for optimization purposes, the generalization question has not been addressed a great deal. The *schema analysis* proposed by J. Holland (1975) can be used as a basis for associating combinations of attributes with the potential for improving current individual performances. Schemas provide a way of decomposing a complex search problem into a hierarchy of progressively simpler ones in which the simplest level consists of single variables assignments. The idea is that a GA tackles the simpler problems first and that these partial solutions are then combined, especially through recombination, into more complex solutions until the complete (or generalized) problem is solved. From a pattern recognition perspective, the problem formulation can be viewed as a string-matching task, in which the GA aims at discovering sets of common schemas that collectively match (cover) a different set of strings. In this case, the generalization issue arises when there are not enough individuals in the population to assign one individual (or subpopulation) to each task, niche, or fitness peak. Generalization in a GA is equivalent to the detection of common schemas shared among many individuals of the population to be recognized (Forrest *et al.*, 1993).

6.4.11. Non-Linearities

The non-linearities in AIS appear mainly in the use of binding functions to define a binding value between two attribute strings proportionally to their affinity (Section 3.5, see Figure 3.11). Some immune network models, such as the second generation immune networks use Gaussian-like functions (Figure 3.22) to make the maturation and proliferation probabilities dependent on the degree of connectivity of an immune cell with the current network configuration.

Non-linearities in artificial neural networks reside basically in the activation functions of individual neurons (see Figure 6.10). The combined operation of several non-linear neural units results in a network with great potential to perform nonlinear approximations. These activation functions can assume several shapes, like sigmoid (Cybenko, 1989), Gaussian (Chen *et al.*, 1991; Freeman & Saad, 1995), hermite polynomials (Hwang *et al.*, 1994; Von Zuben & Netto, 1997), and others.

A standard evolutionary algorithm does not present any explicit non-linearity. However, one can assume the selective advantage of an individual based on its fitness as a type of non-linearity. The fittest individuals have higher probabilities of being selected and thus propagating their genetic information. Under this perspective, an affinity proportionate selection also corresponds to another form of non-linearity in AIS. Evolutionary algorithms that alter the fitness value of an individual, like fitness sharing strategies that in most cases use a non-linear sharing function as the one presented in Equation (6.7), have explicit non-linearity.

6.4.12. Characterization

The classification of these three biologically inspired computing approaches can be made according to different aspects. For example, AIS can be classified according to their structure as population-based or network-based. They can also be classified based upon their paradigm as an evolutionary or a learning system. Table 6.3 depicts two possible characterizations for AIS contrasting them with ANN and EA.

Table 6.3.   Possible characterizations of AIS, ANN and EA.

	Characterization		
	AIS	**ANN**	**EA**
Structure	Population-based or network-based	Network-based	Population-based
Paradigm	Learning and/or evolutionary	Learning	Evolutionary

6.4.13. Summary of Similarities and Differences

Table 6.4 summarizes the discussion presented so far about the similarities and differences among the standard versions of the three biologically motivated computing paradigms reviewed: AIS, ANN, and EA.

Table 6.4.   Contrasting AIS, ANN, and EA.

	AIS	ANN	EA
Components	Attribute string in S	Artificial neurons	Strings representing chromosomes
Structure	Set of discrete or networked elements	Networked neurons	Discrete chromosomes
Knowledge storage	Attribute strings/ connection strengths	Connection strengths	Chromosomal strings
Dynamics	Learning/evolution	Learning	Evolution
Metadynamics	Elimination/ recruitment of components	Constructive/pruning algorithms	Elimination/ recruitment of chromosomes
Interaction with other components	Through recognition of attribute strings or network connections	Through network connections	Through recombination operators and/or fitness function
Interaction with the environment	Recognition of an input pattern or evaluation of an objective function	Input units receive the environmental stimuli	Evaluation of an objective function
Threshold	Influences the affinity of elements	Influences neuron activation	Influences genetic variation mechanisms
Robustness	Population/network of components	Network of individuals	Population of components
Generalization capability	Cross-reaction	Network extrapolation	Detection of common schemas
Non-linearity	Binding function	Neuronal activation function	Not explicit
Paradigm	Evolutionary and/or learning	Learning	Evolutionary

6.5   A Survey of Hybrids: AIS+ANN and AIS+EA

The idea of integrating different computational intelligence paradigms in order to create hybrids combining the strengths of the different approaches is not new. Soft Computing (SC) was the term coined to address a new trend of co-existence and integration that reflects a high degree of interaction among several computational intelligence approaches like artificial neural networks, evolutionary algorithms, and fuzzy systems (Zadeh, 1997). Even engineering principles for the design of hybrid systems can be found in the literature (e.g., Khosla & Dillon, 1997).

In a recent work, de Castro and Timmis (2002) introduced AIS as a new soft computing paradigm. This work summarized the framework described in Chapter 3 and AIS were placed in context with other well-established soft computing approaches such as ANNs, EAs, and fuzzy systems (FS). Generally speaking, AIS, ANN, and EA have great potential to interact with each other in any direction, as suggested in Figure 6.18. Most of the works that try to integrate AIS with ANN and EA, involve artificial neural and immune network models or immune and evolutionary algorithms. This section is an extended version of that paper and reviews these hybrid approaches focusing on how one strategy was used in order to improve the performance of the other.

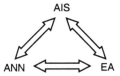

Figure 6.18.   Multidirectional interaction among AIS, ANN, and EA.

6.5.1. AIS and Artificial Neural Networks

Section 5.4 identified several similarities, differences, and pathways of interaction between the nervous and the immune system. In the last section, a comparison between their artificial counterparts (AIS and ANN) was presented. This section reviews the works from the literature concerning hybrids between neural networks and artificial immune systems.

An Unorthodox Neural Network

Hoffmann (1986) and Hoffmann *et al.* (1986) used the analogy between the immune network theory and the central nervous system to formulate a neural network model they classified as unorthodox. Their neural network was based upon a variation of Farmer's mathematical immune network model, discussed in Section 3.5, interpreted in the context of neural networks. This network was composed of a set of N neurons in a system of N coupled ordinary differential equations.

The authors demonstrated that this network was capable of learning without explicitly changing the values of synaptic connection strengths. The main rule of their learning algorithm is that one may select which stimulus is applied to the network at any time and with which strength. Thus, learning involves varying the strength of the input stimuli instead of the strengths among neurons.

The immune system was viewed as an N-dimensional system containing a very large number of singular points representing attractors. The memory capacity of this system was directly related to the existence of a large number of attractors. Learning corresponded to transitions to stable steady states in the network dynamics. Nothing else changed: the strength of interaction between any network element remained fixed. This is in contrast with the traditional view of learning in the central nervous system and most ANN models, which involves the alteration of the strengths of synaptic connections among neurons. This feature led to the denomination 'unorthodox neural network'. Table 6.5 presents a mapping between the unorthodox neural network proposed and the immune system.

Table 6.5.   Mapping from the immune system to the unorthodox neural network model.

Immune System	Neural Network Model
Clone	Neuron
Size of a clone	Rate of firing a neuron
Number of clones	Number of neurons
Stimulation/suppression of a clone	Stimulation/suppression of a neuron
Stable steady states (long-term immunity)	Singular points (attractors)

A Multi-Epitope Approach

Vertosick and Kelly (1989) conjectured that the immune system may represent a good source of inspiration for the development of novel neural network architectures. Based on the Parallel Distributed Processing (PDP) theory (Rumelhart *et al.*, 1986), they attempted to incorporate the immune network theory into a PDP immune network.

It was argued that B-cells (or lymphocyte clones) could act as the units that compose a PDP network in the sense that they receive inputs (from APCs, antigens and/or cytokines), generate outputs (antibodies), remember antigenic patterns, and convert inputs (antigenic stimulation) into output (antibody secretion) in a quantitative fashion. The PDP immune network architecture could be multi-layered, where lymphocytes would correspond to input units, plasma cells would be output units, and lymphocytes producing anti-idiotypic antibodies would serve as examples of hidden units. The definition of the connection weights within the immune network would depend upon the definition of the units. The connection weights between two lymphocytes could be defined in terms of the affinities between their immune receptors. However, if the units were defined as clones, then both the affinity and the relative sizes of two clones would have to be considered in the definition of the weight between them.

The model also included cytokines, which were responsible for the clonal expansion of the populations and subsequent alteration of the connection strengths of a PDP network composed of clonal units. Another possible role of cytokines was related to the network temperature. A simulated annealing of a PDP network was used to find the lowest energy configuration of the network by altering the shape of the activation functions of the units. No learning algorithm was explicitly presented, though the authors strongly suggested that the learning behavior of the immune system uses an unsupervised local learning rule.

Related Works from the Authors

Vertosick, F. T. & Kelly, R. H. (1991), "The Immune System as a Neural Network: A Multi-epitope Approach", *J. theor. Biol.*, **150**, pp. 225-237.

Vertosick, F. T. (1992), "The Immune System as a Neural Network: An Alternative Approach to Immune Cognition", *SigBio Newsletter*, **12**, pp. 4-6.

Vertosick, F. T. (1994), "Fluid Neural Networks as a Model of Intelligent Biological Systems", In *Computing with Biological Metaphors*, R. Paton (ed.), Chapman & Hall, pp. 156-165.

Application of a PDP Model to Immune Networks

Fujita and Aihara (1989) made use of the similarities between neural and immune networks in order to modify a PDP model to simulate immune idiotypic networks. The modifications introduced that are peculiar to the immune networks were the introduction of time delays and bilateral and asymmetric interactions between units. Like Vertosick and Kelly (1989), the authors regarded the immune system, particularly the immune networks, as a parallel distributed processor system.

This PDP model of the immune network follows the same standard network dynamics and metadynamics as the one proposed in Equation 3.20. The concentration of a given network cell at a given time step was proportional to the network activation and suppression among cells, the antigenic stimuli, and a threshold of activation.

Competitive Networks

In the work presented by de Castro *et al.* (2002), the authors developed a growing Boolean competitive network, named ABNET for AntiBody NETwork, based on the clonal selection and affinity maturation principles of the immune system. The main features of the proposed algorithm are competitive learning, automatic generation of the network architecture, and binary representation in the Hamming shape-space of the connection strengths or weights. Table 6.6 summarizes the metaphors employed by the authors to develop a competitive neural network using ideas from immunology.

The weight updating procedure corresponds to a guided search simulating the affinity maturation process of the antibody repertoire (Section 3.4), such that the weights (antibodies) iteratively become a more perfect complement of the antigens. This process is equivalent to a multi-point mutation usually employed in evolutionary algorithms. The hypermutation rate is directly related to the capability and speed of maturation of a given antibody. The cells with larger stimulation levels (the cells with higher affinity and subject to the highest concentration of antigens) are candidates to suffer clonal expansion. Additionally, the least stimulated cells are removed from the network.

Note that this network learning algorithm incorporates adaptive processes in two different levels: the weights (dynamics) and the network architecture (metadynamics). As argued by the authors, this algorithm brings interesting insights into how to develop new, constructive, self-organized neural network models employing ideas from the immune system.

Table 6.6.   Mapping from the immune system to competitive neural networks.

Immune System	Competitive Neural Network
Antibody	Neuron
Affinity maturation	Weight updating
Most stimulated antibody	Winner neuron
Non-stimulated antibody	Inactive neuron
Cloning	Splitting
Apoptosis	Pruning

Neural Network Initialization

As a practical aspect of neural network training discussed in Section 6.2, the initial weight vector to be used in supervised learning for multilayer feedforward neural networks has a strong influence in the learning speed and in the quality of the solution obtained after convergence. An inadequate initial choice may cause the training process to get stuck in a poor local minimum or to face abnormal numerical problems. A novel approach to create a simulated annealing algorithm based on the immune metaphor has been proposed by de Castro and Von Zuben (2001b) and applied to the problem of initializing feedforward neural networks.

The authors argued that the correlation between the quality of initial network weights and the quality of the network output could be likened to the quality of the initial antibody repertoire and the quality of the immune responses. The authors extracted the metaphors of creating antibody diversity and the idea of a Euclidean shape-space to propose an algorithm called SAND (Simulated ANnealing for Diversity). The aim of the algorithm was to generate a set of initial weight vectors, to be used in feedforward ANN training, that are diverse enough to reduce the likelihood of the neural network to converge to a poor local optimum. In SAND, an antibody was considered to be a vector of weights of a given neuron and an antigen was the input pattern presented to the neural network. By the use of an energy function that maximizes the Euclidean distance among antibodies, a diverse population of antibodies, thus weight vectors, was generated. The empirical results demonstrated that the spread of the weight vectors used to initialize multilayer feedforward neural networks increases, on average, their learning speed.

RBF Neural Network

As another aspect related to the practical application of artificial neural networks, the appropriate operation of a radial basis function (RBF) neural network depends strongly upon an adequate choice of the number of basis functions and their associated parameters, such as their positions and dispersions.

The immune network model described in Section 3.5 was employed by de Castro and Von Zuben (2001c) to implement an unsupervised approach to select radial basis function centers. The main objective of this work was to cluster and filter unlabeled numerical data sets. As important results, the method proposed was capable of reducing redundancy and incorporating the statistical distribution of the data set structure, including the shape of the existing clusters. As in the previous model, the authors employed a Euclidean shape-space to represent the molecules, where an antibody corresponded to a candidate center for the RBF neural network and an antigen corresponded to an input pattern. Clonal expansion, affinity maturation, and selection were used to generate populations of increasingly better individuals with relation to the input data set. Immune network interactions, in contrast, were used to control the final number of cells in the network, so that parsimonious networks could be automatically generated.

Related Works from the Authors

de Castro, L. N. & Von Zuben, F. J. (2001), "An Immunological Approach to Initialize Centers of Radial Basis Function Neural Networks", *Proc. of the Brazilian Congress on Neural Networks*, pp. 79-84.

6.5.2. AIS and Evolutionary Algorithms

The majority of the immune algorithms currently developed have an evolutionary-like type of learning or embodied process. This section reviews the works in which techniques from one strategy have been used to enhance another. The focus here is given mainly to immune algorithms that account for the formation of niches, species, and diverse populations, that integrate with genetic programming, and that contribute to handle constraints in evolutionary algorithms.

Niches, Species and Diversity in Artificial Immune Systems

Forrest *et al.* (1993) employed a binary Hamming shape-space to model the immune system. The goal was to study the pattern recognition and learning that takes place at the individual and species level of this artificial immune system. In their model a population of antibodies was evolved in order to recognize a given population of antigens. A genetic algorithm was used to study the maintenance of diversity and generalization capability of their AIS, where generalization means the detection of common schemas shared among many antigens. The affinity function between an antibody and an antigen was evaluated by summing the number of complementary bits between their attribute strings (Hamming distance, given by Equation 3.3). This way, it was possible to study the ability of a GA in the detection of common patterns (schemas) in the antigen population and to discern and maintain a diverse population of antibodies.

As a result of their study about diversity in a model of the immune system, the authors proposed a hybrid immune algorithm that has been used in important applications of AIS, such as computer network security (Kim & Bentley, 1999) and job-shop scheduling (Hart & Ross, 1999); this case study on job-shop scheduling is undertaken in Chapter 7. The authors proposed the following hybrid immune algorithm:

1. Build random populations of antigens and antibodies;
2. Match antibodies against antigens;
3. Score the antibodies according to their affinity; and
4. Evolve the antibody repertoire using a standard GA.

The authors argued that this model allows the study of how the immune system learns which antibodies are useful for recognizing the given antigens. In addition, it was suggested that changing details such as the shape-space used and the sampling methods for the antibody molecules could create several interesting variations of this algorithm. In order to evolve a population of antibodies that maintains diversity under the GA, a fitness measure accounting for the following immune properties was developed:

- Antigens are typically encountered sequentially;
- An immune system responds with only a subset of its lymphocytes that come in contact with the antigen;
- There is competition among lymphocytes for antigenic recognition, so that the cells that bind the antigen with higher affinities are selected to proliferate;
- Antibodies are improved by somatic hypermutation during the affinity maturation process.

The resulting fitness scheme proposed works as follows:

1. Choose an antigen randomly;
2. Choose, without replacement, a random sample of μ antibodies;
3. Match each antibody against the selected antigen using Equation 3.3 (Hamming distance);
4. Add the match score of the highest affinity antibody to its fitness maintaining the fitness of all other antibodies fixed; and
5. Repeat this process for many antigens (typically three times the number of antibodies).

Note that the features stressed in this algorithm can be added to those covered by the clonal selection algorithm and lead to another immune algorithm that combines the strength of both methods: sampling of the antigen space and affinity proportional selection and mutation.

The results presented showed that by matching an antigen with multiple antibodies and then giving the fitness score to the best-matched antibody, an antibody population could be evolved and maintained by the GA containing representatives of different antibodies. Thus, multiple peaks could be discovered and maintained in this population with this matching and scoring schemes, demonstrating that this algorithm is capable of performing a form of *implicit fitness sharing*. When compared with the *explicit fitness sharing* discussed previously, it was shown that the sample set size μ of the antibody population plays a role analogous to the σ_{share} parameter used in the explicit fitness sharing (Equation (6.7)).

The authors' strategy was theoretically and empirically compared with the explicit fitness sharing in another paper (Smith *et al.*, 1993). They reported that the antibody sampling mechanism promoted a niching strategy of the artificial immune system whose generalization was controlled by the antibody sample size μ. Decreased sample sizes resulted in more generalist antibodies, whilst increased sample sizes resulted in more specific antibodies.

Related Works from the Authors

Forrest, S. & A. Perelson (1992), "Computation and the Immune System", *SIGBIO Newsletter, Association for Computing Machinery*, **12**(2), pp. 52-57.

Forrest, S. & A. Perelson (1990), "Genetic Algorithms and the Immune System", *Proc. of the Parallel Problem Solving from Nature*, G. Goos & J. Hartmanis (eds.), Springer-Verlag, pp. 320-325.

Mori *et al.* (1993) proposed an immune algorithm that attempted to model mathematically immune diversity, network theory and clonal selection, as a multimodal function optimization problem. They introduced an index of diversity for an antibody population and kept the multiple solution attribute strings as memories of the system. Like Forrest's immune algorithm, Mori's algorithm has also been broadly used by other researchers in the field of AIS. The immune algorithm to be reviewed below is a more recent version of the one cited above and can be found in (Fukuda *et al.*, 1999). The metaphors extracted to propose the AIS are summarized in Table 6.7.

Assume an antibody repertoire composed of a set of N molecules in an L-dimensional shape-space (Ab$_i \in S^L$, $i = 1,...,N$) in which individual molecules are represented by attribute strings defined over a finite alphabet of length k. The authors proposed the function $H_j(N)$ as a measure of the informative entropy of locus j in the antibody repertoire

$$H_j(N) = -\sum_{i=1}^{k} p_{i,j} \log p_{i,j}, \tag{6.9}$$

where $p_{i,j}$ is the probability that locus j is allele i. The mean of the informative entropy among all the antibodies in the repertoire is then given by

$$H(N) = \frac{1}{L}\sum_{j=1}^{L} H_j(N), \tag{6.10}$$

Table 6.7.   Immune metaphors proposed by Fukuda *et al.* (1999).

Immune System	AIS
Antigen	Problem to be solved
Antibodies	Solution vectors
Recognition of antigen	Identification of the optimization problem
Production of antibodies from memory cells	Recalling past successful solutions
Calculation of affinity	Search for optimal solutions
Lymphocyte proliferation	Reproduction of antibodies with high antigenic affinity
Lymphocyte differentiation	Maintenance of good solutions (memory antibodies)
Lymphocyte suppression	Elimination of surplus candidate solutions
Diversity introduction	Use of genetic variation operators from a GA to create new antibodies

The proposed immune algorithm is implemented as follows:

1. Identify the optimization problem (function to be optimized);
2. Generate random candidate solutions (antibodies);
3. Calculate the affinity $ay_{v,w}$ between two antibodies v and w according to

$$ay_{v,w} = \frac{1}{1 + H(2)}, \tag{6.11}$$

where $H(2)$ evaluates the diversity between two antibodies according to Equation (6.10) for $N = 2$. This mutual recognition scheme simulates the immune network.

4. Calculate the affinity ax_v between an antibody v and an antigen according to Equation (6.12).

$$ax_v = opt_v, \tag{6.12}$$

where opt_v corresponds to the evaluated (decoded) value of the function being optimized (it corresponds to the affinity between an antigen and the antibody v).

5. Determine the concentration (number) c_v of each antibody in the repertoire

$$c_v = \frac{1}{N} \sum_{w=1}^{N} ac_{v,w},$$

$$ac_{v,w} = \begin{cases} 1 & ay_{v,w} \geq \delta_1 \\ 0 & \text{otherwise} \end{cases} \tag{6.13}$$

where δ_1 is a pre-specified threshold and $ay_{v,w}$ is the affinity between antibodies v and w given by Equation (6.11). If c_v is greater than a given threshold δ, then this antibody is suppressed (eliminated) from the repertoire; else, it becomes a memory antibody. The goal of this step is to eliminate surplus solution candidates.

6. Calculate the expected value e_v of the proliferation of the antibody according to Equation (6.14). This equation regulates the concentration and variety of the

antibodies. Antibodies presenting high affinities with an antigen (ax_i) are selected to proliferate, while antibodies with high concentrations (c_v) are suppressed.

$$e_v = \frac{ax_v \prod_{j=1}^{N} (1 - as_{v,j})}{c_v \sum_{i=1}^{N} ax_i},$$

$$as_{v,j} = \begin{cases} ay_{v,j} & ay_{v,j} \geq \delta_2 \\ 0 & \text{otherwise} \end{cases}$$

(6.14)

7. To allow for a response to unknown antigens (introduce diversity), generate new antibodies by using genetic variation operators, such as crossover and mutation, and replace the antibodies eliminated in the previous steps by the new antibodies.

The authors argued that the main characteristics of their method were the diversity among the candidate solutions and an efficient parallel search. The block diagram for this algorithm is summarized in Figure 6.19.

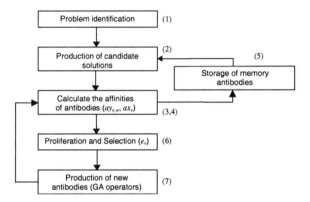

Figure 6.19. Flow chart of the immune algorithm proposed by Fukuda *et al.* (1999).

Related Works from the Authors

Mori, M., Tsukiyama, M. & Fukuda, T. (1996), "Multi-Optimization by Immune Algorithm with Diversity and Learning", *Proc. of the 2nd Int. Conf. on Multi Agent Systems, Workshop Notes on Immunity-Based Systems*, pp. 118-123.

Mori, M., Tsukiyama, M. & Fukuda, T. (1993), "Immune Algorithm with Searching Diversity and Its Application to Resource Allocation Problem", *Trans. IEE Japan*, **113**-**C**(10), pp. 872-878.

AIS and Genetic Programming

Nikolaev *et al.* (1999) proposed a hybrid of an immune network approach to Genetic Programming (GP). In this immune GP version (iGP), the search was controlled by a dynamic fitness function based on an analogy with a continuous immune network model. The approach was that of reinforcement learning where the programs evolved are reinforced with a rewarding signal when they are run and the output satisfies a given criterion. The fitness function consisted of two dynamic models that exerted influence on each other: 1) a model for propagating programs that recognized more important examples, and 2) a model for changing the importance of examples in relation to the number of programs that recognize it. The mapping proposed between the genetic programming and the immune system is presented in Table 6.8.

The authors applied their method to a machine learning task and a time series prediction problem. The machine learning problem considered was one of finding a function f from a given set of examples $\{(x_1,y_1),..., (x_M,y_M)\}$, and the time series prediction was regarded as the inductive problem of identifying regularities among a given series of points: $...,x(t), x(t+1),...$ sampled at discrete time intervals. The performance of the proposed algorithm was compared with a traditional GP system that uses trees as representation models. The only difference between the two methods is that the iGP uses a dynamic fitness measure inspired by a continuous immune network model. The results presented demonstrated that the immune version attained fitter programs maintaining higher population diversity on the machine learning and time series prediction problems tested.

Table 6.8.   Analogy between the immune system and genetic programming.

Immune System	Genetic Programming
Antigen	Example
Antigen concentration	Importance of an example
Lymphocyte clone	Program
Concentration of a clone	Fitness of the program
Interaction between two antigens	Complementarity in the recognition potential of two programs
Clonal selection process	Fitness proportional selection

Constrained Genetic Search via an AIS

In a constrained genetic search optimization, the population of individuals should not only exhibit fitness from the standpoint of the objective function value, but must also be feasible, i.e., satisfy some constraints. Thus, the evolution towards the optimum may be regarded as co-adapting the population of individuals to two distinct criteria. Traditional methods to handle constraints usually add a penalty term, which accounts for constraint violation, in the objective function to be optimized. Hajela and Yoo (1999) proposed an immune network model to handle design constraints in evolutionary algorithms.

The authors employed a binary Hamming shape-space to model the components of their hybrid AIS. Unfeasible designs were likened to the repertoire of antibodies that have to be evolved toward the feasible designs, which were likened to antigens. The evolutionary process co-adapts the unfeasible designs (antibodies) to the structure of the feasible designs (antigens), thus resulting in a process that reduces constraint violations. An interesting aspect of their simulation is that the evolutionary algorithm used, in particular a GA, relies on a unconstrained scalar function to define fitness. The objective function to be optimized is used to define the fitness of the individuals of the GA population. In their algorithm, an initial population of designs is generated at random and evaluated to compute its objective function value and a cumulative measure of constraint violation. Feasible and unfeasible designs are separated, and a fraction of the feasible designs is selected and denoted as the antigen population. Using these antigens and the unfeasible designs as an initial population of antibodies, antigens and antibodies are matched against each other in order to evolve a set of antibodies corresponding to constrained designs. Figure 6.20 summarizes the process of handling constraints in a GA using ideas from immune networks.

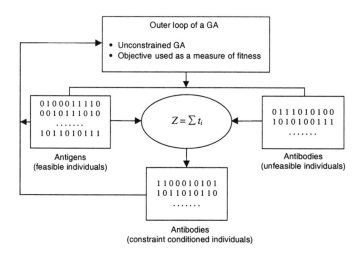

Figure 6.20.   Procedure for constraint handling using an immune system simulation (reproduced with permission from [Hajela & Yoo, 1999]. © *McGraw-Hill, 1999*).

Related Works from the Authors

Yoo, J. & Hajela, P. **(1999)**, "Enhanced GA Based Search through Immune Network Modeling", *Proc. of 3rd World Congress on Structural and Multidisciplinary Optimization* (CD-ROM).

Yoo, J. & Hajela, P. **(1999)**, "Immune Network Simulations in Multicriterion

Design", *Structural Optimization*, **18**, 2/3, pp. 85-94, 1999.

Yoo, J. & Hajela, P. **(1999)**, "Multicriterion Design of Fuzzy Structural Systems Using Immune Network Modeling", *Proc. of the AIAA/ASME/ASCE/AHS SDM Meeting*, AIAA 99-1425, pp. 1880- 1890.

Hajela, P., Yoo, J. & Lee, J. (1997), "GA Based Simulation of Immune Networks - Applications in Structural Optimization", *Engineering Optimization*, **29**, pp. 131-149.

Hajela, P., & Lee, J. (1996), "Constrained Genetic Search via Schema Adaptation: An Immune Network Solution", *Structural Optimization*, **12**(1), pp. 11-15.

6.5.3. A Summary of the Integrative Benefits

As could be observed in this section, the integration of various aspects of artificial immune systems, such as immune network models, clonal selection models, etc., with neural networks and evolutionary algorithms, can allow for the improvement of the individual paradigms and can broaden their applicability. Table 6.9 summarizes the main outcomes of integrating AIS with ANNs and AIS with EAs, as reviewed from the literature. It was also observed that AIS have been used to tackle the practical aspects of ANNs and EAs. For example, new learning algorithms for ANNs including constructive and pruning algorithms were proposed for feedforward and RBF neural networks based on AIS. The problem of ANN initialization has also been studied using AIS. In the case of EAs, AIS have been broadly used to generate and maintain subpopulations of individuals capable of finding a large number of optima solutions.

Table 6.9. Outcomes of integrating AIS, ANN and EA.

Hybrid	Outcome
AIS + ANN	• AIS have suggested new ANN models, architectures, and learning algorithms; • AIS provided increased memory capacities for ANN; • AIS were used to develop new initialization techniques for ANN.
AIS + EA	• AIS have been used to promote and maintain niches, species, and diversity in evolutionary algorithms; • An immune version of genetic programming was proposed; and • AIS have been used to handle constraints in GAs.

6.6 AIS in Context with Other Approaches

In the discussions so far, investigations into the similarities, differences and integrative benefits of the currently most influential biologically motivated computing paradigms, ANN and EA, have been undertaken placing them in context with AIS. However, artificial immune systems have also been widely used in conjunction and/or compared with other computational intelligence paradigms, such as Case-Based Reasoning (CBR), Classifier Systems (CS), and Fuzzy Systems (FS). A novel computing paradigm, for instance DNA Computing, has also been used to implement immune algorithms.

With the exception of the fuzzy systems, these approaches are basically compared with AIS instead of hybridized with them. It is appropriate that a review of these works is made to allow the reader to appreciate where AIS fits in comparision to these other paradigms. A brief introduction to all the strategies outlining their main components and basic operations will be presented. Then, a review of literature with works that relate these computational intelligence paradigms will be given. In the particular case of DNA computing, the only work known from the literature proposing a DNA implementation of the negative selection algorithm will be reviewed. Additionally, a tentative comparison between DNA computing and AIS will be presented, bearing in mind they constitute distinct paradigms.

6.6.1. AIS and Case-Based Reasoning

Problem solving in *case-based reasoning* (CBR) uses knowledge from previously experienced problem situations, named *cases*. A new problem (case) can be solved by finding a similar past case within a *case-base*. This can then be used for suggesting a solution to the current problem or evaluating the proposed solution. The case-base can then be updated from this experience (new case). CBR, therefore, allows the retention (storage) of new experiences each time a problem has been solved. Thus, it presents an incremental, sustained learning strategy.

Aamodt and Plaza (1994) described a general cycle for a CBR system as depicted in Figure 6.21. A new problem (case) is used to *retrieve* a case from the case-base by performing a match against the cases in the case-base. The retrieved case is combined with the new case through *reuse* and presented as a solved case, which constitutes a candidate solution to the initial problem. Then, a *revision* process tests the proposed solution for success (e.g., by applying it to evaluate cases, or by evaluating a given performance measure) and repairs if it failed. During *retain*, useful experience(s) is (are) retained for future reuse, and the new case-base is updated by a new learned case or by modifying an existing case.

Work in (Hunt *et al.*, 1995) presented a novel approach to case-base organization and case retrieval inspired by an immune network model. The authors illustrated how the immune system is inherently case-based, and how it relies on a content-addressable memory, together with an affinity measure, to help to identify new antigens (cases) that are similar to antibodies (past cases). They constructed a case memory based on the immune network model proposed by Farmer *et al.* (1986) and described how some operations of this immune network model, such as pattern recognition, learning, and memory, could support a CBR system.

An antigen corresponded to a new case, or problem to be solved, while an antibody was each past case from the case-base. The "immune-based case memory" was responsible for maintaining a set of cases and links among cases. The antigens and antibodies (cases) composing their AIS were represented using a Symbolic shape-space, and the degree of matching between two cases (antigen-antibody) was evaluated using the multiple-contiguous bit rule. An illustrative Symbolic shape-space representation for the immune version of CBR, and how the affinity was evaluated, is presented in Figure 6.22.

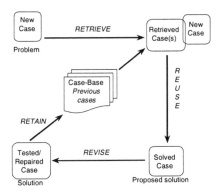

Figure 6.21. Case-Based Reasoning (CBR) cycle.

In a highly simplified form, the immune version of case-based reasoning works as follows. Given a case base (immune network) and a new case (antigen), *retrieve* the best matching case (antibody) according to the multiple-contiguous bit rule (Figure 6.22). If the affinity of the antibody with the antigen is above a certain threshold, the antigen may be able to bind to the current antibody, and its stimulation level is determined. This new case is *retained* in the case-base (added to the immune network) in a region of the network close to those cases with which it has a high affinity.

The stimulation level of a case (antibody) is determined by an equation similar to Equation 3.15 and is proportional to how well this case matches the new situation and its affinity to its neighbor antibody in the network. This mechanism is important to control the dimension of the network, once low stimulated antibodies (cases) are purged from the network. Table 6.10 summarizes how the authors proposed to alleviate the CBR problems of case memory organization and case retrieval by taking inspiration from the immune system.

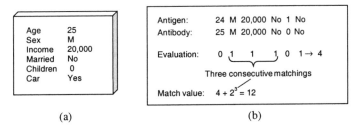

(a)   (b)

Figure 6.22. An example of a hybrid encoding for the artificial immune system applied in conjunction to case-based reasoning. (a) Structure of a case, where an antigen corresponds to the present case, and an antibody corresponds to a case in the case base. (b) Case matching through the multiple continuous bit rule.

Table 6.10.   Mapping from the immune system to case-based reasoning.

Immune System	Case-Based Reasoning
Antigen	New case (problem)
Antibodies	Past cases (problems)
Immune network that maintains a current set of antibodies and links among them	Case-base
Antibody-Antigen binding	Case matching
Secondary immune response	Case retrieval
Recruitment of novel antibodies into the network	Case insertion
Elimination of non-stimulated antibodies	Case forgetting

According to the authors, the main advantage of their method was the emergence of an immune network-like structure for the case-base without the need for a detailed domain analysis to define and maintain the memory organization (case-base). In a later work, Hunt and Fellows (1996) applied this immune version of CBR to a data mining problem.

6.6.2. AIS and Classifier Systems

Classifier systems (CS) can be defined as parallel, message-passing, rule-based systems, where all rules have the same form (Booker *et al.*, 1989). In the simplest form of a CS the messages are binary strings of length L built out of an alphabet containing the symbols $\{0,1,\#\}$ (# represents a "don't care"). The rules have the form *condition/action*, where the condition part specifies the messages that satisfy (activate) the rule and the action part specifies which message is going to be sent when the rule is satisfied. In addition, the rules might also contain a *strength*, which is an assigned number indicating its value to the system. A classifier system consists of the four basic parts illustrated in Figure 6.23:

- *Input interface*: receives information from the environment and transforms it into messages;
- *Classifiers*: rules containing information about the possible response of the system;
- *Message list*: contains all current messages generated from the inputs and the satisfied rules and provides a forum for the rules to communicate and interact with each other; and
- *Output interface*: translates some messages into effector actions.

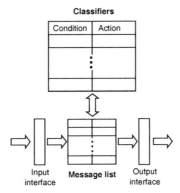

Figure 6.23.   Basic parts of a classifier system (reproduced with permission from [Booker *et al.*, 1989]. © *Elsevier Science, 1989*).

A CS operates according to the following cycle. The messages are read from the input interface and added to the message list. Then, all messages from the message list are compared to all conditions of all classifiers, and the matches (satisfied conditions) are recorded. For each set of matches satisfying the condition part of some classifier, post the message specified by its action part to a list of new messages and replace all messages from the message list by these new messages. Finally, translate these new messages on the message list to produce the output of the system.

The strength of a rule is used as a basis for competition. If a rule contributes to a useful response its strength is increased, otherwise it is decreased. At each time step, each satisfied rule makes a *bid* based on its strength, and only the highest bidding rules get their messages on the message list for the next time step. If a rule is allowed to post a message, it must *pay* the rule that supplied the message that it matched to. This procedure is called *bucket brigade* (BB) and is responsible to *assign credit* (*credit assignment stage*) to the useful rules. It is established by means of a mock economy, in which the rules *pay* each other for information.

As one last aspect, it is important to raise the question about how the classifier systems, as described here, can discover new rules by simply reading and posting messages, and altering their strengths. Indeed, these processes are not enough to cope with a dynamical environment. Unless the best rules are already contained in the system, its behavior will not be optimal. As a solution to this problem of *rule discovery*, one can employ a genetic algorithm, which will bias the accumulated experience of the system during the process of generating new candidate rules for the CS. This way, it is possible to identify three levels of activity when looking at learning and information processing in a CS. At the lowest level is the *performance system* (classifier system) responsible for the direct interaction with the environment. At the second level there is the *credit assignment* (bucket brigade) stage used to evaluate and alter the strength of the rules. Finally, there is the *rule discovery system* (genetic algorithm) in the highest level, required to maintain the diversity of the set of rules keeping track of previous relevant rules.

Although the four steps described above and the basic cycle are somewhat general for classifier systems, different approaches can be used to implement one. For example, rule discovery and credit assignment can be performed using different paradigms or variations of the suggested ones (GA and BB). The same is true concerning immune system models and artificial immune systems.

To make the analogy between a classifier system and the immune system, Farmer *et al.* (1986) represented the CS in the form of a dynamical system. This resulted in an equation of motion similar to that proposed in their immune network model discussed in Section 3.5. The authors found close analogies between the resultant two systems, as summarized in Table 6.11. Although the authors did not hybridize their immune network model with learning classifier systems, they were emphatic in suggesting that the close correspondence between these two models could account for universal approaches to the design of efficient learning systems with great potentialities for problem solving. As an example, they suggested that changing the structure of epitopes and paratopes from one-dimensional strings to two-dimensional matrices could result in a pattern recognizer with potential application to character recognition in a noisy background.

Table 6.11.   Comparison of the major components of a classifier system and a dynamic immune network model (reproduced with permission from [Farmer *et al.*, 1986]. © *Elsevier Science, 1986*).

Classifier Systems	**Immune Network Model**
Classifier	Antibody
Condition	Epitope
Action	Paratope
Strength	Concentration
Payoff	Antigen reduction
External message	Antigen
Message list	All paratopes and antigens
Economy	Concentration update rule
Performance function	Rate of antigen removal
Genetic operators to generate new rules	Genetic operators to generate new antibody types

Hofmeyr and Forrest (2000) also pointed out a set of similarities and differences between their artificial immune system for network intrusion detection described in Section 7.3, and the learning classifier systems. The reader is encouraged to refer to this section before going into the comparison between their AIS and CS. Although the authors suggested that the mapping between their AIS and classifier systems is not one to one, a tentative comparison was performed. They argued that the architecture of both systems (AIS and CS) resembles each other, and the self/nonself discrimination can be likened to a CS first classifying a message as self or nonself. In their analogy, a classifier condition corresponds to a detector, the matching between 1, 0 and # (don't care) is performed via the r-contiguous bit rule, the specificity of a rule in classifier system was likened to the specificity r of a detector (cross-reactivity threshold). The strength of a classifier corresponds to the state of a detector (immature, mature, activated or memory detector), the message list is the network traffic (data-path triples), the competition for packets is equivalent to the bidding for messages, and the message intensity is the sensitivty level. Finally, the bucket brigade algorithm was said to perform affinity maturation.

6.6.3. AIS and Fuzzy Systems

The concept of a *fuzzy set* was introduced by L. A. Zadeh in 1965. In the mid sixties, Zadeh observed that the technological resources available were not capable of automating the activities related to industrial, biological, or chemical problems involving ambiguous situations. This implied that they could not be processed through the computational logic of Boolean algebra. In order to solve these problems, Zadeh published a paper summarizing the concepts of fuzzy sets, thus promoting a revolution with the creation of *fuzzy systems* (FS). Fuzzy inference involves the capture, representation, and operation with *linguistic variables* and *fuzzy sets* (Pedrycz & Gomide, 1998). Fuzzy sets appeared as a new paradigm to represent uncertainties and have been widely used in real-world applications, mainly in conjunction with other methodologies such as artificial neural networks (e.g., Kwan & Cai, 1994; Pal *et al.*, 2000), evolutionary algorithms (e.g., Chan *et al.*, 1997; Shi *et al.*, 1999), and more recently artificial immune systems (e.g., Krishnakumar *et al.*, 1995).

Logic refers to the formal principles that sustain the rules of thinking or reasoning and mirrors the fundamentals of several science and engineering fields of research. Systems with a two-valued logic (binary logic) deal with sentences whose values are *true* or *false*. In multi-valued logic, a sentence might be *true*, *false* or can assume any *intermediate truth-value*. *Fuzzy logic* goes far beyond multi-valued logic and admits truth-values that are fuzzy sets of the unit interval. The truth-values might be seen as linguistic characterizations of numerical truth-values. Thus, fuzzy logic deals with the principles of approximate reasoning.

In Section 3.5, a binding value between two molecules proportionally to their affinity was defined. This binding value is dependent upon an activation function that can allow crisp or fuzzy values. In the immune system, antigenic recognition is approximate, i.e., an immune response can be elicited even when the binding between an antigen and an antibody is not perfect; an approximate binding may suffice. Together with cross-reactivity, these characteristics stress the presence of "fuzzy activities" within the immune systems, suggesting that fuzzy logic might be appropriate to model several aspects and mechanisms of biological immune systems. Consequently, fuzzy and artificial immune systems might provide powerful interactions, as will be demonstrated in the following examples from the literature and further discussed in the next section.

Krishnakumar *et al.* (1995) proposed what he called an immunized computational system employing immune metaphors and several computational intelligence techniques. One of their aims was to reproduce the adaptability and robustness of the immune system. The proposed hybrid system, briefly described in Section 4.8, could be composed of artificial neural networks, fuzzy systems, and evolutionary algorithms, according to the problem under study. The performance of their approach was evaluated in an autonomous aircraft control problem.

In the works of Lee *et al.* (1999) and Jun *et al.* (1999) (Section 4.7), the authors used different types of antibodies, each with a specific task. In these papers, the stimulation level of a given antibody was a function of its percentage of success in the execution of a given task, according to a function similar to the one presented in Figure 6.24. This function is typical in fuzzy systems, where the universe of discourse of a variable (in this case the percentage of success) is partitioned into several intervals, leading to an approximate representation (fuzzyfication) of the phenomenon under study.

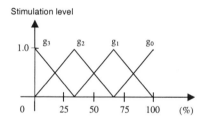

Figure 6.24.   Function that determines the stimulation level of a given antibody.

Based on the immune feedback mechanism identified by Takahashi and Yamada (1997) and briefly discussed in Section 4.8, Ding and Ren (2000) derived a universal controller structure suitable for high and low order plants. The controller includes a basic fuzzy self-tuning immune controller and an incremental block with the aim of treating the order of the plants. The performance of their approach was examined by designing a fuzzy self-tuning PID-type immune controller for the control of tissue hyperthermia. Their immune feedback law involved the interactions of B-cells, T-helper, and T-suppressor cells.

In (de Castro and Von Zuben, 2001d), the authors proposed an artificial immune network model to perform data analysis, in particular information compression and data clustering (Sections 3.5 and 4.2). In that paper, the representation of clusters by their centroids allowed the specification of membership levels to each immune network cell in relation to the determined clusters, yielding a fuzzy clustering scheme. Their fuzzy clustering network extended the notion that each network cell belonged to a single cluster and associated each cell with every network cluster using a fuzzy membership function.

In the neural network context, de Castro and Von Zuben (2001c) used their artificial immune network model to define the number and positions of a set of basis functions for radial basis function neural networks. The authors concluded their work suggesting that the way their algorithm defines the parameters for the radial basis functions would also be appropriate to automatically define parameters for fuzzy systems, like number and position of membership functions in fuzzy rules. The authors used as arguments similar approaches from the literature that employ different paradigms such as competitive learning (Caminhas *et al.*, 1995).

Related Works from the Authors

Nagano, S., Iwasaki, Y. & Yonezawa, Y. (1996), "Immuno Fluctuate Model as Defense System Included Complexity Process", *Proc. of the 7ᵗʰ International Symposium on Micro Machine and Human Science*, pp. 257-263.

Nagano, S. & Yonezawa, Y. (1999), "DNA Evolutionary Process Simulated with Self-Nonself Recognition Based on Immuno-Function Mechanism", *Proc. of the 3ʳᵈ Workshop on Orders and Structures in Complex Systems*, pp. 117-130.

6.6.4. AIS and DNA Computing

The basic idea underlying *DNA Computing*, also termed *(bio)molecular computing*, is the use of the information processing capabilities of organic DNA molecules in computers to replace, or at least supplement, the current digital primitives. The two fundamental features of DNA computing are: 1) the massive parallelism of DNA strands, and 2) the Watson-Crick complementarity.

A molecule of DNA (*DeoxyriboNucleic Acid*) consists of *polymer chains*, usually referred to as *DNA strands*. A chain is composed of nucleotides that may differ only by their *bases*. There are four bases: A (adenine), C (cytosine), G (guanine), and T (thymine). A *double helix of DNA* is a result of the bonding of two separate strands as illustrated in Figure 6.25.

The Watson-Crick complementarity plays an important role in the formation of the double strands of DNA. A binding between two bases only occurs according to the following pair wise attraction: A with T, and C with G. DNA computing involves not only new data structures (DNA molecules), but also operations used by nature to manipulate the strands, such as cut and paste, adjoining, and deletion. The use of these operations, together with DNA molecules as alternative data structures, result in DNA computing as a new computing paradigm rather different from the classical Turing machines. There are several basic operations found in DNA (Păun *et al.*, 1998):

- *Melting (denaturation)*: separation of a double stranded DNA into two single strands;

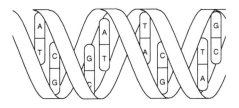

Figure 6.25.   The double helix of DNA.

- *Annealing (hybridization)*: fusion of two single stranded molecules by Watson-Crick complementary base pairings. This operation is the reverse of denaturation and, thus, is sometimes referred to as renaturation;
- *Splice*: to cut two strings at points specified by given substrings and to concatenate the obtained fragments crosswise;
- *Amplify*: application of a technique called *Polymerase Chain Reaction* (PCR) that doubles the number of strands at each iteration, resulting in an exponential growth of the number of strands;
- *Merge*: the union of different sets of DNA strands;
- *Separate*: given a set of strands and a specific referential strand s_1, this operation identifies and separates all strands from the set that contains s_1 as a substrand;
- *Detect and Length-separate*: detect the presence of DNA strands and separate all strands with length less than or equal to a given length. Both processes are performed using a technique called *gel electrophoresis*.

As discussed, there is a fundamental philosophical difference between DNA computing and the biologically motivated paradigms reviewed so far (AIS, ANN, and EA). While DNA computing proposes the actual use of DNA computations (operations, as described above) as a novel computing paradigm, the other approaches extract ideas or metaphors from the biological systems to develop computational algorithms for problem solving. However, the data structures employed in DNA computing (DNA strands) can be seen as a special case of a Symbolic shape-space represented by the quaternary alphabet {A,C,G,T}. This particular shape-space could be named *DNA shape-space*. If we make an analysis of the operations involved in DNA computing, we can identify similar operations in the immune system at the cellular level, such as the amplification via PCR might be regarded as a "DNA cloning". In Table 6.12 we propose a high-level abstraction from the DNA computing data representation and operations into the domain of artificial immune systems.

Table 6.12.   Mapping AIS into DNA computing.

	AIS	**DNA computing**
Encoding	Attribute strings in S that represent immune cells and molecules	DNA strands composed of the nucleotides {A,C,G,T}
Processing	Immune algorithms or processes	DNA computing operations
Recombination	Mutation and gene rearrangement	Annealing
Binding	Shape complementarity in S	Watson-Crick complementarity
Reproduction	Clonal expansion	Amplification via PCR
Antigen processing and presentation	Antigen fragmentation and presentation via APC	Operations: melting, separate, detect and length-separate

Although DNA computing might be seen basically as a novel computing paradigm, we decided to include it in this section about computational intelligence approaches for two reasons. First, it can be used to solve complex problems such as in the pioneer work presented by Adleman (1994), where he applied DNA computing to solve the Hamiltonian path problem. This problem belongs to the NP-hard category, is of combinatorial nature, and resembles the travelling salesman problem. Second, there is one paper in the literature that proposes a DNA implementation of the negative selection algorithm, and there are some AIS in the literature that use a DNA shape-space to manipulate DNA sequences, as will be reviewed now.

A *promoter* is a region of the DNA to which RNA (*RiboNuleic Acid*) polymerase binds before initiating the transcription of DNA into RNA. The RNA structure and base sequence are determinants for protein synthesis and for the transmission of genetic information. Cooke and Hunt (1995) used an artificial immune network model to recognize promoters in DNA sequences. Like in DNA computing, their encoding scheme (antigens and antibodies) was created by copying the mRNA following the Watson-Crick complementarity: T→A, A→T, C→G and G→C, which corresponds to the complementary binding of these bases in DNA. Note that this representation is equivalent to the quaternary DNA shape-space discussed above. Although the authors employed this DNA-based encoding scheme, their approach consisted of using an AIS to solve a real-world problem and is not necessarily a hybrid of an AIS with a DNA computing strategy.

In the paper presented by Nagano and Yonezawa (1999) (Section 4.7), DNA sequences were used to represent the self and nonself elements of a self-recognition system. The dynamics of the system was controlled by an evolutionary algorithm, more specifically a genetic algorithm, instead of DNA computing operations.

Deaton *et al.* (1997) proposed to implement the negative selection algorithm, described in Section 3.5, in a DNA-based computer. The fusion of two single stranded molecules by Watson-Crick complementarity was viewed as a string matching reaction similar to that performed in AIS. The idea was to implement the censoring and monitoring parts of the negative selection algorithm in DNA computers using techniques from molecular biology. The DNA negative selection algorithm is illustrated in Figure 6.26, and works as follows:

- *Censoring*: generate a random set of single stranded DNA molecules of length L. The self strings are encoded into DNA strands, and a self set is constructed from the Watson-Crick complements of the encoded strands. From many copies of the random and self sets, *melting* and *annealing* operations are used so that the strands in the random set hybridize with their Watson-Crick complements in the self set. Since the self set was composed of the Watson-Crick complements of the self strands, the random strands that have hybridized correspond to the self strands. Finally, the *splice* operation is used to effectively remove the self strands from the whole mix. This process is repeated until all self strands have been removed, and the remaining strands represent the set of detector strands;
- *Monitoring*: given a set of protected strands (labeled with fluorescent markers), try to hybridize them with the detector strands, and in case the strands fuse (hybridize), a nonself strand is detected.

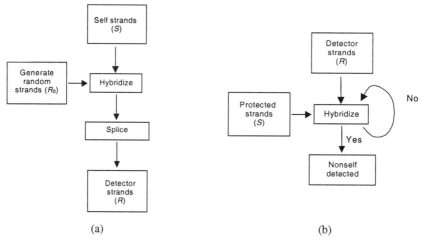

(a)   (b)

Figure 6.26. DNA implementation of the negative selection algorithm. (a) *Censoring*: the operations hybridize and splicegenerate the set of detector strands. (b) *Monitoring*: if a protected strand hybridizes with a detector strand, then nonself is detected (reproduced with permission from [Deaton *et al.*, 1997]. © *IEEE, 1997*).

6.6.5. Summary

This section has attempted to highlight the use and/or similarities between AIS and other computational paradigms, in particular case-based reasoning, classifier systems, fuzzy systems, and DNA computing. As has been discussed, there are several similarities between AIS, CBR, and CS, which may help the reader understand where AIS fits in the wider picture of computational intelligence. Work has also shown that DNA computing can be used as an alternative to implement AIS, and fuzzy systems can be used as an approach to manipulate uncertainties in AIS. Table 6.13 provides a summary of AIS in context with CBR and CS, and Table 6.14 presents a summary of AIS in context with DNA Computing and FS.

Table 6.13.   AIS in context with CBR and CS.

Paradigm	Outcome
AIS + CBR	• Immune networks as a novel approach to case organization and retrieval • The immune system is inherently case-based
AIS + CS	• Continuous immune network models are similar to CS represented in the form of dynamical systems • An AIS for distributed computer network intrusion detection has similarities with CS

Table 6.14.   AIS in context with fuzzy systems (FS), and DNA Computing.

AIS + FS	• Use of fuzzy logic as a means to provide approximate representations for the components of an AIS • Fuzzy clustering of the components of an artificial immune network model • Use of immune networks to automatically define parameters for fuzzy systems
AIS + DNA Computing	• Immune networks used to recognize patterns in DNA sequences • DNA sequences used to represent self and nonself components of an AIS • DNA computing implementation of AIS algorithms and processes

6.7   Future Trends: Hints and Speculations

By placing artificial immune systems in context with ANNs and EAs, it can be seen that most of the hybrids were aimed at creating systems with improved practical applications. In addition, it was observed that AIS are naturally suitable to create and maintain stable subpopulations of individuals; a property interesting for applications such as multimodal search, and that provides some indication that our argument of Section 5.5 that the immune system maintains niches of antibodies is reasonable.

To provide the reader with some insights into new ways of hybridizing AIS with ANNs and EAs, and the benefits of this integration, their practical aspects and how each of these paradigms has been hybridized with each other will be discussed. Additionally, fuzzy systems will be added to the list of approaches, as it is one of the three most used computational intelligence paradigms to date. The discussion to be presented here is based on the proposal by (de Castro & Timmis, 2002), and a set of references will be provided as a guide to the reader.

As evolutionary algorithms constitute very good search strategies, they have been widely used to model selection and parameter setting for other approaches. For example, they have been used to evolve artificial neural network architectures (Harrald & Kamstra, 1997; Maniezzo, 1994; Friedrich & Moraga, 1996; Opitz & Shavlik, 1997) or to design fuzzy systems (Chan *et al.*, 1997; Shi *et al.*, 1999; Belarbi & Titel, 2000). Neurofuzzy systems, i.e., the combination of ANN with fuzzy systems, usually have the advantage of allowing an easy translation of the final system into a set of if-then rules, and the fuzzy system can be viewed as a neural network structure with knowledge distributed throughout connection strengths (Kosko, 1992). Several examples of neurofuzzy systems can be found in the literature (e.g., Kuo *et al.*, 1993; Kwan & Cai, 1994; Chiang & Gader, 1997; Juang, 2000; Pal *et al.*, 2000). More complex hybrids, combining fuzzy, neural, and evolutionary algorithms are also available in the literature (e.g., Krishnakumar *et al.*, 1995; Iyoda *et al.*, 1999).

All these works suggest that evolutionary algorithms can also be used to search for an adequate model selection and automatic parameter definition for artificial immune systems. Also, the integration of fuzzy logic with AIS may lead to hybrid systems that are more biologically plausible, that can be expressed in the form of a set of if-then rules, and that can compute with fuzzy or incomplete information. Neural networks can provide alternative learning algorithms, network architectures, types of cells, and non-linearities for immune networks, and vice-versa.

The problem of model selection in ANN can be dealt with through several approaches, among which constructive (Kwok & Yeung, 1997; Fritzke, 1994) and pruning strategies (Reed, 1993; de Castro & Von Zuben, 1999) are the most common. Evolutionary algorithms with adaptive population sizes can also be found in the literature (e.g., Arabas *et al.*, 1994; Krink *et al.*, 1999). Automatic methods to define the number of partitions and their respective positions for linguistic variables in fuzzy systems can be found in (Caminhas *et al.*, 1995). Strategies to automatically determine user-defined parameters have also been implemented in all strategies (e.g., Yu & Chen, 1997; Lobo, 2000; Angeline, 1995). It is possible that all these techniques applied to other approaches may shed some light into the solution of the respective problems in AIS: model selection and parameter setting. Although we did not discuss much about parameter setting in AIS, it is clear from Section 3.5 that most algorithms require a number of its features to be defined a priori, such as affinity thresholds, selection mechanisms, and so on.

Another question to be raised is "How equivalent are AIS with other computational intelligence and search methods?" This is an interesting and intriguing matter that requires exploration not yet undertaken. Works can be found in the literature drawing parallels between evolutionary and gradient-based search strategies (e.g., Salomon, 1998) and fuzzy systems with specific neural network architectures and other systems (e.g., Jang & Sun, 1993; Hunt *et al*, 1995; Hunt & Cooke, 1996; Li & Chen, 2000) suggesting that similar equivalencies could be made between AIS and these paradigms. This is still an open question even for the more established fields of research.

Finally, inspired by the DNA computing implementation of the negative selection algorithm, it is possible to suggest a DNA implementation of all the other algorithms and processes of the framework to design AIS. This would lead to a new computational paradigm merging potentialities of DNA computing with AIS.

6.8   Chapter Summary

This chapter has covered a vast amount of material, ranging from artificial neural networks to evolutionary algorithms to the combination of these techniques with AIS. The whole purpose of this chapter was to show the reader the context of computational intelligence in which AIS should be placed. The chapter began by reviewing different computational intelligence paradigms such as artificial neural networks and evolutionary algorithms. It is always important to remember that AIS is another paradigm and is not going to be suitable for all problems. Therefore, through an understanding of other computational intelligence approaches, the reader should be able to judge the validity of the AIS approach, identify strengths and weakness within it, and see how these may be used or overcome through the combination of the many paradigms.

A pressing question when comparing AIS with other approaches, is 'Where are AIS better than other approaches?' Basically, are there certain types of problems that AIS are more suited to than others? Again, it is the authors' opinion that this question is of paramount importance to be raised for researchers in AIS and has yet to be addressed in any meaningful way. It implies that researchers need to investigate what is it that makes the immune system different from other biological systems and how is it possible to exploit that for computation. This is a challenge for AIS, but a necessary step of the field in the direction of its maturion. By contrasting AIS with ANNs and EAs, we believe we have taken the first steps in this direction.

References

Aamodt, A. & Plaza, E. (1994), "Case-Based Reasoning: Foundational Issues, Methodological Variations, and System Approaches", *AI Communications*, 7(i), pp. 39-59.

Adleman, L. M. (1994), "Molecular Computation of Solutions to Combinatorial Problems", *Science*, 266, pp. 1021-1024.

Angeline, P. J. (1995), "Adaptive and Self-Adaptive Evolutionary Computations", In *Computational Intelligence: A Dynamic Systems Perspective*, M. Palaniswami, Y. Attikiouzel, R. Marks, D. Fogel & T. Fukuda (eds.), Piscataway, NJ:IEEE Press, pp. 152-163.

Arabas, J., Michalewicz, Z. & Mulawka, J. (1994), "GAVaPS – A Genetic Algorithm with Varying Population Size", *Proc. of the Conference on Evolutionary Computation*, pp. 73-78.

Beasley, D., Bull, D. R. & Martin, R. R. (1993), "A Sequential Niche Technique for Multimodal Function Optimization", *Evolutionary Computation*, 1(2), pp. 101-125.

Belarbi, K. & Titel, F. (2000), "Genetic Algorithm for the Design of a Class of Fuzzy Controllers: An Alternative Approach", *IEEE Trans. on Fuzzy Systems*, 8(4), pp. 398-405.

Booker, L. B., Goldberg, D. E. & Holland, J. H. (1989), "Classifier Systems and Genetic Algorithms", *Artificial Intelligence*, 40, pp. 235-282.

Caminhas, W. M., Tavares, H. M. F. & Gomide, F. (1995), "Competitive Learning of Fuzzy, Logical Neural Networks", *Proc. of the 5th Int. Fuzzy Systems Association World Congress*, 2, pp. 639-642.

Chan, K. C. C., Lee, V. & Leung, H. (1997), "Generating Fuzzy Rules for Target Tracking Using a Steady-State Genetic Algorithm", *IEEE Trans. on Evolutionary Computation*, 1(3), pp. 165-178.

Chen, S., Cowan, C. F. N. & Grant, P. M. (1991), "Orthogonal Least Squares Algorithm for Radial Basis Function Networks", *IEEE Trans. on Neural Networks*, 2(2), pp. 302-309.

Chiang, J. –H. & Gader, P. D. (1997), "Hybrid Fuzzy-Neural System in Handwritten Word Recognition", *IEEE Trans. on Fuzzy Systems*, 5(4), pp. 497-510.

Cooke, D. E. & Hunt, J. E. (1995), "Recognising Promoter Sequences Using an Artificial Immune System", *Proc. of Intelligence Systems in Molecular Biology*, pp. 89-97.

Cybenko, G. (1989), "Approximation by Superpositions of a Sigmoidal Function", *Mathematics of Control Signals and Systems*, 2, pp. 303-314.

Dasgupta, D. (ed.) (1999), *Artificial Immune Systems and Their Applications*, Springer-Verlag.

Dasgupta, D., (1997), "Artificial Neural Networks and Artificial Immune Systems:

Similarities and Differences", *Proc. of the IEEE System, Man, and Cybernetics Conference*, **1**, pp. 873-878.

Deaton, R, Garzon, M, Rose, J. A., Murphy, R. C., Stevens Jr., S. E. & Franceschetti, D. R. (1997), "A DNA Based Artificial Immune System for Self-Nonself Discrimination", *Proc. of the IEEE System, Man, and Cybernetics*, pp. 862-866.

Deb, K. (1989), *Genetic Algorithms in Multimodal Function Optimization*, Masters Dissertation, University of Alabama, TCGA Report 89002.

de Castro, L. N. & Von Zuben, F. J. (1999b), "An Improving Pruning Technique with Restart for the Kohonen Self-Organizing Feature Map", *Proc. of the Int. Joint Conf. on Neural Networks*, **3**, pp. 1916-1919.

de Castro, L. N. & Von Zuben, F. J. (2001a), "Immune and Neural Network Models: Theoretical and Empirical Comparisons", *International Journal of Computational Intelligence and Applications (IJCIA)*, **1**(3), pp. 239-259.

de Castro, L. N. & Von Zuben, F. J. (2001b), "An Immunological Approach to Initialize Feedforward Neural Network Weights", *Proc. of the Int. Conf. on Artificial Neural Networks and Genetic Algorithms*, pp. 126-129.

de Castro, L. N., & Von Zuben, F. J., (2001c), "Automatic Determination of Radial Basis Function: An Immunity-Based Approach", *International Journal of Neural Systems*, Special Issue on Non-Gradient Learning Techniques, **11**(6), pp. 523-535.

de Castro, L. N. & Von Zuben, F. J. (2001d), "aiNet: An Artificial Immune Network for Data Analysis", In *Data Mining: A Heuristic Approach*, H. A. Abbass, R. A. Sarker, and C. S. Newton (eds.), Idea Group Publishing, USA, Chapter XII, pp. 231-259.

de Castro, L. N., Von Zuben, F. J. & de Deus Jr., G. A. (2002), "The Construction of a Boolean Competitive Neural Network Using Ideas From Immunology", *International Journal of Neurocomputing* (in print).

de Castro, L. N. & Timmis, J. I. (2002), "Artificial Immune Systems as a Novel Soft Computing Paradigms", *Soft Computing Journal* (in print).

de Jong, K. A. (1994), "Genetic Algorithms: A 25 Year Perspective", *Computational Intelligence: Imitating Life*, IEEE Press, pp. 125-134.

de Jong, K. A. (1975), *An Analysis of the Behavior of a Class of Genetic Adaptive Systems*, Ph.D. Thesis, University of Michigan, Michigan/U.S.A.

Ding, Y. & Ren, L. (2000), "Fuzzy Self-Tuning Immune Feedback Controller for Tissue Hyperthermia", *Proc. of the 9th IEEE Int. Conf. on Fuzzy Systems*, **1**, pp. 534-538.

Eiben, Á. E., Hinterding, R. & Michalewicz, Z. (1999), "Parameter Control in Evolutionary Algorithms", *IEEE Trans. on Evol. Comp.*, **3**(2), pp. 124-141.

Farmer, J. D., Packard, N. H. & Perelson, A. S. (1986), "The Immune System, Adaptation, and Machine Learning", *Physica 22D*, pp. 187-204.

Fogel, L. J., Owens, A. J. & Walsh, M. J. (1966), *Artificial Intelligence Through Simulated Evolution*, Wiley, New York.

Fogel, D. B. (1994), "An Introduction to Simulated Evolutionary Optimization", *IEEE Trans. on Neural Networks*, **5**(1), pp. 3-14.

Fogel, D. B. (1991), *System Identification through Simulated Evolution: A Machine Learning Approach to Modeling*, Ginn Press, Needham Heights.

Forrest, S., Javornik, B., Smith, R. E. & Perelson, A. S. (1993), "Using Genetic Algorithms to Explore Pattern Recognition in the Immune System", *Evolutionary Computation*, **1**(3), pp. 191-211.

Freeman, J. A. S. & Saad, D. (1995), "Learning and Generalization in Radial Basis Function Networks", *Neural Computation*, **7**, pp. 1000-1020.

Friedrich, C. M. & Moraga, C. (1996), "An Evolutionary Method to Find Good

Building-Blocks for Architectures of Artificial Neural Networks", *Proc. of the IPMU'96*, pp. 951-956.

Fritzke B. (1994), "Growing Cell Structures – A Self-Organizing Network for Unsupervised and Supervised Learning", *Neural Networks*, 7(9), pp. 1441-1460.

Fukuda, T., Mori, K. & Tsukiama, M. (1999), "Parallel Search for Multi-Modal Function Optimization with Diversity and Learning of Immune Algorithm", In D. Dasgupta (ed.), *Artificial Immune Systems and Their Applications*, Springer-Verlag, pp. 210-220.

Fujita, H. & Aihara, K. (1989), "Application of the PDP Model with a Logistic Activation Function to Immune Networks", *Trans. of IEICE*, E 72(4), pp. 416-421.

Goldberg, D. E. & Richardson, J. (1987), "Genetic Algorithms With Sharing for Multimodal Function Optimization", *Genetic Algorithms and Their Applications: Proc. of the II ICGA*, pp. 41-49.

Hajela, P., & Yoo, J. S. (1999), "Immune Network Modeling in Design Optimization", In *New Ideas in Optimization*, D. Corne, M. Dorigo & F. Glover (eds.), McGraw Hill, London, pp. 203-215.

Harrald, P. G. & Kamstra, M. (1997), "Evolving Artificial Neural Networks to Combine Financial Forecasts", *IEEE Trans. on Evolutionary Computation*, 1(1) pp. 40-52.

Hart, E. & Ross, P. (1999), "An Immune System Approach to Scheduling in Changing Environments", *Proc. of the Genetic and Evolutionary Computation Conference*, pp. 1559-1566

Haykin S. (1999), *Neural Networks – A Comprehensive Foundation*, Prentice Hall, 2nd Ed.

Hoffmann, G. W. (1986), "A Neural Network Model Based on the Analogy with the Immune System", *J. theor. Biol.*, 122, pp. 33-67.

Hoffmann, G. W., Benson, M. W., Bree, G. M. & Kinahan, P. E. (1986), "A Teachable Neural Network Based on an Unorthodox Neuron", *Physica 22D*, pp. 233-246.

Hofmeyr S. A. & Forrest, S. (2000), "Architecture for an Artificial Immune System", *Evolutionary Computation*, 8(4), pp. 443-473.

Holland, J. H. (1987), "Genetic Algorithms and Classifier Systems: Foundations and Future Directions", *Proc. of the Int. Conf. on Genetic Algorithms*, pp. 82-89.

Holland, J. H. (1975), *Adaptation in Natural and Artificial Systems*, MIT Press.

Hopfield, J. J. (1982), "Neural Networks and Physical Systems with Emergent Collective Computational Capabilities", *Proc. Natl. Acad. Sci. USA*, 79, pp. 2554-2558.

Hunt, J. E. & Cooke, D. E. (1996), "Learning Using an Artificial Immune System", *Journal of Network and Computer Applications*, 19, pp. 189-212.

Hunt, J. E. & Fellows, A. (1996), "Introducing an Immune Response into a CBR system for Data Mining", *Research and Development in Expert Systems XIII*, pp. 35-42.

Hunt, J. E., Cooke, D. E. & Holstein, H. (1995), "Case Memory and Retrieval Based on the Immune System", *I ICCBR*, Published as Case-Based Reasoning Research and Development, Ed. Manuela Weloso and Agnar Aamodt, Lecture Notes in Artificial Intelligence 1010, pp 205 -216.

Hunt, K. J., Haas, R. & Murray-Smith, R. (1996), "Extending the Functional Equivalence of Radial Basis Function Networks and Fuzzy Inference Systems", *IEEE Trans. on Neural Networks*, 7(3) 776-781.

Hwang, J. N., Lay, S. R., Maechler, M., Martin, R. D. & Schimert, J. (1994), "Regression Modeling in Back-Propagation and Projection Pursuit Learning", *IEEE Trans. on Neural Networks*, 5(3), pp. 342-353.

Inman, J. K. (1978), "The Antibody Combining Region: Speculations on the Hypothesis of General Multispecificity", *Theoretical Immunology*, (Eds.) G. I. Bell,

A. S. Perelson & G. H. Pimbley Jr., Marcel Dekker Inc., pp. 243-278.

Iyoda, E. M., de Castro, L. N., Gomide, F. A. C. & Von Zuben, F. J. (1999), "Evolutionary Design of Neuro-Fuzzy Networks for Pattern Classification", *Proc. of the IEEE Congress on Evolutionary Computation*, **2**, pp. 1237-1244.

Jones, G., Brown, R. D., Clark, D. E., Willet, P. & Glen R. C. (1993), "Searching Databases of Two-Dimensional and Three-Dimensional Chemical Structures Using Genetic Algorithms", *Proc. of Int. Conf. on Genetic Algorithms*, pp. 597-602.

Juang, J. –G. (2000), "Fuzzy Neural Network Approaches for Robot Gait Synthesis", *IEEE Trans. on Systems, Man, and Cybernetics, Part B: Cybernetics*, **30**(4), pp. 594-600.

Jang, J. S. R. & Sun, C. T. (1993), "Functional Equivalence Between Radial Basis Function Networks and Fuzzy Inference Systems", *IEEE Trans. on Neural Networks*, **4**(1) 156-158.

Jun, J.-H., Lee, D.-W. & Sim, K.-B., (1999), "Realization of Cooperative and Swarm Behavior in Distributed Autonomous Robotic Systems Using Artificial Immune System", *Proc. of the IEEE System, Man, and Cybernetics*, **4**, pp. 614-619.

Khosla, R. & Dillon, T. (1997), *Engineering Intelligent Hybrid Multi-Agent Systems*, Kluwer Academic Publishers.

Kim, J. & Bentley, P. (1999), "Negative Selection and Niching by an Artificial Immune System for Network Intrusion Detection", *Proc. of the Genetic and Evolutionary Computation Conference*, pp. 149-158.

Kinnear Jr., K. E. (1994), *Advances in Genetic Programming*, MIT Press.

Kohonen T. (1982), "Self-Organized Formation of Topologically Correct Feature Maps", *Biological Cybernetics*, **43**, pp. 59-69.

Kosko B. (1992), *Neural Networks and Fuzzy Systems – A Dynamical Systems Approach to Machine Intelligence*, University of Southern California, Prentice-Hall International, Inc.

Koza, J. R. (1992), *Genetic Programming: On the Programming of Computers by Means of Natural Selection*, MIT Press.

Krink, T., Mayoh, B. H. & Michalewicz, Z. (1999), "A Patchwork Model for Evolutionary Algorithms with Structured and Variable Size Populations", *Proc. of the Genetic and Evolutionary Computation Conference*, **2**, pp. 1321-1328.

Krishnakumar, K. Satyadas, A. & Neidhoefer, J. (1995), "An Immune System Framework for Integrating Computational Intelligence Paradigms with Applications to Adaptive Control", In *Computational Intelligence A Dynamic System Perspective*, M. Palaniswami, Y. Attikiouzel, R. J. Marks II, D. Fogel and T. Fukuda (Eds.), IEEE Press, pp. 32-45.

Kuo, Y. –H., Kao, C. –I. & Chen, J. –J. (1993), "A Fuzzy Neural Network Model and Its Hardware Implementation", *IEEE Trans. on Fuzzy Systems*, **1**(3), pp. 171-183.

Kwan, H. K. & Cai, Y. (1994), "A Fuzzy Neural Network and its Application to Pattern Recognition", *IEEE Trans. on Fuzzy Systems*, **2**(3), pp. 184-193.

Kwok T. Y., & Yeung. D. Y. (1997), "Constructive Algorithms for Structure Learning in Feedforward Neural Networks for Regression Problems", *IEEE Trans. on Neural Networks*, **8**(3), pp. 630-645.

Lee, D-W., Jun, H-B. & Sim, K-B. (1999), "Artificial Immune System for Realization of Cooperative Strategies and Group Behavior in Collective Autonomous Mobile Robots", In *Proc. of the AROB'99*, pp. 232-235.

Li, H. –X. & Chen, C. L. P. (2000), "The Equivalence Between Fuzzy Logic Systems and Feedforward Neural Networks", *IEEE Trans. on Neural Networks*, **11**(2), pp. 356-365.

Lobo, F. (2000), *The Parameter-less Genetic Algorithm: Rational and Automated Parameter Simplified Genetic Algorithm Operation*, Dissertation from the University of Lisbon, Portugal.

Maniezzo, V. (1994), "Genetic Evolution of the Topology and Weight Distribution of Neural Networks", *IEEE Trans. on Neural Networks*, **5**(1), pp. 39-53.

McCulloch W. & Pitts W. (1943), "A Logical Calculus of the Ideas Immanent in Nervous Activity", *Bulletin of Mathematical Biophysics*, **5**, pp. 115-133.

Michalewicz, Z. (1996), *Genetic Algorithms + Data Structures = Evolution Programs*, Springer-Verlag, 3rd Ed.

Mitchell, M. (1998), *An Introduction to Genetic Algorithms*, The MIT Press.

Mori, M., Tsukiyama, M. & Fukuda, T. (1993), "Immune Algorithm with Searching Diversity and its Application to resource Allocation Problem", *Trans. of the Institute of Electrical Engineers of Japan*, (in Japanese), **113-C**(10), pp. 872-878.

Nagano, S. & Yonezawa, Y., (1999), "Generative Mechanism of Emergent Properties Observed with the Primitive Evolutional Phenomena by Immunotic Recognition", *Proc. of the IEEE System, Man, and Cybernetics*, **I**, pp. 223-228.

Nikolaev, N. I., Iba, H. & Slavov, V. (1999), "Inductive Genetic Programming with Immune Network Dynamics", *Advances in Genetic Programming 3*, MIT Press, pp. 355-376.

Opitz, D. W. & Shavlik, J. W. (1997), "Connectionist Theory Refinement: Genetically Searching the Space of Network Topologies", *Journal of Artificial Intelligence Research*, **6**, pp. 177-209.

Pal, S. K., De, R. K. & Basak, J. (2000), "Unsupervised Feature Evaluation: A Neuro-Fuzzy Approach", *IEEE Trans. on Neural Networks*, **11**(2), pp. 366-376.

Păun, G., Rozenberg, G. & Salomaa, A. (1998), *DNA Computing*, Springer-Verlag.

Pedrycz, W. & Gomide, F. A. C. (1998), *An Introduction to Fuzzy Sets Analysis and Design*, MIT Press.

Perelson, A. S. & Weisbuch, G. (1997), "Immunology for Physicists", *Rev. of Modern Physics*, **69**(4), pp. 1219-1267.

Potter, M. A. & de Jong K. A. (1998), "The Coevolution of Antibodies for Concept Learning", *Proc. of the 5th Int. Conference on Parallel Problem Solving from Nature*, pp. 530-539.

Prechelt L. (1998), "Automatic Early Stopping Using Cross Validation: Quantifying the Criteria", *Neural Networks*, **11**(4), pp. 761-767.

Rechenberg, I. (1973), *Evolutionsstrategie: Optimierung Technischer Systeme Nach Prinzipien der Biologischen Evolution*, Frommann-Holzboog, Stuttgart.

Reed R. (1993), "Pruning Algorithms – A Survey", *IEEE Trans. on Neural Networks*, **4**(5), pp. 740-747.

Rumelhart, D. E., McClelland, J. L. & The PDP Research Group, Eds. (1986), *Parallel Distributed Processing*, Cambridge MIT Press.

Salomon, R. (1998), "Evolutionary Algorithms and Gradient Search; Similarities and Differences", *IEEE Trans. on Evolutionary Computation*, **2**(2), pp. 45-55.

Schwefel, H. –P. (1965), *Kybernetische Evolutionals Strategie der Experimentellen Forschung in der Stromungstechnik*, Diploma Thesis, Technical University of Berlin.

Shi, Y., Eberhart, R. & Chen, Y. (1999), "Implementation of Evolutionary Fuzzy Systems", *IEEE Trans. on Fuzzy Systems*, **7**(2), pp. 109-119.

Smith, D. J., Forrest, & Perelson, S. A. (1993), "Searching for Diverse, Cooperative Populations with Genetic Algorithms", *Evolutionary Computation*, **1**, pp. 127-149.

Sutton, R. S. & Barto, A. G. (1998), *Reinforcement Learning an Introduction*, A Bradford Book.

Takahashi, K. & Yamada, T. (1997), "A Self-Tuning Immune Feedback Controller for Controlling Mechanical Systems", *IEEE/ASME International Conference on Advanced Intelligent Mechatronics*, CD-ROM#101.

Vertosick, F. T. & Kelly, R. H. (1989), "Immune Network Theory: A Role for Parallel Distributed Processing?", *Immunology*, **66**, pp. 1-7.

Von Zuben, F. J. & Netto, M. L. A. (1997), "Projection Pursuit and the Solvability Condition Applied to Constructive Learning", *Proc. of the IEEE Int. Joint Conference on Neural Networks*, 2, pp. 1062-1067.

Yu, X.-H. & Chen, G.-A. (1997), "Efficient Backpropagation Learning Using Optimal Learning Rate and Momentum", *Neural Networks*, 10(3), pp. 517-528.

Zadeh, L. A. (1997), "What is Soft Computing", *Soft Computing*, 1, pp. 1.

Further Reading

Theory of Soft Computing

Bonissone, P. P. (1997), "Soft Computing: The Convergence of Emerging Reasoning Technologies", *Soft Computing*, 1(1), pp. 6-18.

Novák, V. (1998), "Towards Formal Theory of Soft Computing", *Soft Computing*, 2(1), pp. 4-6.

Introduction to Artificial Neural Networks

Bishop. C. M. (1996), *Neural Networks for Pattern Recognition*, Oxford University Press.

Fausett, L. (1994), *Fundamentals of Neural Networks, Architecture, Algorithms, and Applications*, Prentice Hall International.

Freeman, J. A. (1991), *Neural Networks, Algorithms, Applications, and Programming Techniques*, Addison-Wesley.

Kosko B. (1992), *Neural Networks and Fuzzy Systems – A Dynamical Systems Approach to Machine Intelligence*, University of Southern California, Prentice-Hall International, Inc.

Medsker, L. R. & Jain, L. C. (2000), *Recurrent Neural Networks: Design and Applications*, CRC Press.

Poggio, T. & Girosi, F. (1990), "Networks for Approximation and Learning", *Proc. of the IEEE*, 78(9), pp. 1481-1497.

Saarinen S., Bramley R., e Cybenko G. (1992), "Neural Networks, Backpropagation, and Automatic Differentiation", In *Automatic Differentiation of Algorithms: Theory, Implementation, and Application*, Philadelphia, PA, pp. 31-42.

Practical Aspects of Neural Network Training

Anders, U. & Korn, O. (1999), "Model Selection in Neural Networks", *Neural Networks*, 12, pp. 389-323.

Battiti R. (1992), "First- and Second-Order Methods for Learning: Between Steepest Descent and Newton's Method", *Neural Computation*, 4, pp. 141-166.

Bauer, H.-U & Villmann, Th. (1997), "Growing a Hypercubical Output Space in a Self-Organizing Feature Map", *IEEE Trans. on Neural Networks*, 8(2), pp. 218-226.

Castellano, G., Fanelli, A. M. & Pelillo, M. (1997), "An Iterative Pruning Algorithm for Feedforward Neural Networks", *IEEE Trans. on Neural Networks*, 8(3), pp. 519-531.

Chen, S., Chng, E. S. & Alkadhimi, K. (1995), "Regularized Orthogonal Least Squares Algorithm for Constructing Radial Basis Function Networks", *Int. J. of Control*, 64, pp. 829-837.

Cho S.-B. (1997), "Self-Organizing Map with Dynamical Node Splitting: Application to Handwritten Digit Recognition", *Neural Computation*, 9, pp. 1345-1355.

de Castro, L. N. & Von Zuben, F. J. (1999), "Neural Networks with Adaptive

Activation Functions: A Second Order Approach", *Proceedings of SCI/ISAS'99*, **3**, pp. 574-581.

de Castro, L. N. & Von Zuben, F. J. (1999), "An Improving Pruning Technique with Restart for the Kohonen Self-Organizing Feature Map", *Proc. of the Int. Joint Conference on Neural Networks*, **3**, pp. 1916-1919.

de Castro, L. N. & Von Zuben F. J. (1998), "A Hybrid Paradigm for Weight Initialization in Supervised Feedforward Neural Network Learning", *Proceedings do ICS'98, Workshop on Artificial Intelligence*, pp. 30-37, Taipei/Taiwan, R.O.C.

Erwin, E., Obermayer, K. & Schulten, K. (1992), "Self-Organizing Maps: Ordering, Convergence Properties and Energy Functions", *Biol. Cybern.*, **67**, pp. 47-55.

Fahlman S. E., & Lebiere C. (1990), "The Cascade Correlation Learning Architecture", *Advances in Neural Information Processing Systems 2*, pp. 524-532.

Fritzke B. (1994), "Growing Cell Structures – A Self-Organizing Network for Unsupervised and Supervised Learning", *Neural Networks*, **7**(9), pp. 1441-1460.

Haese, K. (1998), "Self-Organizing Maps with Self-Adjusting Learning Parameters", *IEEE Trans. on Neural Networks*, **9**(6), pp. 1270-1278.

Hopfield, J. J. (1984), "Neurons with Graded Response Have Collective Computational Properties Like Those of Two-State Neurons", *Proc. Natl. Acad. Sci. USA*, **81**, pp. 3088-3092.

Kwok T. Y., & Yeung. D. Y. (1997), "Constructive Algorithms for Structure Learning in Feedforward Neural Networks for Regression Problems", *IEEE Trans. on Neural Networks*, **8**(3), pp. 630-645.

Lehtokangas, M. (1999), "Modeling with Constructive Backpropagation", *Neural Networks*, **12**, pp. 707-716.

Lehtokangas, M., Saarinen, J., Kaski, K. & Huuhtanen, P. (1995), "Initializing Weights of a Multilayer Perceptron by Using the Orthogonal Least Squares Algorithm", *Neural Computation*, **7**, pp. 982-999.

Moody, J. & Darken, C. (1989), "Fast Learning in Networks of Locally-Tuned Processing Units", *Neural Computation*, **1**, pp. 281-294.

Reed R. (1993), "Pruning Algorithms – A Survey", *IEEE Trans. on Neural Networks*, 4(5), pp. 740-747.

Ritter, H. & Schulten, K. (1988), "Convergence Properties of Kohonen's Topology Conserving Maps: Fluctuations, Stability, and Dimension Selection", *Biol. Cybern.*, **60**, pp. 59-71.

Shepherd, A. J. (1997), *Second-Order Methods for Neural Networks – Fast and Reliable Methods for Multi-Layer Perceptrons*, Springer-Verlag.

Stäger, F. & Agarwal, M. (1997), "Three Methods to Speed up the Training of Feedforward and Feedback Perceptrons", Neural Networks, **10**(8), pp. 1435-1443.

Thimm, G. & Fiesler, E. (1997), "High-Order and Multilayer Perceptron Initialization", *IEEE Trans. on Neural Networks*, **8**(2), pp. 349-359.

Verma, B. (1997), "Fast Training of Multilayer Perceptrons", *IEEE Trans. on Neural Networks*, **8**(6), pp. 1314-1320.

Yu, X.-H. & Chen, G.-A. (1997), "Efficient Backpropagation Learning Using Optimal Learning Rate and Momentum", *Neural Networks*, **10**(3), pp. 517-528.

Introduction to Evolutionary Algorithms

Angeline, P. J. (Ed.) (1997), *Evolutionary Programming VI: 6th International Conference, EP97*, Springer.

Bäck, T., Fogel, D. B. & Michalewicz, Z. (2000a), *Evolutionary Computation 1*

Basic Algorithms and Operators, Institute of Physics Publishing (IOP), Bristol and Philadelphia.

Bäck, T., Fogel, D. B. & Michalewicz, Z. (2000b), *Evolutionary Computation 2*

Advanced Algorithms and Operators, Institute of Physics Publishing (IOP), Bristol and Philadelphia.

Bäck, T. (1996), *Evolutionary Algorithms in Theory and Practice: Evolution Strategies, Evolutionary Programming, Genetic Algorithms*. Oxford University Press.

Bäck, T. & Schwefel, H. –P. (1993), "An Overview of Evolutionary Algorithms for Parameter Optimization", *Evolutionary Computation*, 1(1), pp. 1-23.

Bäck, T., Hammel, U., & Schwefel, H. –P. (1997), "Evolutionary Computation: Comments on the History and Current State", *IEEE Trans. on Evol. Comp.*, vol. 1, no. 1, pp. 3-17.

Banzhaf, W., Nordin, P., Keller, R. E. & Francone, F. D. (1998), *Genetic Programming: An Introduction. On the Automatic Evolution of Computer Programs and Its Applications*, Morgan Kaufmann.

Fogel, D. B. (1995), *Evolutionary Computation: Toward a New Philosophy of Machine Intelligence*, IEEE Press.

Fogel, D. B. (Ed.) (1995), *Evolutionary Computation: The Fossil Record*, IEEE Press.

Goldberg, D. E. (1989), *Genetic Algorithms in Search, Optimization and Machine Learning*, Addison-Wesley Reading, Massachusetts.

Koza., J. R. (1994), *Genetic Programming II: Automatic Discovery of Reusable Programs*, MIT Press.

Michalewicz, Z. (1996), *Genetic Algorithms + Data Structures = Evolution Programs*, Springer-Verlag, 3rd Ed.

Rechenberg, I. (1973), *Evolutionsstrategie: Optimierung Technischer Systeme Nach Prinzipien der Biologischen Evolution*, Frommann-Holzboog, Stuttgart.

Schwefel, H.-P. (1995), *Evolution and Optimum Seeking*, Wiley.

Niches and Species in Evolutionary Algorithms

Deb, K. (1989), *Genetic Algorithms in Multimodal Function Optimisation*, Master's Dissertation, University of Alabama; TCGA Report 89002.

Goldberg, D. E., Deb, K. & Horn, J. (1992), "Massive Multimodality, Deception, and Genetic Algorithms", In *Parallel Problem Solving from Nature 2*, R. Männer & B. Manderick (eds.), pp. 37-46.

Goldberg, D. E. & Richardson, J. (1987), "Genetic Algorithms with Sharing for Multimodal Function Optimization", *Genetic Algorithms and Their Applications: Proc. of the II Int. Conference on Genetic Algorithms*, pp. 41-49.

Mahfoud, S. W. (1995), *Niching Methods for Genetic Algorithms*, Ph.D. Dissertation, Illinois Genetic Algorithms Laboratory, University of Illinois at Urbana-Champaign.

Perry, Z. A. (1984), *Experimental Study of Speciation in Ecological Niche Theory Using Genetic Algorithms*, Doctoral Thesis, University of Michigan.

Pétrowski, A. & Genet, M. G. (1999), "A Classification Tree for Speciation", *Proc. of the IEEE Congress on Evolutionary Computation*, pp. 204-211.

Pétrowski, A. (1996), "A Clearing Procedure as a Niching Method for Genetic Algorithms", *Proc. of the IEEE Congress on Evolutionary Computation*, pp. 798-803.

Porter, B. & Xue, F. (2001), "Niche Evolution Strategy for Global Optimization", *Proc. of the IEEE Congress on Evolutionary Computation*, pp. 1086-1092.

Sareni, B. & Krähenbühl, L. (1998), "Fitness Sharing and Niching Methods Revisited", *IEEE Trans. on Evolutionary Computation*, 2(3), pp. 97-106.

Practical Aspects of Evolutionary Algorithms

Angeline, P. J. (1995), "Adaptive and Self-Adaptive Evolutionary Computations", In *Computational Intelligence: A Dynamic Systems Perspective*, M. Palaniswami, Y. Attikiouzel, R. Marks, D. Fogel & T. Fukuda (eds.), Piscataway, NJ:IEEE Press, pp. 152-163.

Arabas, J., Michalewicz, Z. & Mulawka, J. (1994), "GAVaPS – A Genetic Algorithm with Varying Population Size", *Proc. of the IEEE Congress on Evolutionary Computation*, pp. 73-78.

Bäck, T. (1992), "The Interaction of Mutation Rate, Selection and Self-Adaptation Within a Genetic Algorithm", In *Parallel Problem Solving from Nature*, 2, pp. 85-94.

Grefenstette, J. J. (1986), "Optimization of Control Parameters for Genetic Algorithms", *IEEE Trans. on Systems, Man, and Cybernetics*, 16(1), pp. 122-128.

Hinterdirg, R., Michalewicz, Z. & Eiben, A. E. (1997), "Adaptation in Evolutionary Computation: A Survey", *Proc. of the 4th IEEE Conference on Evolutionary Computation*, pp. 420-429.

Krink, T., Mayoh, B. H. & Michalewicz, Z. (1999), "A Patchwork Model for Evolutionary Algorithms with Structured and Variable Size Populations", *Proc. of the Genetic and Evolutionary Computation Conference*, 2, pp. 1321-1328.

Lobo, F. (2000), *The Parameter-less Genetic Algorithm: Rational and Automated Parameter Simplified Genetic Algorithm Operation*, Dissertation from the University of Lisbon, Portugal.

Other Computational Intelligence Paradigms

Condon, A. & Rozenberg, G. (Eds.) (2001), *DNA Computing*, Springer-Verlag.

Garzon, M. H. & Deaton, R. J., (1999), "Biomolecular Computing and Programming", *IEEE Trans. on Evol. Computation*, 3(3), pp. 236-250.

Giles, C. L., Sun, R. & Zurada, J. M. (eds.) (1998), *IEEE Transaction on Neural Networks*, Special Issue on Neural Networks and Hybrid Intelligent Approaches, 9(5).

Holland, J. H. (1986), "Escaping Brittleness: The Possibilities of General Purpose Learning Algorithms Applied to Parallel Rule-Based Systems", In *Machine Learning 2*, R. S. Michalski, J. G. Carbonell & T. M. Mitchell (eds.), Morgan Kauffman, pp. 593-623.

Holland, J. H. (1987), "Genetic Algorithms and Classifier Systems: Foundations and Future Directions", *Proc. of the Int. Conf. on Genetic Algorithms*, pp. 82-89.

Kolodner, J. (1993), *Case-Based Reasoning*, Morgan-Kauffman.

Leake, D. B. (1996), *Case-Based Reasoning, Experiences, Lessons & Future Directions*, AAAI Press/The MIT Press.

Leondes, C. T. (1999), *Fuzzy Theory Systems*, Academic Press.

Pedrycz, W. & Gomide, F. A. C. (1998), *An Introduction to Fuzzy Sets Analysis and Design*, MIT Press.

Watson, I. & Marir, F. (1994), "Case-Based Reasoning: A Review", *The Knowledge Engineering Review*, 9(4), pp. 327-354.

Zadeh, L. A. (1965), "Fuzzy Sets", *Information and Control*, 8, pp. 338-353.

Chapter 7

Case Studies

> *...scientists have come up with solutions to certain problems only to find that the biological world got there first*
>
> – R. Paton

7.1 Introduction

Chapter 4 presented a broad survey of artificial immune systems, focusing primarily on metaphors employed by researchers and how these works could be considered in light of the framework proposed in Chapter 3. The reviews in Chapter 4 were intentionally brief and aimed at providing the reader with an overview of the major application domains and research schools on AIS; this was a different approach from the one adopted in this chapter. Here it is the intent to present more detailed descriptions of four different types of applications of AIS: 1) autonomous navigation, 2) computer network security, 3) job-shop scheduling, and 4) data analysis and function optimization. These reviews will provide the reader with a more in-depth understanding of AIS applications, which could not realistically be undertaken in Chapter 4. These applications were selected to illustrate the variety of application areas of AIS and the use of different immune algorithms and shape-spaces. The reader may wish to review Chapter 3 again, particularly Section 3.5 on engineering AIS. This process is used in this chapter as a basis to describe each application of AIS.

This chapter is organized as follows. Section 7.2 reviews the works of Watanabe *et al.* (1999) on autonomous robotic navigation. In Section 7.3 an application of computer network security as proposed by Hofmeyr and Forrest (2000) is discussed. Section 7.4 describes the application of an artificial immune system to a job-shop scheduling problem as found in the works of Hart and Ross (1999). Finally, in Section 7.5 we review the works of de Castro and Von Zuben (2001) and de Castro and Timmis (2002) that employ an artificial immune network model to perform data analysis and multimodal function optimization. The chapter is summarized in Section 7.6.

7.2 Autonomous Navigation

Section 4.7 provided descriptions of applications of artificial immune systems to the field of robotics. That section reviewed approaches to two different problems. First, a review of works on AIS applied to the emergent collective behavior of a set of robots was presented. This was followed by a review of works applying AIS to create a walking robot with six legs. This section reviews the works of Watanabe *et al.*,

(1999) where the authors employ a continuous immune network model for an autonomous navigation problem. In this situation, the application domain corresponds to a robot whose goal it is to navigate autonomously throughout a closed environment in order to collect garbage.

7.2.1. Problem Description

The problem under examination is as follows. A robot is required to collect garbage (from various locations within the environment) and to place that garbage into a can, without total depletion of its energy E (Figure 7.1). The robot is equipped with a set of sensors that allow it to obtain information about the environment in which it is placed, such as its distance from garbage and from the home base. An initial amount of energy is given to the robot before it is placed in the environment, with one of the robot's sensors being capable of measuring the internal energy level.

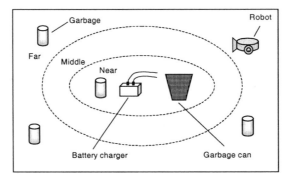

Figure 7.1.   Environment for an autonomous robot navigation problem (reproduced with permission from [Ishiguro *et al.*, 1996]. © *Akio Ishiguro, 1996*).

7.2.2. Immune Principles

In order to govern the behavior of the AIS, continuous immune network models were adapted and employed. The dynamic equation proposed by Farmer and collaborators (Farmer *et al.*, 1986) was modified to control the number of antibodies in the network. This was coupled with a sigmoid function that guaranteed the stability of the number of antibodies. Additionally, each antibody had its network sensitivity assessed by an equation similar to the one introduced by Varela and Coutinho (1991) (Equation (3.17), Section 3.5). This equation was used to govern the metadynamics of the AIS.

7.2.3. **Engineering the AIS**

To accomplish its task of collecting garbage without running out of energy, it is necessary to monitor the energy level of the robot, which depends upon four parameters:

1. The energy level at the previous iteration (time step), $E(t - 1)$;
2. The energy consumption at each iteration, E_m;
3. The additional energy consumed when the robot carries garbage, E_g;
4. The energy loss when the robot collides with any obstacle (e.g., garbage or wall), E_c;

The energy level of the robot at each iteration t, $E(t)$, is given by the following expression:

$$E(t) = E(t - 1) - E_m - k_1 E_g - k_2 E_c.$$ (7.1)

where,

$$k_1 = \begin{cases} 1 & \text{if carrying garbage} \\ 0 & \text{otherwise} \end{cases},$$

$$k_2 = \begin{cases} 1 & \text{if collides with wall/garbage} \\ 0 & \text{otherwise} \end{cases}.$$

At each time step, the energy level of the robot is reduced by a fixed amount of energy E_m. Constants k_1 and k_2 indicate that energy will be additionally consumed only if the robot is currently carrying garbage and/or if it collides with an obstacle.

Immune Components and their Representations

The robot sensors receive the environmental stimuli (including its internal energy level) and transform them into a *condition* that represents the current *state* of the robot, e.g., *obstacle on the right* and/or *low energy level*. The robot contains a set of *state/action* (or *condition/action*) rules that will be matched against the information received from the sensors in order to decide an appropriate action to be taken.

This system then is composed of sets of antigens and antibodies. The current *state* of the robot is read from its sensors and corresponds to an antigen. A predefined behavior (condition/action rule) is part of an antibody and can be used as a response to an antigen. Each antigen is composed of four attributes that represent the state of the robot as follows:

1. *Direction of garbage*: F (front), R (right), L (left), N (none), H (in hand, i.e., carrying garbage);
2. *Direction of obstacle*: F (front), R (right), L (left), N (none);
3. *Location of home base*: F (front), R (right), L (left), N (none), Nr (near), Md (middle), Fr (far); and
4. *Energy level*: Hi (high), Lo (low).

Each antibody is modeled in a Symbolic shape-space under the form of a *rule* composed of three parts, as illustrated in Figure 7.2.

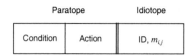

Figure 7.2.   Structure of a network antibody molecule.

1. *State* or *condition*: Information contained in the paratope of the antibody, which is linked to a given *action*. It contains the same structure displayed by the antigens;
2. *Action*: a response to a given *state*;
3. *ID number and stimulation*: indicates with which network antibody it interacts and to what degree.

Six different actions were selected to compose the action part of the antibodies: F (move forward), R (turn right), L (turn left), Sh (search for home base), C (catch garbage), and E (explore). As can be seen from Figure 7.2, the antibody molecule was divided into a paratope and an idiotope. The paratope contains the set of rules condition/action, and the idiotope contains additional parameters such as the ID number of the stimulating antibody and its stimulation level $m_{i,j}$.

The dynamic behavior of the system is based upon a "matching" of the current state of the robot (antigen) with a set of candidate states of the robot (antibodies). These candidate states are associated with a set of appropriate behaviors.

Network Structure

The problem of selecting which action to take, or behavior to adopt, is now reduced to the problem of matching the information (state) obtained from the sensors of the robot with the condition parts of the antibodies. As proposed in the immune network theory, the idiotope of each antibody is capable of recognizing the paratope of another antibody and vice-versa. These recognition events allow the immune network to select antibodies from the whole antibody repertoire. As an illustration, consider the example depicted in Figure 7.3. Suppose that four antigens could be used to represent the state of the robot: Ag_1, Ag_2, Ag_3 and Ag_4. These antigens select four antibodies: Ab_1, Ab_2, Ab_3 and Ab_4. Note that each antigen matches the condition part of a single antibody, and the antibodies interact with themselves. The recognition of a paratope by an idiotope is always stimulating for the antibody that recognizes the idiotope, and suppressing for the recognized antibody. For example, as Ab_1 recognizes the idiotope in Ab_3, Ab_3 stimulates Ab_1, while Ab_1 suppresses Ab3.

In immune network models, usually two parameters influence the selection of a cell to become an effector or a memory cell: 1) its concentration level, and 2) its affinity with an antigen and other cells in the network. In this approach, as a result of the interaction among antibodies, each antibody will have its concentration altered according to Equation (7.2), which is a differential equation similar to the one proposed by Farmer *et al.* (1986) and discussed in Section 3.5 (Equation (3.15)).

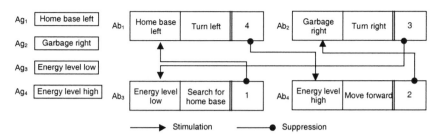

Figure 7.3. Example of interactions among antibodies in an immune network for autonomous robot navigation.

Dynamics

Once the antibodies have recognized the antigens, they will compete with each other to specify a single action to be taken by the robot, i.e., a single antibody will be selected and have its action performed. This *competition* to perform an action is based upon the concentration level of each of the selected antibodies. The concentration level of an antibody is dependent upon its affinity with other antibodies in the network and with the antigen. Assume the selection of N antibodies with concentration c_i, $i = 1,...N$. The differential equation governing the dynamics of the concentration of antibodies is given by:

$$\frac{dc_i}{dt} = \sum_{j=1}^{N} m_{j,i} c_i c_j - k_3 \sum_{k=1}^{N} m_{i,k} c_i c_k + k_4 m_i c_i - k_5 c_i, \qquad (7.2)$$

where $m_{j,i}$ and m_i correspond to the affinity between Ab_j and Ab_i, and between Ab_i and the detected antigen respectively (compare this equation with Equations 3.15 and 3.20). The first term, from left to right, represents the stimulation of the paratope of Ab_i by the idiotope of Ab_j. The second term represents the suppression of Ab_i when its idiotope is recognized by the paratope of Ab_k. The third term corresponds to the antibody stimulation by the antigen. Finally, the fourth term models the tendency of antibodies to die in the absence of any interaction. The parameter k_3 is a positive constant aiming at representing a possible inequality between stimulation and suppression. Parameter k_4 weights the influence of the antigenic recognition in the overall network behavior, and parameter k_5 quantifies the death rate of non-stimulated antibodies.

To ensure the stability of the concentration of antibodies, a squashing function is applied:

$$c_i = \frac{1}{1 + \exp(0.5 - c_i)}. \qquad (7.3)$$

Once the concentration of each antibody Ab_i, $i = 1,...N$ is determined, the selection is performed using a Roulette-Wheel algorithm (Section 6.3).

Adapting the Idiotopes

In order to evaluate Equation (7.2), it is necessary to determine the idiotopes of all antibodies as depicted in Figure 7.2; these are composed of an ID number and a stimulation level $m_{i,j}$. The authors proposed an on-line adjustment mechanism that initially starts with all idiotopes undefined and obtains their values using *reinforcement signals*. Two types of reinforcement signals were suggested: 1) a *reward signal* and 2) a *penalty signal*.

Reward:

- Robot recharges with low energy level; and
- Robot catches garbage with high energy level.

Penalty:

- Robot catches garbage with low energy level; and
- Robot collides with an obstacle.

Assume that two antigens match the condition part of two antibodies Ab_i and Ab_j of the initial population with undefined idiotopes. As the initial values of the idiotopes are unknown, an antibody Ab_i is selected randomly and receives a reinforcement signal according to the result of its action.

- If this signal is a *reward*, then the ID number of Ab_i, i.e., i, is recorded in the idiotope of Ab_j, and the affinity $m_{j,i}$ of Ab_j with Ab_i is increased.
- If this signal is a *penalty*, then the ID number of Ab_j, i.e., j, is recorded in the idiotope of Ab_i, and the affinity $m_{i,j}$ of Ab_i with Ab_j is increased.

Note that an increase in the affinity (stimulation) of a specific antibody forces the robot to select this antibody when the same (or a similar) antigen invades the robot. The modification of the affinity is performed according to the following expression:

$$m_{i,j} = \frac{T_p^{Ab_i} + T_r^{Ab_j}}{T_{Ab_j}^{Ab_i}}, \tag{7.4}$$

where $T_p^{Ab_i}$ and $T_r^{Ab_i}$ correspond to the number of times antibody Ab_i receives penalty and reward, respectively. Parameter $T_{Ab_j}^{Ab_i}$ denotes the number of times both antibodies, Ab_i and Ab_j, are activated by their respective antigens.

Some interesting features can be observed from the above procedure. First, the selection of antibodies by antigens results in a natural interconnection among the antibodies defined by the ID numbers of antibodies placed in the idiotopes of other antibodies. Second, by dynamically adjusting the affinity of each antibody, through penalty or reward, it is possible to determine relative *priorities* (stimulation) between antibodies.

Metadynamics

With the procedures described so far, it is possible to design an artificial immune system modeled as an immune network for the autonomous garbage-collecting robot. The only pre-requisite is to specify an initial population of antibodies (condition/action rules) capable of covering adverse environmental conditions. An alternative approach would be to devise a strategy that appropriately generates antibodies (condition/action rules) for the robot; these would then be selected and adapted by the procedures presented. Nevertheless, the pre-specification of a set of condition/action rules might be too restrictive, prohibiting the robot from being 'creative'. Introducing a mechanism to generate candidate antibodies to enter the network can alleviate this limitation.

Using a bone marrow model, random sets of antibodies (condition/action rules) can be generated by gene recombination. Given a set of conditions and a set of actions, recombine them such that different condition/action rules are generated to form the paratopes of the antibodies. Then, it is necessary to select which antibodies are going to be incorporated into the network and which are going to die.

To determine if one of the generated antibodies is going to be allowed to enter the network, it is necessary to determine the *sensitivity* (stimulation and suppression) level of each new antibody in relation to the antibodies already in the network. This can be performed using the following equations:

$$\sigma_i = \sum_{j=1}^{N} m_{j,i} c_j,$$

$$\delta_i = \sum_{j=1}^{N} m_{i,j} c_j,$$

(7.5)

where σ_i is the sum of stimulation from the network over Ab_i, and δ_i is the sum of suppression from the network over Ab_i. Note that these equations follow Equation (3.17) proposed by Varela and Coutinho (1991).

Given the total stimulation and/or suppression of a given antibody, it will be allowed to be incorporated or not in the network. The authors suggested that the candidate antibody satisfying max σ_i, or max $|\sigma_i - \delta_i|$ would be selected to enter the network.

In addition to allowing new antibodies to be inserted into the network, it is necessary to eliminate those antibodies that are not useful, i.e., that are never selected or that receive a large number of penalty signals. The absence of selection or the excess of penalty will result in the decay of the antibody concentration c_i according to the following equation:

$$\frac{dc_i}{dt} = k_6 \Delta c_i - k_7 c_i,$$

(7.6)

where k_7 is a dissipation factor, Δc_i is the variation in the concentration c_i from the last to the previous iteration, and k_6 is given by

$$k_6 = \begin{cases} -1 & \text{if the antibody is selected and penalized} \\ 0 & \text{if the antibody is not selected} \\ 1 & \text{if the antibody is selected and rewarded} \end{cases}.$$

Equation (7.6) incorporates the notion of age of an antibody. If it is never selected, then it tends to die because its concentration is iteratively reduced. If it is constantly penalized, then it dies even quicker; and if it is rewarded, it has its life span increased. If the concentration of an antibody falls below a given threshold (default 0), then this antibody is removed form the network.

7.2.4. Performance Evaluation

The authors used the *Khepera* robot to evaluate their immune network model. The robot has a gripper to catch the garbage. It is equipped with 8 infrared proximity sensors, 8 photo sensors, and one color CCD camera. Each infrared sensor detects garbage or a wall in its corresponding direction. The photo sensors recognize the direction of an electric-light bulb that indicates the home base. The CCD camera detects the current position of the robot, supplying it with information about its distance to the home base.

A number of 24 antibodies were prepared a priori, in which the paratope and idiotope were described. The robot began with a maximum energy level of 1000, and the following values for the energy parameters: $E_m = 1$, $E_g = 3$, and $E_c = 5$ were used. These values indicate that the robot collision results in an energy consumption greater than the energy consumed when it is simply carrying garbage.

The authors reported the following typical behaviors for the robot. While the energy level is not low, the robot tries to collect garbage and deposits it into the home base. If the energy level is low, the robot tends to select an antibody with an action part of type *go to home base* and/or *search for home base*. After reaching the home base and recharging, the robot starts to explore the environment again.

7.2.5. Some Remarks

Table 7.1 summarizes the main features of the proposed artificial immune system for autonomous navigation mapping each of these features into their corresponding biological counterparts.

Note that there are many similarities between this system and the learning classifier systems briefly reviewed in Section 6.6. The classifier rules that measure the performance of the system in relation to the environmental stimuli and determine and post an action in the output of the system perform the same role as the antibodies. The bucket brigade algorithm that assigns a credit to each rule can be equated to the reinforcement signals that adapt the idiotopes of individual antibodies. Finally, the network metadynamics, which generates and selects the paratopes of antibodies, can be likened to the process of rule discovery usually performed by a genetic algorithm in classifier systems.

The dynamic behavior of the system is based upon a "match" of the current state of the robot (antigen) with a set of candidate states of the robot (antibodies). These candidate states are therefore associated with a set of appropriate behaviors. Due to this fact, it is not unreasonable to ask what is the difference between this artificial immune system model and a standard rule-based system. In this case, the difference is clear: this AIS model relies mainly in the idiotypic part of the antibody. This part is responsible for coordinating the immune network interactions and, hence, the dynamics and metadynamics of the sets of condition/action rules (antibodies).

Table 7.1. Main features the AIS for autonomous navigation and their corresponding biological counterparts.

Immune System	Artificial Immune System
Robot	Organism
Antigen	State of the robot read from its sensors
Antibody	Condition/action rule plus an ID number and a stimulation level
Paratope	Condition/action part of an antibody
Idiotope	ID number and stimulation level parts of an antibody
Network dynamics	Differential equation governing the concentration of antibodies
Network metadynamics	Insertion and elimination of antibodies from the network
Antibody sensitivity	Stimulation and/or suppression of each candidate antibody to enter the network
Antibody selection	Roulette Wheel on the antibody concentration
Maturation of antibodies	Reinforcement signals

The idiotope part of the antibodies allow antibodies to interact with each other, which would be compared to having a set of rules in a rule-based system with knowledge of each other. This is an additional level of knowledge embodied in the system and leads to interesting patterns of behaviors.

Related Works from the Authors

Ishiguro, A., Watanabe, Y. & Kondo, T. (1997), "A Robot with a Decentralized Consensus-Making Mechanism Based on the Immune System", *Proc. ISADS'97*, pp. 231-237.

Ishiguro, A., Kondo, T., Watanabe, Y. & Uchikawa, Y. (1997), "Emergent Construction of Artificial Immune Networks for Autonomous Mobile Robots", *Proc. of IEEE System, Man, and Cybernetics Conference*, pp. 1222-1228.

Ishiguro, A. Watanabe, Y., Kondo, T., Shirai, Y. & Uchikawa, Y. (1996), "Immunoid: A Robot with a Decentralized Behavior Arbitration Mechanisms Based on the Immune System", *Proc. of the*

ICMAS Workshop on Immunity-Based Systems, pp. 82-92.

Ishiguro, A., Watanabe, Y. & Uchikawa, Y. (1995), "An Immunological Approach to Dynamic Behavior Control for Autonomous Mobile Robots", In *Proc. of IROS'95*, 1, pp. 495-500.

Ishiguro, A., Kondo, T., Watanabe, Y. & Uchikawa, Y. (1995), "Dynamic Behavior Arbitration of Autonomous Mobile Robots Using Immune Networks", *Proc. of the Int. Conference on Evolutionary Computation*, 2, pp. 722-727.

Ishiguro, A., Kondo, T., Watanabe, Y. & Uchikawa, Y. (1994), "Immunoid: An Immunological Approach to Decentralized Behavior Arbitration of Autonomous Mobile Robots", *Lecture Notes in Computer Science*, **1141**, Springer-Verlag, pp. 666-675.

Watanabe, Y., Ishiguro, A., Shirai, Y. & Uchikawa, Y. (1998), "Emergent Con-struction Behavior Arbitration Mechanism Based on the Immune System", *Proc. of the Int. Conference on Evolutionary Computation*, pp. 481-486.

7.3 Computer Network Security

The use of immune metaphors for the development of computational security systems has been very popular. Section 4.3 reviewed a number of works on this topic. Indeed, when one considers AIS, it is usually the first area of application that comes to mind. This section describes in detail the work of Hofmeyr and Forrest (2000), that was applied to the field of computer network security.

7.3.1. Problem Description

Consider the problem of protecting a local area broadcast network of computers (LAN) from network-based intrusions. Broadcast LANs have the property that every computer in the network has access to each packet passing through the LAN. The aim of the artificial immune system for network security is to monitor the network traffic through the network connections. A connection is defined in terms of its *data-path triple*: the source internet protocol (IP) address, the destination IP address, and the service (port) by which the computers communicate (Figure 7.4).

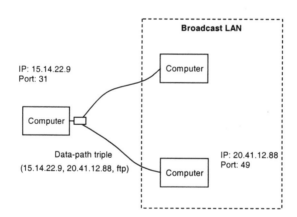

Figure 7.4. Example of a broadcast LAN and a connection.

7.3.2. Immune Principles

The negative selection algorithm was the main immune principle employed in this application. However, several other concepts were also incorporated such as co-stimulation, MHC peptide presentation, B-cells and T-cells, and variable and constant regions of antibody molecules.

7.3.3. Engineering the AIS

Immune Components and their Representations

Each data-path triple corresponds to a network connection and is represented using a binary string of length $L = 49$ in a binary Hamming shape-space. Each bitstring in this shape-space is unique to each connection. Self is defined as the set of normally occurring connections observed over time on the LAN. Thus, self depends upon frequencies: it is assumed that any connection that occurs frequently over a long time period is part of the self. Nonself is also a set of connections, but in contrast to self, nonself consists of those connections not normally observed on the LAN.

The environment is modeled using a graph $G = (V,E)$, where each vertex $v \in V$ corresponds to an internal computer of the broadcast LAN, and the whole network represents a fully connected graph. The connections among these vertices are the edges $e \in E$ of the graph.

In this case, the AIS is required to learn to discriminate between what is self (normally occurring connections) and what is nonself (intrusions). Given the universe set U of all possible bitstrings of length $L = 49$, 2^{49}, this universe has to be partitioned into two disjoint subsets: the self-set S and the nonself set N ($U = S \cup N$, $S \cap N = \varnothing$).

Applying Immune Principles

The self-set can be defined dynamically while the network is being monitored and is based upon a single type of mobile *detector*. This detector combines immune properties of B-cells, T-cells, and antibodies and is allowed to migrate from one vertex of the graph to the next via the edges (i.e., move from one computer to another).

The detector (self) set is generated based upon the negative selection algorithm as follows. Each binary string of length $L = 49$ representing a detector is created randomly and remains immature for a time period t, known as the tolerization period. During this period, the detector is exposed to the environment (self and nonself strings), and if a recognition occurs it is eliminated. If it does not recognize any string during tolerization, it becomes a mature detector. Mature detectors need to exceed a cross-reactivity threshold (r-contiguous bits) in order to become activated; this increases its life span. Recognition is quantified by matching two strings using the r-contiguous bit rule.

These nonself detectors are constantly being matched against the bitstrings representing the data-path triples that correspond to the connections in the network. Each detector is allowed to accumulate matches through a *match count* (m), which itself decays over time. In order for a detector to become activated, it has to match at least δ strings within a given time period; this threshold δ was termed the *activation threshold*. Once a detector has been activated, its match count is reset to zero. Each detection node has a local sensitivity level ω, which subtracts its activation threshold δ, i.e., the higher the local sensitivity, the lower the local activation threshold. This mechanism ensures that disparate nonself strings will still be detected, providing they occur in a short period of time.

When a new packet (bitstring) enters the network, several different detectors are activated with distinct degrees of match (through the r-contiguous bit rule). The best matching detectors become memory detectors (memory cells). These memory detectors make copies of themselves that are then spread out to neighboring nodes in the network. Consequently, a representation of the memory detector is distributed throughout the graph, accelerating future (secondary) responses to this specific nonself bitstring. As another aid to increase the speed of response of memory detectors, they have their activation thresholds reduced.

When a detector is activated, it sends an initial signal that an anomaly has been detected. As in the biological immune system, the detection of an anomaly is not enough to promote an immune response; a co-stimulatory signal is required from an accessory cell. The authors simulated the co-stimulatory (or second) signal by using a human operator, who is given a time period t_s to decide if the detected anomaly is really nonself. If the operator decides that this anomaly is indeed nonself, then a second signal is returned to the detector that identified it. This second signal increases the life span of this detector, maintaining it as a memory detector. The recognition of an anomaly in the absence of the second signal causes the death of a detector and its replacement by a new one.

Figure 7.5 summarizes the life cycle of a detector. A detector consists of randomly generated bitstrings that are immature during the tolerization period (negative selection). If it recognizes (matches) any bitstring during tolerization it is rejected and replaced by a new randomly generated detector. If it survives tolerization, it becomes a mature, naïve detector that lives for a certain period of time. If a detector accumulates enough matches m to exceed the activation threshold δ, then it is activated. If the activated detector does not receive co-stimulation, it is rejected (dies). If it receives co-stimulation, then it enters a competition to become a memory detector. Memory detectors have indefinite life spans and require the recognition of a single bitstring, i.e., a single match, to become activated.

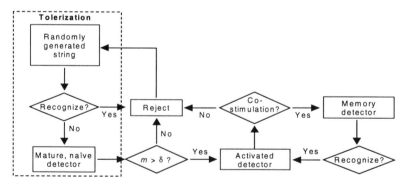

Figure 7.5. Life cycle of a detector. (Note that the negative selection algorithm is embodied in the tolerization period.)

In an attempt to employ another immune property in the AIS the authors proposed the use of so-called *permutation masks* as a way to protect the population of individuals from *holes* in the detection coverage of nonself. A hole corresponds to a nonself string for which no valid detector can be generated. The permutation masks are said to model MHC peptide presentation (Section 2.8), in which different ways of representing peptides on an APC surface increases the probability of a T-cell to recognize an antigen hidden within one of our body cells. The permutation masks are randomly generated and applied to the detectors. This way, the "shape" (attribute string) of the detector is changed, while the shape of the self-set is kept constant. As a consequence, one node in the network graph could fail to detect the intrusion, while another node would succeed.

Table 7.2 summarizes the mapping between the immune system and the artificial immune system for network intrusion detection described in this section.

Table 7.2. Comparison between the immune system and the artificial immune system proposed in Hofmeyr and Forrest (2000).

Immune System	Artificial Immune System
B-cell, T-cell, antibody	Detector represented as a bitstring
Memory cell	Memory detector
Antigen	(Nonself) bitstring
Binding	String matching via the *r*-contiguous bit rule
MHC	Representation parameters
Tolerization	Negative selection algorithm
Co-stimulation: signal one	A match exceeding the activation threshold
Co-stimulation: signal two	Human operator
Cell cloning	Detector replication
Antigenic detection/response	Recognition/response to a nonself bitstring

7.3.4. Performance Evaluation

To evaluate the performance of this AIS, the system was implemented and tested using real data collected on a sub-network of 50 computers at the Computer Science Department of the University of New Mexico. Two data sets were collected: a self-set composed of normal network traffic and a nonself set consisting of traffic generated during network intrusions.

The self set was collected in a period of 50 days, during which a total of 2.3 million TCP connections were logged, each of which is a data-path triple. These 2.3 million data-paths were filtered down to 1.5 million data-paths. The filtering aimed at removing several classes of noisy traffic sources, and after filtering a self set containing 3900 unique bitstrings of length $L = 49$ was defined. The nonself set was comprised of only seven different intrusions.

The results reported correspond to off-line simulations of the network with 50 detection nodes (computers). The elapsed time is reported in days, where one day is equivalent to 25000 time-steps in the simulation. At each time step t, a bitstring was randomly drawn from the set of self-strings.

In summary, the authors adopted the following parameters for the simulation. String length $L = 49$ bits, cross-reactivity threshold $r = 12$ bits, activation threshold $\delta = 10$ matches, match decay period $1/\gamma_{match} = 1$ day, sensitivity decay period $1/\gamma_\omega = 0.1$ day, tolerization period $t = 4$ days, co-stimulation delay $t_s = 1$ day, life expectancy $1/p_{death} = 14$ days, and number of detectors per node $n_d = 100$. All detectors start the simulation as immature detectors and have to survive negative selection (tolerization period) for 30 simulated days of normal (self) traffic. After these 30 days, the AIS was challenged with the intrusion; these were presented one after the other separated by a buffer zone of a simulated day's self traffic.

The authors reported a rate of 1.76 ± 0.2 false positives averaged over the last 20 days. A false positive occurs when a self-string is classified as anomalous (nonself). They argued this value is encouraging, since in the intrusion detection community less than 10 false positives per day is regarded as very low. Finally, the AIS proposed was capable of correctly detecting all the seven intrusions tested.

Related Works from the Authors

Forrest, S. & Hofmeyr, S. A. (2000), "Immunology as Information Processing", In *Design Principles for the Immune System and Other Distributed Autonomous Systems*, I. Cohen & L. A. Segel (Eds.), Oxford University Press, pp. 361-387.

Forrest, S. & Hofmeyr, S. A. (1999), "John Holland's Invisible Hand: An Artificial Immune System", *Presented at the FESTSCHIRIFT for John Holland*.

Forrest, S., Somayaji, A & Ackley, D. H. (1997), "Building Diversity Computer Systems", *Proc. of the 6th Workshop on Hot Topics in Operating Systems*, pp. 67-72.

Forrest, S., Hofmeyr S. A. & Somayaji A. (1997), "Computer Immunology", *Communications of the ACM*, **40**(10), pp. 88-96.

Forrest, S., A. Perelson, Allen, L. & Cherukuri, R. (1994), "Self-Nonself Discrimination in a Computer", *Proc. of the IEEE Symposium on Research in Security and Privacy*, pp. 202-212.

Hofmeyr S. A. & Forrest, S. (2000), "Architecture for an Artificial Immune System", *Evolutionary Computation*, **7**(1), pp. 45-68.

Hofmeyr S. A. & Forrest, S. (1999), "Immunity by Design: An Artificial Immune System", *Proc. of the Genetic and Evolutionary Computation Conference (GECCO'99)*, pp. 1289-1296.

Hofmeyr S. A. (1999), *An Immunological Model of Distributed Detection and its Application to Computer Security*, Ph.D. Thesis, Computer Science Department, University of New Mexico.

7.4   Job-Shop Scheduling

Work in Hart and Ross (1999) described the application of an artificial immune system to a job-shop scheduling problem. In this application, sudden changes in the scheduling environment require rapid production of new schedules. The system operates in two phases. In the first phase, a genetic algorithm is used to detect common patterns among scheduling sequences frequently used by a factory. In the second phase, these common patterns will correspond to the gene segments; these will compose the gene libraries to be used in a bone marrow model to produce new schedules.

7.4.1. Problem Description

The authors argued that data related to scheduling problems of real companies reveal that although deviations in the scheduling process occur, the situations leading to the deviations are often predictable and there are generally known methodologies for dealing with them. Thus, it is reasonable that in many real-life situations a set of historical complete or partial schedules is available for use when trying to reschedule. Additionally, this set of schedules reveals that various patterns occur in subsets of schedules. Based upon this argument, the authors claim that a set of common patterns, or parts of schedules, can be built up using the knowledge encapsulated in past schedules. These patterns could then be utilized as libraries of gene segments (building blocks or gene libraries) to construct new schedules, similarly to the way performed by the immune system.

In the first phase of this AIS, the gene libraries are evolved and stored in order to capture information (common patterns) contained in the past schedules. These are then used, in phase two, to construct new schedules.

The description below assumes the simple scheduling scenario where there are j jobs, each with different arrival dates, due-dates, and processing times, all of which have to be scheduled on a single machine m.

7.4.2. Immune Principles

For this work, two simple ideas are employed from the immune system. The first is that the gene segments to be used in the construction of antibody molecules evolve, so as to capture information about genes that occur with higher frequencies in the antigenic universe. The second idea employed is that the bone marrow combines these gene segments together in order to generate final antibody molecules.

7.4.3. Engineering the AIS

Immune Components and their Representations

An antigen is represented as an integer string of length j in an Integer shape-space, where j is the number of jobs to be scheduled on the machine, with each element of the string corresponding to the identity of a given job to be scheduled.

A gene is a sequence of DNA occupying a given locus in a chromosome. Within this AIS, an Integer shape-space is employed and therefore, a gene segment is represented by a sequence of l integers, where $l \ll j$. A gene is also allowed to contain a don't care symbol "#" which can match any job. The don't care symbol has the advantage that if many of the common job-sequences are shorter than the chosen length l of the gene segment, a partially matching gene segment will have high fitness. The initial population of gene segments is generated randomly, but duplicate jobs are not permitted. Table 7.3 summarizes the metaphors extracted by the authors in the development of their AIS for scheduling.

Table 7.3.   Mapping between the immune system and the artificial immune system proposed in Hart and Ross (1999).

Immune System	Artificial Immune System
Antigen	Sequence of jobs on a particular machine, given a particular scenario
Antigenic universe	Collection of antigens that define a particular scheduling
Gene segment	Short sequence of jobs that is common to more than one schedule
Antibody	Schedule
Matching	Degree of interaction between a gene segment and an antigen, given a particular affinity measure
Match-score	Number of matches between an antigen and an antibody gene

Applying Immune Principles

In order to determine the fitness of the gene segments, which allowed for the evolution of these segments towards the antigens, the authors proposed a variation of the implicit fitness sharing algorithm of Forrest *et al.* (1993) reviewed in Section 6.5. The authors were interested in two features of the gene libraries: overlap (or cross-reactivity) and redundancy (or niche formation). It is important to find patterns (job sequences) that are common to as many schedules as possible (overlap). It is also advantageous to maintain sub-populations of dissimilar genes that recognize the same antigen (redundancy).

The modified implicit fitness-sharing algorithm works as follows:

1. Choose a sample of antigens of size τ at random, without replacement;
2. Choose, without replacement, a random sample of μ gene segments;

3. Determine the affinity of each gene segment in relation to each antigen selected. A match-score is assigned to the gene segment equal to the sum of its affinity with each of the antigens. The affinity measure is described below;

4. The gene segment with highest match-score has its match-score added to its fitness. The fitness of all other gene segments remains fixed;

5. Repeat Steps (1) to (4) for typically three times the number of antigens.

The affinity between a gene segment and an antigen is evaluated by aligning the two strings. If the gene segment is shorter than the antigen, then a match-score is calculated for every possible alignment, and the highest score found corresponds to their affinity. A possible alignment is one in which every gene of the gene segment is aligned with every gene of the antigen. The match-score is calculated by counting the number of matches between the gene segment and the antigen. An exact match contributes to a score of 5, whereas a don't care match contributes to a score of 1, preventing the evolution of gene segments containing all don't care genes. This is illustrated in Figure 7.6.

After evolving the gene segments to compose the gene libraries, the second phase of the algorithm corresponds to the reconstruction of schedules (antibodies) from these libraries. Assume that the gene libraries contain n gene segments and that a minimum of s gene segments is required to generate an antibody (schedule). The role of the AIS is now to recombine genes from the libraries in order to complete the schedules. The inputs to the system are a set of gene segments each of length l and a partial schedule of length $l_p < j$ that has to be completed. Three mechanisms for recombining gene segments are employed:

• *Simple recombination*: a gene segment is selected randomly from the evolved libraries that contain those gene segments in which every job in the segment has not yet been scheduled in the partially completed schedule;

• *Somatic recombination*: a gene segment is selected among those that overlap with the current partially completed schedule. An overlap is said to occur if the first n jobs in the gene segment are equal to the last n jobs in the partially complete schedule, where $n \leq l$, and the remaining $(l - n)$ jobs in the gene segment do not occur in the partial schedule. The partial schedule is thus extended by $(l - n)$ jobs;

• *Single job addition*: a single job can be selected from the set of all jobs that do not occur in any of the gene segments evolved in the previous phase of the algorithm; these are then added to the end of the partial schedule. This allows the construction of a complete schedule when the gene libraries lack an instance of a given job.

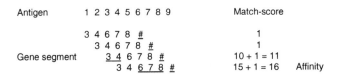

Figure 7.6. Integer encoding for the gene segments and antigens and their affinity measure.

7.4.4. Performance Evaluation

Ten test-scenarios were generated from a base problem containing 15 jobs. Each job has a different arrival date, due date and processing time, with the aim being to minimize the maximal tardiness of a job T_{max}. The test-scenarios were produced by applying a mutation operator with probability 0.2 to each of the arrival dates given in the base problem. The mutation operator randomly changes the arrival date, with the restriction that the new arrival date is at least p_t days before the expected due date, where p_t is the processing time of the job.

Implementation Details

The evolution of the gene libraries in the first phase of the AIS was performed using a genetic algorithm based on GENESIS (Grefenstette, 1984). The recombination of gene segments was done via one of three crossover operators, depending on the relationship between two parent gene segments:

- Order-based crossover (OX): if the parents are permutations of each other, then use the crossover OX;
- 2pt-crossover: if the parents do not have any genes in common, excluding don't cares, and differ from a randomly chosen cross-segment, use 2-point crossover;
- Overlap crossover: used when one of the parents overlaps the other, i.e., have regions in common. In this case, align the matching regions of the parents and read from the left most position. If only one parent has a gene at a given position, use that in the offspring, else select randomly from either parent. Continue reading from left to right until the offspring has the right length. This process is illustrated in Figure 7.7.

A mutation operator is also applied to each offspring gene segment by randomly mutating a gene with probability $1/l$. The authors reported results for a population of 100 gene segments of length $l = 5$ jobs. Thus, the mutation rate corresponds to $p_m = 1/5 = 0.2$. The crossover rate was set to 0.7.

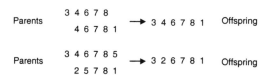

Figure 7.7. Overlap crossover.

Simulation Results

Satisfactory schedules were then evolved using a genetic algorithm for each of the 10 scenarios, and the resulting job-sequences were used as antigens. The 10 resultant antigens defined the antigenic universe.

Results were reported for experiments using gene segments of length $l = 5$, corresponding to 1/3 of the length of an antigen, on one of the $m = 5$ machines. The experiments were performed to identify good settings for three main parameters: the size μ of the samples of gene segments, the antigen sample size τ, and the length of the gene segments l. To simplify the report of results, the authors introduced the concept of binding. A gene segment and an antigen are said to bind if the number of non don't cares in which the antigen and gene segment agree is greater than or equal to a threshold t_m.

As one of the goals of the evolution of gene segments is to evolve diverse segments representing commonly occurring patterns in the antigenic universe, the final population of gene segments evolved by the GA was examined. The results obtained demonstrate that the number of patterns, corresponding to niches of gene segments, decreases as τ increases and increases as μ decreases. It was also verified that for high values of τ a large number of antigens remain unbound, but by setting these three parameters appropriately it is possible to evolve a set of unique gene segments capable of binding to at least one antigen.

To quantify the degree of overlap exhibited by the libraries of gene segments, the authors recorded the number of antigens recognized by each gene segment. The most useful library of gene segments contained segments that have a high degree of general characteristics, i.e., each gene segment recognizes more than one antigen. Additionally, it was verified that more antigens are recognized at high values of τ.

The second phase of the algorithm functions given a partially completed schedule, which may be empty, and a set of gene segments. Gene segments are added to the partial schedules until it either completes an antibody (schedule), or it cannot be extended further by iteratively selecting a gene segment for recombination, with probability p_r for simple recombination, p_{sr} for somatic recombination, and p_a for single job addition.

Considering the case where partial schedules are provided to the system, the authors present results for different lengths of the partial schedules l_p. For $l_p = 7$, 30% of 10 schedules are exactly reconstructed, for $l_p = 8$, 70% of 10 schedules are exactly reconstructed, and for $l_p = 9$, 80% of 10 schedules are exactly reconstructed; all cases averaged over 10 runs.

Related Works from the Authors

Hart, E. & Ross, P. (1999), "The Evolution and Analysis of a Potential Antibody Library for Use in Job-Shop Scheduling", In *New Ideas in Optimization*, D. Corne, M. Dorigo & F. Glover (eds.), McGraw Hill, London, pp. 185-202.

Hart, E., Ross, P. & Nelson, J. (1998), "Producing Robust Schedules Via An Artificial Immune System", *Proc. of the Int. Conference on Evolutionary Computation*, pp. 464-469.

7.5   Data Analysis and Optimization

Chapter 4 and work reviewed in this chapter, make clear the broad applicability of artificial immune systems. It has been shown that the negative selection algorithm is widely used in applications such as anomaly detection, fault diagnosis, and computer security, which are areas far beyond the initial domain in which for which it conceived. Clonal selection has been modeled as an evolutionary-like algorithm to describe the interactions of the elements of the AIS with the environment. In some cases, clonal selection is part of immune network models (continuous and discrete).

This section describes the last case study of this book. To reinforce the idea that the framework proposed in Chapter 3 is generic, the discrete immune network model of de Castro and Von Zuben (2001), originally proposed to perform data compression and clustering, it has been adapted to perform multimodal optimization (de Castro & Timmis, 2002). As the original algorithm was described in Section 3.6, only limited discussion and simulation results for a benchmark problem will be discussed here. However, its adapted version for multimodal function optimization will be fully described, along with an illustration of its performance.

7.5.1. Problem Description

In the case of data analysis, assume a set of unlabeled patterns $\mathbf{X} = \{x_1, x_2, ..., x_M\}$, where each pattern (object, or sample) x_i, $i = 1, ... M$, is described by L variables (attributes or features) in a real-valued space. An immune network can be constructed to answer the following questions: 1) Is there a great amount of redundancy within the data set and, if there is, how can it be reduced? 2) Is there any group or subgroup intrinsic to the data and, if there is, how many are there? and 3) What is the structure or spatial distribution of these data (groups)?

In the multimodal function optimization version of the algorithm assume an objective function $g(\cdot)$ to be optimized, either maximized or minimized. The main goal of the algorithm is to determine and maintain the maximum number of optima solutions possible, including the global optima(l).

7.5.2. Immune Principles

The artificial immune network model to be used is aiNet. This network model employs the clonal selection algorithm CLONALG as a pattern of response to foreign antigens and network interactions to control the number of cells in the network. A full description of the algorithm and immune principles was provided in Section 3.5. However, its main computational steps will be reproduced here, mainly to allow for a comparison with the optimization version. It should be noted that the CLONALG was used as a basis to create an immune network model (aiNet) to perform data clustering – this in itself goes someway to reinforce the generic nature of the AIS framework. To reinforce this even further, aiNet was then taken out of its domain and further adapted for multi-modal optimisation, called opt-aiNet.

7.5.3. Engineering the AIS

Immune Components and their Representations

Each input pattern x_i, $i = 1,...,M$, corresponds to an antigen Ag_i, $i = 1,...,M$, in an Euclidean shape-space. In the data analysis case these are patterns to be recognized and clustered; in the optimization version of the algorithm, each extreme (peak or valley) of the objective function to be optimized is viewed as an antigen and the whole objective function is equivalent to the overall environment in which the network is inserted. As in the biological immune system, the population of immune cells has to be adapted to the whole environment. This means that the AIS has to be capable of detecting all the clusters of antigens (extremes in the case of an optimization application) in the environment.

The aiNet clusters serve as *internal images* responsible for mapping existing clusters in the data set into network clusters. The shape of the spatial distribution of the resulting aiNet antibodies will somehow follow the shape of the data spatial distribution. No distinction between the network cells and their antibodies is made; a cell is equivalent to an antibody and vice-versa. The antigen-antibody (Ag-Ab) and antibody-antibody (Ab-Ab) interactions are quantified via Euclidean distance. The goal is to use this distance metric to generate an antibody repertoire (network) that constitutes the internal image of the antigens to be recognized. The evaluation of the similarity degree among the aiNet antibodies allows the number of antibodies in the network to be controlled. The Ag-Ab affinity is inversely proportional to the distance between them: the smaller the distance, the higher the affinity and vice-versa.

Both, antigens and antibodies are represented as real-valued vectors in an Euclidean shape-space. An aspect that has to be accounted for is the data normalization; antigens and antibodies are normalized over the [0,1] interval. In neither case, (aiNet and opt-aiNet), were the network antibodies encoded as binary strings as in the original version of CLONALG. Instead, they correspond to the normalized real values of the input vectors (data analysis), or real values of the variables of a numerical function to be optimized (multimodal optimization).

Network Structure, Dynamics, and Metadynamics

This artificial immune network model assumes the structure of a *disconnected edge-weighted graph*, composed of a set of *nodes*, called *antibodies* (Ab), and sets of node pairs called *edges* with an assigned number called *weight*, or *connection strength* ($s_{i,j}$), associated with each connected edge.

In order to compare the original version of the aiNet learning algorithm with its optimization version, the algorithm described in Section 3.5 will be reproduced here followed by its modified optimization version.

Original aiNet learning algorithm for data analysis:

1. *Initialization*: create an initial random population of network antibodies;
2. *Antigenic presentation*: for each antigenic pattern, do:

    2.1 *Clonal selection and expansion*: for each network element, determine its affinity with the antigen presented. Select a number of high affinity elements and reproduce (clone) them proportionally to their affinity;

    2.2 *Affinity maturation*: mutate each clone inversely proportional to affinity. Re-select a number of highest affinity clones and place them into a clonal memory set;

    2.3 *Clonal interactions*: determine the network interactions (affinity) among all the elements of the clonal memory set;

    2.4 *Clonal suppression*: eliminate those memory clones whose affinity is less than a pre-specified threshold;

    2.5 *Metadynamics*: eliminate all memory clones whose affinity with the antigen is less than a pre-defined threshold;

    2.6 *Network construction*: incorporate the remaining clones of the clonal memory with all network antibodies;

3. *Network interactions*: determine the affinity (degree of similarity) between each pair of network antibodies;

4. *Network suppression*: eliminate all network antibodies whose affinity is less than a pre-specified threshold;

5. *Diversity*: introduce a number of new randomly generated antibodies into the network;

6. *Cycle*: repeat Steps 2 to 4 until a pre-specified number of iterations is reached.

The optimization version of the aiNet learning algorithm, proposed in (de Castro & Timmis, 2002), can be described as follows:

1. *Initialization*: create an initial random population of network antibodies;

2. *Local search*: while stopping criterion (see below) is not met, do:

    2.1 *Clonal expansion*: for each network antibody, determine its fitness (an objective function to be optimized) and normalize the vector of fitnesses. Generate a *clone* for each antibody, i.e., a set of antibodies which are the exact copies of their parent antibody;

    2.2 *Affinity maturation*: mutate each clone inversely proportionally to the fitness of its parent antibody that is kept unmutated. The mutation follows Equation (7.7). For each mutated clone, select the antibody with highest fitness, and calculate the average fitness of the selected antibodies;

    2.3 *Local convergence*: if the average fitness of the population does not vary significantly from one iteration to the other, go to the next step; else, return to Step 2;

3. *Network interactions*: determine the affinity (similarity) between each pair of network antibodies;

4. *Network suppression*: eliminate all network antibodies whose affinity is less than a pre-specified threshold, and determine the number of remaining antibodies in the network; these are named memory antibodies;

5. *Diversity*: introduce a number of new randomly generated antibodies into the network and return to Step 2;

In this algorithm, a network antibody corresponds to an individual of the population represented as a real-valued attribute string in a Euclidean shape-space. The fitness of an antibody corresponds to the value of the objective function when evaluated for this cell. The affinity between two antibodies corresponds to their Euclidean distance. A clone is equivalent to the offspring antibodies that are the children of a single antibody; they are originally identical to the parent antibody but suffer somatic mutation so that they become slight variations of their parent antibody. The fitness proportional mutation of Step 2.2 is performed according to the following expression:

$$c' = c + \alpha N(0,1),$$
$$\alpha = (1/\beta) \exp(-f^*),$$
(7.7)

where c' is a mutated antibody c, $N(0,1)$ is a Gaussian random variable of zero mean and standard deviation $\sigma = 1$, β is a parameter that controls the decay of the inverse exponential function, and f^* is the fitness of an individual normalized in the interval [0,1]. A mutation is only accepted if the mutated antibody c' is within its range of domain. Figure 7.8 depicts the fitness proportional function α for $\beta = 100$ used in the experiments. Note that this equation is based upon a Gaussian mutation that accounts for the fitness proportional mutation, as discussed in Section 3.6.

The stopping criterion adopted for the algorithm is based upon the cardinality of the memory population. After the network suppression, a fixed number of cells remains and if this number does not vary from one suppression to the other, then the network is said to have stabilized and the remaining cells are all memory cells corresponding to the solutions of the problem. Although this strategy seems rather empirical, the authors claim that simulation results demonstrated its effectiveness for the problems tested.

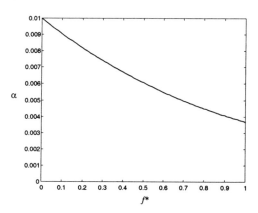

Figure 7.8. Function that performs the fitness proportional mutation.

7.5.4. Performance Evaluation

There are major differences between the data analysis and the optimization versions of aiNet (see the section on "Some Remarks"). In the data analysis case, the following parameters have to be set by the user: n_1 – number of highest affinity antibodies to be selected (Step 2.1); n_2 – number of highest affinity antibodies to be selected after the affinity maturation process (Step 2.2); σ_s – suppression threshold (Steps

2.4 and 4); and d – number of newcomer antibodies (Step 5). In the multimodal optimization version of aiNet there is no selection, all antibodies generate a clone of same size; $n_2 = 1$, which means that the best offspring antibody is selected to replace its parent; and a number of clones Nc is generated per each selected antibody.

The performance of both versions of the algorithm will be illustrated using benchmark tasks. The training parameters adopted for the data analysis problem were: $n_1 = 4$, $n_2 = 10\%$, $d = 10$, and $\sigma_s = 0.02$. In the optimization version, the authors adopted the following parameters: $d = 40\%$, $\sigma_s = 0.1$, $N_0 = 20$ (initial population size), $\beta = 100$, and $Nc = 10$ – number of clones for each antibody.

Data Analysis

After training the aiNet using the algorithm described above, the resultant network of antibodies represent internal images of the antigens to which they are exposed. This implies that the same shape-space representation for antibodies and antigens has to be employed. As a consequence, visualizing the network for antigens (and antibodies) of length greater than 3 can become a difficult task and consequently, interpreting the final network is also difficult. To alleviate this problem, the authors suggested the use of hierarchical clustering and graph theoretical techniques to interpret the generated network.

The *minimal spanning tree* (MST) of a graph was used as a mechanism to search for the network structure. A tree is a *spanning tree* of a graph if it is a subgraph containing all the vertices of the graph. A minimal spanning tree of a graph is a spanning tree with minimum weight, where the weight of a tree is defined as the sum of the weights of its constituent edges.

After tracing the MST among the resultant network cells there is the problem of deleting edges from an MST so that the resulting connected sub-trees correspond to the observable clusters. These network clusters are mirrors of the clusters existing in the input data set. The following criterion is used: an MST edge (i,k) whose weight $s_{i,k}$ is significantly larger than the average of nearby edge weights on both sides of the edge (i,k) is deleted. This edge is called inconsistent. In the present application, the weight of an edge is considered significantly larger than the average of nearby edge weights on both sides of the edge when the ratio r between $s_{i,k}$ and the respective averages is greater than or equal to 2 ($r \geq 2$).

Consider the data set illustrated in Figure 7.9(a) used to evaluate a hierarchical self-organizing map (Costa & Netto, 2001). It aims at demonstrating that even in the presence of very different pattern structures, the aiNet plus MST is capable of reducing redundancy, and detecting and separating clusters. The number of patterns in each class (1 to 8) is 314, 100, 100, 100, 100, 10, 53 and 57 respectively. Classes 2 to 5 were generated by multivariate Gaussian probability distributions. Class 2 is completely enclosed by a circular cluster (class 1). Class 1 is connected to class 5 by a bridge, class 6, which is a chain of intermediate objects. Note that this bridge is not usually regarded as a cluster by a human observer, as can be seen in Figure 7.9(b) that presents a possible conceptualization of the data set of Figure 7.9(a). Although the data set is labeled in the picture, the aiNet learning algorithm is unsupervised, thus the network is presented with the unlabeled data.

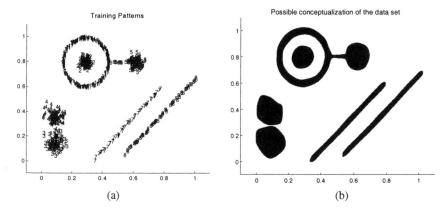

Figure 7.9. Multi-structured benchmark task. (a) Discrete data set with labeled input classes. The input data is taken to be unlabelled. (b) Possible conceptualization of the data set presented in (a).

Out of the 834 patterns, the resultant aiNet contained only 157 antibodies, what corresponds to a compression rate of 81.81%. The algorithm was also capable of detecting the main clusters in the data set, but due to the bridge (class 6) between clusters 1 and 5 it could not separate them. The significance ratio employed was $r = 1.8$. The result presented in Figure 7.10 is consistent with the possible conceptualization proposed for the data set in Figure 7.9(b) where clusters 1, 5 and 6 are fused together.

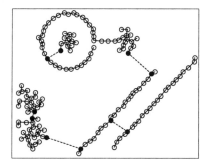

Figure 7.10. Resultant MST traced over all the cells positioned by the aiNet learning algorithm. The dark cells, whose links are dashed lines, correspond to those cells separated by the method presented.

Optimization

The Multi function, described by Equation (7.8), was originally used by de Castro and Von Zuben (2000) to evaluate the performance of CLONALG when applied to multimodal function optimization tasks.

$$g(x,y) = x.sin(4\pi x) - y.sin(4\pi y + \pi) + 1, \quad\quad\quad (7.8)$$

where $x,y \in [-2,2]$.

In (de Castro & Timmis, 2002), the authors used the Multi function, among others, to evaluate the performance of their optimization version of the aiNet learning algorithm. Figure 7.11 illustrates the behavior of the algorithm along the search process. Figure 7.11(a) depicts the initial repertoire of 20 antibodies (dark stars in the picture – only a few of them can be seen, because the others are hidden behind some hills).

Figure 7.11(b) illustrates the initial repertoire after the local search of Step 2 has been performed. Note that all the antibodies are located in a local optimum of the function. As the average fitness of the repertoire does not vary significantly (a variance less than 0.001) from one iteration to the other, a local convergence is assumed and new antibodies are allowed to be inserted into the repertoire. Figure 7.11(c) depicts the antibody repertoire after the fourth local convergence, corresponding to iteration 115. Note that the number of local optima determined has increased significantly from the first local convergence. Figure 7.11(d) depicts the final repertoire of antibodies after thirteen local convergences, and a total number of 366 iteration steps. It is important to note that the algorithm converges automatically according to the two proposed stopping criteria: one for the local convergence that evaluates the stability of the average fitness and the global convergence that evaluates the stability of the number of antibodies in the repertoire. In Figure 7.11(c) there is a total of 45 antibodies in the repertoire, while the final population in Figure 7.11(d) there are 58 antibodies.

Figure 7.12(a) illustrates the behavior of the fitness of the best antibody in the repertoire (solid line) and the average fitness of the repertoire (dashed line). Figure 7.12(b) depicts how the number of memory antibodies increases over the local searches performed by the algorithm. Note that when the number of antibodies in the network stabilizes, the algorithm is said to have converged and the iterative process of adaptation is halted.

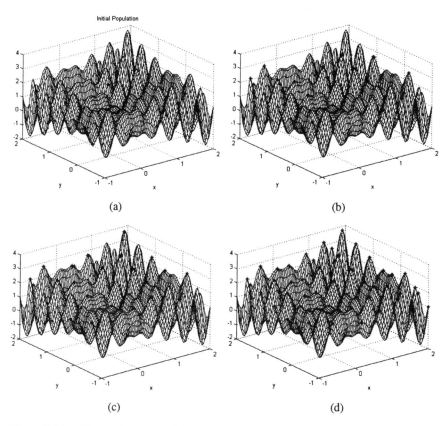

Figure 7.11. The performance of the optimization version of aiNet in the Multi function. (a) Initial repertoire. (b) Antibody repertoire after the first local convergence at iteration 35. (c) Antibody repertoire after the fourth local convergence at iteration 115. (d) Final antibody repertoire after the global convergence at iteration 366.

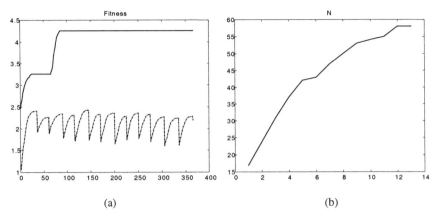

(a)   (b)

Figure 7.12.   Fitness and number of memory antibodies. (a) Fitness of the best individual
of the repertoire (solid line), and average fitness of the repertoire (dashed
line). (b) Number of memory antibodies along the thirteen local searches.

7.5.5. Some Remarks

By comparing the data analysis and the optimization versions of the aiNet learning
algorithm, it is possible to note several major differences. First, in the optimization
algorithm there is no antigen population to be recognized, instead there is an objective function to be optimized. Each antibody in the network corresponds to a candidate variable of this function. The cyclic process of Step 2 corresponds to a local
search evolutionary strategy, in which candidate solutions are reproduced and mutated based upon their fitness. There is no selection for reproduction, all antibodies
in the network are allowed to reproduce and have the same number of offspring.
This is one main characteristic of the multimodal capability of this algorithm, individual antibodies have the same probability of reproducing, thus of exploiting their
surroundings. A criterion to evaluate the convergence of the population of antibodies to local optima is proposed based on the variability of the average fitness of the
best antibodies at each generation within Step 2. Note also the existence of fitness
and affinity measures in this version of the algorithm. This fitness was responsible
for evaluating the individuals according to the external environment (function to be
optimized), and the affinity corresponded to the network interactions that controls
the number of antibodies in the network. Finally, a network is never constructed;
affinity is used for parsimony purposes only.

Any reader familiar with evolution strategies, ES, (Schwefel, 1965) would
promptly notice a number of similarities between these two approaches. The authors
(de Castro & Timmis, 2002) presented a philosophical comparison between these
algorithms. The selection mechanism of opt-aiNet can be equated to the $(\mu + \lambda)$-ES,
where μ parents generate λ offspring, which are reduced again to μ parents. The
selection operates on the joined set of parents and offspring, and parents can survive
until they are superseded by one of their offspring. In opt-aiNet, $\mu = N$ (the whole

population) and $\lambda = Nc$. Both strategies employ Gaussian mutation, with the difference that opt-aiNet has an affinity proportional Gaussian mutation with fixed standard deviation, while ES might use a fixed or time variant standard deviation and is not proportional to fitness. Another major difference between the two strategies is that opt-aiNet has a dynamic adjustment of the population size through metadynamics (diversity introduction) and network suppression, while ESs have a static number of individuals in the population.

7.6   Chapter Summary

The goal of this chapter was to explore four applications of AIS in more depth. The motivation for this was to provide the reader with a more detailed view of the possibilities of employing the immune metaphor and how the framework proposed can be used to design and understand artificial immune systems. Through these, it is possible to explain, in relatively simple terms, the metaphors employed and the approach adopted for building the AIS.

The applications chosen reflect four different immune algorithms: continuous immune networks, negative selection, bone marrow, and discrete immune networks. Through the investigation of these case studies, it has been possible to see how people have taken simple immune algorithms, usefully mapped them into the domain under investigation and produced powerful and feasible AIS. It is not only the immune algorithms that are important; representation and interaction also need to be considered. Here, varying types of shape-spaces have been used, ranging from Integer to Symbolic, with their associated affinity measures. Table 7.4 summarizes the case studies reviewed.

Table 7.4.   Summary of the case studies in the light of the proposed framework.

	Robotics	Network Intrusion	Scheduling	Data Analysis/ Optimization
Shape-space	Symbolic	Hamming	Integer	Euclidean
Main components	Antibodies	B-cell, T-cell	Antibody	B-cell (Antibody)
Algorithms	Continuous network	Negative selection	Bone marrow	Discrete network
Affinity measure	String match	r-contiguous bit	String match	Euclidean distance

Hopefully, this chapter has revealed to the reader the broad applicability of the immune approach. In addition, the view can be taken that although these immune algorithms were conceived in a particular domain, it is possible to assume these algorithms as generic and therefore apply them in domains for which they were not envisaged. This was exemplified in the adaptation of the discrete immune network model, which was originally proposed for machine learning and data analysis and subsequently applied to multimodal optimization.

References

Costa, J. A. F. & Netto, M. L. A. (2001), "Clustering of Complex Shaped Data Sets via Kohonen Maps and Mathematical Morphology", In *Data Mining and Knowledge Discovery: Theory, Tools, and Technology III*, B. Dasarathy (ed.). *Proc. of SPIE*, **4384**, pp. 16-27.

de Castro, L.N & Timmis, J. (2002), "An Artificial Immune Network for Multimodal Optimization", In *2002 Congress on Evolutionary Computation. Part of the 2002 IEEE World Congress on Computational Intelligence*. pp, 699-704.

de Castro, L. N. & Von Zuben, F. J. (2001), "aiNet: An Artificial Immune Network for Data Analysis", In *Data Mining: A Heuristic Approach*, H. A. Abbass, R. A. Sarker, and C. S. Newton (eds.), Idea Group Publishing, USA, Chapter XII, pp. 231-259.

de Castro, L. N. & Von Zuben, F. J. (2000), "The Clonal Selection Algorithm with Engineering Applications", *Proc. of the Genetic and Evolutionary Computation Conference*, Workshop on Artificial Immune Systems and Their Applications, pp. 36-37.

Farmer, J. D., Packard, N. H. & Perelson, A. S. (1986), "The Immune System, Adaptation, and Machine Learning", *Physica 22D*, pp. 187-204.

Forrest, S., Javornik, B., Smith, R. E. & Perelson, A. S. (1993), "Using Genetic Algorithms to Explore Pattern Recognition in the Immune System", *Evolutionary Computation*, **1**(3), pp. 191-211.

Grefenstette, J. (1984), "GENESIS: A System for Using Genetic Search Procedures", *Proc. of a Conference on Intelligent Systems and Machines*, pp. 161-165.

Hart, E. & Ross, P. (1999), "An Immune System Approach to Scheduling in Changing Environments", *Proc. of the Genetic and Evolutionary Computation Conference*, pp. 1559-1566.

Hofmeyr S. A. & Forrest, S. (2000), "Architecture for an Artificial Immune System", *Evolutionary Computation*, **7**(1), pp. 45-68.

Ishiguro, A. Watanabe, Y., Kondo, T., Shirai, Y. & Uchikawa, Y. (1996), "Immunoid: A Robot with a Decentralized Behavior Arbitration Mechanisms Based on the Immune System", *Proc. of the ICMAS Workshop on Immunity-Based Systems*, pp. 82-92.

Schwefel, H. –P. (1965), *Kybernetische Evolutionals Strategie der Experimentellen Forschung in der Stromungstechnik*, Diploma Thesis, Technical University of Berlin.

Varela, F. J. & Coutinho, A. (1991), "Second Generation Immune Networks", *Imm. Today*, **12**(5), pp. 159-166.

Watanabe, Y., Ishiguro, A. & Uchikawa, Y. (1999), "Decentralized Behavior Arbitration Mechanism For Autonomous Mobile Robots Using Immune Network", In *Artificial Immune Systems and Their Applications*, D. Dasgupta (ed.), Springer-Verlag, pp. 187-209.

Chapter 8

Conclusions and Future Trends

The best scientists are their own most severe critics

– I. J. Deary

8.1 Introduction

As is probably apparent, the field of AIS is large and at times quite complex, both in terms of application and inspiration. Certainly, for a novice to immunology, sometimes it can appear quite frightening! With this in mind, we tried to make this new and exciting field of research as accessible as possible. It is our hope that this book has excited you about the field by giving new insights, blowing away some misconceptions maybe reinforcing others, and going some way to develop an understanding of how to build your own AIS or develop new algorithms and representations.

The book started with the following set of questions: "What is an artificial immune system? Where have they been used? What are they for? How can I design my own artificial immune system? What is the difference between an artificial immune system and other computational intelligence paradigms? Is the immune system isolated from other bodily systems? Why artificial immune systems behave the way they do?" Hopefully, the thread of the book has been one that answers these questions. In this final chapter, we will take a reflective look at the material we have covered in this book and point some ways forward with more questions and observations for the future.

This chapter is organized as follows. Section 8.2 presents a general overview of the whole book. Section 8.3 argues why AIS are indeed a new computational intelligence approach, and in Section 8.4 we try to assess the new paradigm of artificial immune systems by discussing their usefulness and presenting a critical overview of them. Section 8.5 suggests several new research trends for AIS, from the proposal of new algorithms to be developed to ways of extending the framework we introduced in Chapter 3. Section 8.6 presents some criticisms about the book itself and how it was written. The book is concluded in Section 8.7 with a brief discussion about the importance of having a multidisciplinary research, some of the topics covered in the text, and the benefits of using biology as inspiration to the development of computational intelligence systems.

8.2 A General Overview

The first chapter's objective was familiarizing the reader with the idea of using biology as inspiration for doing computation. We talked about the reasons why one might consider biology to be a good metaphor for computation. It may be that you are already familiar with bio-inspired computing and so need very little convincing. However, you may have come from a different background and so do need some convincing. We highlighted such areas as the development of bullet proof vests and Velcro as two examples of manufactured items inspired by biology. It also has to be said that biology seems to do a very good job in maintaining life and is good at solving problems, such as fighting against diseases. Therefore, the argument is simple, if biology is good at maintaining life and solving problems, can we somehow capture some of those processes and use them as sources of inspiration for the development of computational systems?

Some thought was also given to the nature of interdisciplinary research. By undertaking work in AIS, you are experimenting a little with the word of biology, in particular immunology. How much immunology do you need to know? That depends on what you want to do. If you want to simply use the ideas of the framework to construct an AIS, then not that much, just an awareness of what the processes are and what they are used for may be sufficient. However, if you wish to develop your own immune algorithms, for example, then a deeper understanding is required. If one can see the immune system as a kind of computational system, then it is not so difficult to make the jump from the biological to the artificial world.

We then followed with Chapter 2. Here we presented the basic concepts of the immune system on a high-level, from an information processing perspective. This chapter is needed to provide an understanding of where the inspiration for the AIS originated and an appreciation of the fact that when developing immune algorithms it is necessary to have a reasonable understanding of what is going on in the biological system. During the survey of the research papers on AIS, we found, in places, inaccuracies of immune system understanding, such as authors suggesting the clonal expansion of B-cells involving the crossing over of genetic material. The focus of the chapter was on what we felt was useful immunology and importantly, the immunological concepts that have been used to develop AIS. Very little was said about other properties of the immune system, some of which will be explored in the development of AIS.

When discoursing about the development of AIS, it was important to understand which features of the immune system are worth considering to create simple, yet useful systems. Chapter 3 began by highlighting some of these features, such as distributability, adaptability, diversity, and so on. Artificial immune systems were defined as adaptive systems inspired by theoretical immunology and observed immune functions, principles, and models, which are applied to problem solving. This definition draws a fine line between the pure theoretical models in immunology and algorithms in AIS: one of being their rationales. The field of AIS has not only borrowed a number of ideas and models from theoretical immunology, but it also borrowed its name. While discussing some landmarks on the development of AIS, the first paper to use the terminology of AIS was by the theoretical immunology community. Maybe they were more accurate in using AIS as an expression to name a model of the immune system than we are in using it as a description of applied computational systems inspired by the immune system. Nevertheless, AIS seems to be the name that has been adopted by the field and once a name has been established, it is very hard to change it. Other alternatives are immune-based systems and immunological computation, and certainly other books will follow this one addressing the same subject but may choose to adopt an alternative, maybe more accurate, name for the field.

Once the necessary immunology had been discussed, we then moved onto the idea of AIS themselves. In order to explain AIS, we proposed a framework with which one could both describe and build an AIS. The philosophy of the proposed framework for artificial immune systems is simple in nature. First, one is faced with the application domain. This will have an impact on the type of representation for the components of the system (shape-space) and also the type of algorithm to be used. Within the framework, there are a variety of shape-spaces. These were reviewed from the literature and extended for the creation of abstract models of immune cells and molecules. Simple shape-spaces assume that the portions of the immune cells and molecules responsible for their interactions with each other and the environment can be represented as attribute strings. These strings correspond not only to the "shapes" of the molecules, but also to everything that is necessary to quantify the immune interactions (e.g., electrical charges and chemical interactions). We claimed that a 'shape' could be abstractly viewed as anything that might correspond to the binding portions of an immune cell or molecule. This could be a symbolic attribute string (Symbolic shape-space), an amino-acid sequence (DNA shape-space), a mixture of some of them (Messy shape-space), and others. We then moved onto outline a number of immune algorithms that are present in the literature and presented them as generic algorithms, rather than the specific domain algorithms they were created as. There have been a number of immune system processes abstracted for AIS: lymphocyte receptor production (bone marrow models), negative selection, clonal selection, and immune networks. Chapter 3 then followed with some general guidelines for engineering AIS. The use of the guidelines was illustrated with a simple example of two AIS applied to a pattern recognition problem. It was also argued that these guidelines (when employed with the framework) show some flexibility, illustrated in Chapters 4 and 7 with different applications being surveyed and case studies described using only slight variations of the general steps of the guidelines. The framework also allows for easy incorporation of new representations, algorithms, and domain-specific knowledge into the algorithms. For example, one could include the use of multiple-contiguous bit affinity measures that account for sequence of attributes in the input patterns.

According to our proposed definition and "birth date" for AIS, the field is now around 15 years old. In its early years, there were a small number of publications and a slowly increasing recognition of the field. However, the last five years have seen a burst of interest within research communities and industrial parties for the study and application of AIS. Even so, we estimate that the number of published works on AIS (not including pure immunology) is around two hundred, and may well double in the next couple of years. An attempt was made to survey the whole field in Chapters 4 and 6, with the survey being based on the perspective of artificial immune systems as proposed in Chapter 3. The main research schools, application domains, and authors were identified, with at least one of their works being reviewed. Further reading was provided, including papers in languages other than English and those we could not locate but of whose existence we were aware. The rationale of this chapter was not to undertake an in-depth analysis of each application, but rather to alert the reader to the kind of work being studied within AIS and emphasize the generality of AIS, which is exemplified with the diverse range of application domains. If we have missed anyone in this review, then we offer our sincere apologies.

Attention was then turned back to the biology in Chapter 5 by reviewing the fundamentals of the nervous and endocrine systems. An attempt was made to place the immune system in context with both these systems and to draw out some of their similarities and differences. The motivation for this chapter was to provide some biological background for the discussion on neural networks, evolutionary algorithms, and other topics covered in Chapter 6. Additionally, we believe that by discussing the interactions of these systems it was possible to see how it makes sense to bring together different biological inspired techniques to interact for the development of novel hybrid paradigms. Topics such as the Baldwin effect, species and niches, coevolution and predator-prey interactions were also discussed. These discussions were important as they provided explanations as to some of the behaviors of the immune system and, thus, artificial immune systems.

We first argued the fact that an adaptive immune response follows the same evolutionary pattern of a neo-Darwinian theory of evolution. This is one reason why it might be sometimes difficult to find differences between an artificial immune system and an evolutionary algorithm. There is however, one important conceptual difference residing in the fact that in an evolutionary algorithm the theory of evolution is used as the metaphor for its implementation. In an artificial immune system, by contrast, an immune principle (e.g., clonal selection) is used to generate an immune algorithm that can be characterized as an evolutionary algorithm. Thus, in the latter approach, evolution is used to explain how the system behaves not as an inspiration to develop the system. Work has seemed to indicate that although these approaches may at first seem similar, they perform slightly differently. Two other aspects were also discussed concerning the immune system and evolutionary biology. It was argued that the immune system might contribute to natural selection by reducing the survival probabilities of those individuals whose survival compromises the life of other members of the species. Secondly, the immune system was demonstrated to be capable of maintaining stable sub-populations of cells and molecules that cover a wide range of different antigenic patterns. This way, the immune system has a natural capacity of identifying and maintaining diverse species of cells and molecules. Therefore, one could argue that it is not surprising that immune system models have been successful in the development and maintenance of diverse populations of individuals covering most of the peaks of an affinity landscape.

Chapter 5 concluded with a discussion of immune cognition. Immune cognition was divided into two perspectives. The first one corresponded to the viewpoint that the immune system is a cognitive system that involves the search for a context (when to act), the signal extraction from noise (how to focus), and a response (what to do). The immune properties of recognition, response, learning, and memory were regarded as its most important cognitive characteristics. The second perspective on immune cognition posed it as an indispensable system for complementing nervous cognition. This is due to the fact that without the immune system, our organisms would not be capable of detecting non-physiologic stimuli, such as viruses and bacteria. The nervous system receives the physiologic stimuli from our physiologic sensors (hearing, sight, smell, taste, and touch), while the immune system converts some non-physiologic stimuli into "signals" that can be perceived by the nervous system. As an outcome, AIS that involve basic cognitive processing like recognition, learning, and memory can be classified as cognitive in the same way neural networks are sometimes addressed as cognitive models of the brain.

This book would not have been complete without a comparison of AIS with other computational intelligence paradigms. In order to achieve this, Chapter 6 presented the fundamentals of neural networks, evolutionary algorithms, case-based reasoning, classifier systems, DNA computing, and fuzzy systems with the primary focus being on the first two approaches. Artificial immune systems were divided into population-based and network models, with similarities and differences between AIS, ANN and EA being presented. In our opinion, AIS possess great potential for being integrated with the different paradigms in order to improve the practical applicability of individual approaches. Indeed, some work has already begun on this, and hybrid approaches in the literature were reviewed, complementing the survey list of Chapter 4. Some aspects concerning the practical implementation of neural networks and evolutionary algorithms were discussed as the hybrids reviewed in this chapter were proposed as ways of overcoming these limitations or improving the performance of the original algorithms.

Finally, four case studies were carefully chosen and presented in order to illustrate some aspects of AIS and the book itself. As stated earlier, Chapter 4 could not provide great depth, so to overcome this, Chapter 7 was provided. Here we emphasized the interdisciplinary characteristic of the field by reviewing works applied to a number of different areas: robotics, computer security, data analysis, optimization, and scheduling. The discussion was based on the framework introduced for the design of AIS, and the case studies were described in full, including some simulation results.

8.3   AIS as a New Computational Intelligence Approach

In the summer of 1956, on the campus of Dartmouth College in Hanover, New Hampshire, scholars gathered together in order to discuss the possibilities of creating computer programs that could behave or think like human beings, i.e., with "intelligence". Among the participants, some of them came to play leading roles in the development of the field of Artificial Intelligence, such as John McCarthy (who is considered to have coined the term AI), Marvin Minsky, Herbert Simon, and Allen Newell.

The development of AI did not come in isolation. It happened only a few weeks before the symposium "Cerebral Mechanisms in Behavior," which is said to have given rise to the cognitive sciences (Section 5.7). It was interesting to note that these symposia had some participants and ideas in common. While the cognitive sciences were mostly concerned with the analysis of human knowledge and intelligence, the field of AI was interested in their synthesis.

In this section we do not intend to discuss every stream of artificial intelligence. Instead, we shall focus on the origins of two of the most predominant artificial intelligence paradigms in computer science: expert systems and neural networks. Our aim at discussing the origins of AI is mainly to place it in context with the so-called computational intelligence, which was briefly introduced in Chapter 1. This will then go to give support to our claim that artificial immune systems are not only a novel computational intelligence paradigm, but also a novel soft-computing paradigm.

By the time of the Dartmouth summer school, Newell and Simon had already developed a program, named Logic Theorist (LT), which could manipulate symbolic expressions in order to prove theorems in logic. The LT was developed in a top-down manner, i.e., by looking at how humans solve problems and trying to "program" these problem-solving procedures into a computer. For instance, among the methods used by the LT are substitution of expressions and syllogistic reasoning such as "if *a* implies *b*", and "if *b* implies *c*", then "*a* implies *c*". In further research, these scientists tried the more ambitious goal of developing a 'General Problem Solver' (GPS), which was also based on a top-down approach. A key notion of this type of paradigm, known as a knowledge-based or expert system, is the existence of a knowledge base or production system containing a great deal of knowledge about a given task provided by an expert. In these systems, an action is taken if a certain specific condition is met. A set of these production systems result in an 'intelligent' system capable of inferring an action based on a set of input conditions. Knowledge-based systems were rooted on a philosophy inspired by cognitive theories of the information processes involved in problem solving. With a different perspective, the emerging field of artificial neural networks (Section 6.2) was inspired by the theories of neural information processing, i.e., how the nervous system works. Artificial neural networks, in contrast to knowledge-based systems, constitute a bottom-up approach in which the processing of information is performed by a set of interconnected "artificial neural units" that receive and process environmental stimuli. The network outcome "emerges" from the collective action of network neurons.

After a number of early attempts to develop systems capable of solving a wide range of problems, scientists realized some of the limitations of their approaches and research became more focused on goal-directed problem solving, instead of the development of general problem solvers or complete models of nervous cognition. In the mid sixties, new systems started being developed by looking at some forms of "intelligent behavior" other than human brains and also by trying to model the uncertainties of the natural language. As results, evolutionary algorithms (Section 6.3) and fuzzy systems (Section 6.6) were developed. Even more recently, in the mid nineties, algorithms inspired by the social behavior of insects (Bonabeau *et al.*, 1999) and the simulation of social processes (Kennedy *et al.*, 2001) have been developed; these are termed *swarm intelligence*.

Some of the disagreements between the traditional knowledge-based artificial intelligence paradigms and mainly neural networks were a result of disputes for funding, and individual lack of success in providing their promised end results. For instance, leading figures in traditional AI, such as Marvin Minsky and Seymour Papert published a book (Minsky & Papert, 1968) demonstrating the limitations of one of the first neural network models, known as a *perceptron*, introduced by Frank Rosenblatt. This resulted in an almost complete cessation of funding for research on artificial neural networks for around twenty years. This continued until Rumelhart and collaborators released their book on parallel-distributed processors (Rumelhart *et al.*, 1986). They demonstrated ways of overcoming the limitations of the perceptrons by reviewing the error backpropagation algorithm.

After this, there was a desire to dissociate the research on neural networks from that on knowledge-based systems. The older paradigms based mainly on symbolic, top-down, processing remained as artificial intelligence, while the newer paradigms of neural networks, evolutionary computation, and fuzzy systems composed the younger field of *computational intelligence* (CI). As with every new field (and also several well-established fields), the definition of CI is not unique. It varies among authors and a consensus is not usually agreed upon. In Chapter 1 we defined computational intelligence in the light of Fogel's definition (Fogel, 2000) as being composed of those systems capable of adapting their behavior to the environment in order to solve a particular problem. Note that by paying careful attention to this definition, one realizes that fuzzy systems do not fit into this classification of a CI paradigm. Fuzzy systems are reasoning systems based upon fuzzy logic (Section 6.6). There is no inherent adaptation in fuzzy systems; it constitutes a novel paradigm to compute with imprecise and linguistic information - a new form of computing (reasoning). Nevertheless, fuzzy systems do allow computers to reason (solve problems) more flexibly, in a way that resembles more our own information processing capabilities. Reasoning with imprecise information is one of our most remarkable capabilities, thus fuzzy systems do constitute a computational intelligence paradigm, even if not presenting adaptation.

Artificial immune systems as a field of research is much younger than all these others with the exception of the swarm paradigm proposed in the mid nineties. We traced its origins to the year 1986 with the publication of Farmer's paper (Farmer *et al.*, 1986) on adaptation and machine learning based on an immune network model. We defined AIS as adaptive systems inspired by theoretical immunology and the immune system aiming at problem solving. We could have simply defined AIS as adaptive systems inspired by the immune system, but we wanted to alert the readers about the existence of the already mature field of research on theoretical immunology, which is distinct from AIS for its rationale. Note that our definition of AIS adds an immune inspiration to the concept of computational intelligence, and therefore allows it to be classified as such.

However, it is our opinion that artificial immune systems are not restricted to being a computational intelligence paradigm. The term soft computing (SC) was coined by Lotfi Zadeh to describe computational systems capable of dealing with imprecise, uncertain, and partial information. Initially composed of only fuzzy systems, SC soon embraced other computational intelligence paradigms, such as neural networks and evolutionary algorithms. Its scope now focuses on the combination of one or more of these paradigms in order to create hybrid systems capable of providing better solutions to problems. In light of this, artificial immune systems can be said to have almost emerged as a soft-computing paradigm. In the paper by Farmer and collaborators, an extensive comparison was made between an immune network model and learning classifier systems (which can also be considered as belonging to SC), though no real integration of these approaches was ever performed. Chapter 6 of this book serves to illustrate that AIS are (and can be) related to and hybridized with many other soft computing approaches in several ways.

When addressing the concept of adaptability, the potential of artificial immune systems is remarkable. By their very nature, AIS can account for double plastic mechanisms of adaptation, namely dynamics and metadynamics. The immune system extracts information from the environment by altering the number of individual cells and molecules in the repertoire (metadynamics) and also by altering their genetic composition (dynamics). By having taken inspiration from the immune system, a great number of artificial immune systems are naturally composed of populations of individuals with varying sizes and attributes.

Compared with other computational intelligence approaches, the distinction between AIS and evolutionary algorithms is sharp. For example, AIS can be population or network-based; they can also present an evolutionary or learning (or a mixture of both) type of adaptation. In Section 6.4 we highlighted a number of similarities and differences between AIS, neural networks, and evolutionary algorithms. Together with Sections 3.5 and 7.5 we discussed that although some AIS might share a number of similarities with other strategies, they still differ for their source of inspiration and consequently some processing steps. This distinction is less clear when comparing algorithms like CLONALG and opt-aiNet with some particular types of EAs. In these particular cases, it is possible to see a similar effect as the one occurring with many evolutionary computation techniques (evolution strategies, genetic algorithms, and evolutionary programming): they are becoming ever more similar. Indeed, a soft-computing perspective on the merging of strategies is almost nearly unavoidable with the improvement of the research on computational intelligence.

8.4   Assessment of Artificial Immune Systems

The assessment of a particular algorithm is usually done by evaluating its performance when applied to a given problem and then analyzing its computational complexity, feasibility and other available measures. Assessing a whole field of research, i.e., a paradigm, in contrast cannot be done in such a restricted way. For example, one cannot say that an evolutionary algorithm is the best strategy to be applied to a given search problem, even if this problem presents features that make it suitable for the application of an EA strategy, such as a large and highly multimodal search space. This has been demonstrated with a theorem known as "no free lunch theorem" (Wolpert & Macready, 1997), which says that no algorithm can perform better than any other when averaged over all cost functions.

We believe that the 'no free lunch theorem' is valid not only for search applications, but also for other types of problems tackled by artificial immune systems, such as control, emergence of dynamic behaviors and anomaly detection. Thus, to quantify the motivation behind the study of this novel approach, we must pursue the contributions of the field as a whole. We do not see artificial immune systems though simply as another alternative problem solving technique. To date, many of the applications of AIS have been to the same problems as those studied by other people employing biologically inspired techniques. For such a new field, this is to be forgiven; "we must walk before we run!" However, maybe it is time for attention to be turned to areas where AIS can be used and other techniques are either not suitable, not good enough, or where AIS techniques can bring a useful new perspective on the same problem. The following section highlights some of the more interesting features of the immune system that have been employed within AIS, but still offer a great deal for a researcher to exploit.

8.4.1. Usefulness of the AIS Approach

Applications of artificial immune systems have been seen in the most diverse domain areas. From pattern recognition, to computer security, anomaly detection and fault diagnosis, from optimization to machine learning and robotics, from control to scheduling to associative memories, and from production systems to diversity models and intelligent buildings. What is incorporated, then, in artificial immune systems that make them so broadly applicable?

One of the most remarkable features of AIS is their potential for hybridization with other techniques. By reading through Chapters 4, 6, and 7, it can be seen that a great number of computational intelligence systems were developed as hybrids of well-known strategies with an immune principle or metaphor or with an immune algorithm. This raises another question: what does the immune system have (or AIS have) that makes it so suitable for hybridization with other methodologies? All the immune features described in Section 3.2 serve as answers to this question.

Each individual has an immune system that somehow carries "historical" information about the environment in which it has already been, i.e., microorganisms it has already been challenged with. This suggests that artificial immune systems are strategies capable of coping with novel situations and of "learning" and/or "evolving" so as to become more adapted to the environment in which they are inserted. This is linked to the idea of a dynamic adaptive system. The immune system by its very nature continually learns and adapts to new stimuli. From a computational perspective, if one could harness that process in an automatic way, continual learning algorithms could be created for use in various situations. Some work has already begun on this with many of the algorithms described in this book, but the field still beckons for more research.

Each individual organism has the knowledge about itself. In contrast to the most obvious view of self-knowledge, the individual identity is also embodied in other places than the brain. The immune system also knows itself, or more specifically, the immune system "knows what we are composed of". A number of AIS try to model and incorporate this notion of self-knowledge, endowing them with the capability of performing self-nonself discrimination. Self-nonself discrimination is the process by which the immune system generates a set of cells and molecules capable of identifying the elements of the organism itself (e.g., cells, molecules, and tissues) and distinguishing them from those elements that do not originally belong to the organism (e.g., pathogenic microorganisms and grafted tissues). Self-nonself discrimination thus provides at least two novel types of immune algorithms. The first one, named positive selection, is an algorithm that allows the storage of information (recognition) of the organism itself, or self. The other algorithm, called negative selection, stores information about (recognizes) patterns that are not the self, i.e., that deviate from a standard known pattern and as such allows the AIS to detect anomalies or novelties.

Immune cells and molecules have to be highly diverse to cope with an almost limitless range of possible malefic invaders. This high diversity is achieved by the immune system through a number of highly evolved mechanisms. One of them is the generation of immune receptors through the recombination of genes from individual libraries. This is so that from a finite genome, the immune systems generate a nearly infinite set of different types of receptors. The capability of the immune system to dynamically manipulate its repertoires of cells, i.e., to dynamically add new cells and remove useless ones, is also important for the maintenance of diversity. This process is termed metadynamics in immune network models, but the terminology can be used for the immune system as a whole. Artificial immune systems that incorporate metadynamics usually present diverse and plastic populations of individuals and are also capable of performing a broad coverage of the search space.

Together with the diverse nature of the immune receptors is their capability of covering almost entirely the universe of antigens. After infections, the immune system builds up and maintains a set of cells that are specialized in recognizing the known infections. This is a process similar to the formation of "niches" and "species" of cells within the immune system of each individual. Indeed, the capability of generating and maintaining stable sub-populations of individuals that cover diverse peaks of an affinity landscape is a remarkable feature intrinsic to almost all AIS models.

Unlike the nervous system, where its central portion (central nervous system) is responsible for coordinating the behavior of the whole organism, the immune system is not centralized. Most artificial immune systems are composed of a distributed set of cells (or sets of cells) that interact with each other and the environment. This suggests a few things. First, those AIS are suitable for being modeled or simulated by approaches such as agent-based and cellular automata. This is because these strategies naturally assume a set of "agents" or cells interacting with each other and the environment. If we consider that immune cells and molecules usually behave according to local rules and disturbances, the similarities and potentiality for modeling becomes even more striking for agents and automata, as in their most standard formats, they have similar structures.

The dynamics of repertoires of cells and molecules is in itself a novel approach for computing. It was discussed that most immune network models follow a pattern of behavior similar to predator-prey models used to describe the dynamics of interacting species in ecological systems. The immune system is in a constant fight against invading items. To this end, preys (antigens) reproduce, and new predators are produced (antibodies) in response, as well. This battle between the two can be thought of in co-evolutionary terms, and may provide a useful model for this area.

Also, it is not surprising then that AIS are being proposed to study ecosystem management.

The fact that the immune system has defenses on different levels inspired the development of AIS with several functional layers. This was exemplified in the early work on virus detection by Kephart as discussed in Section 4.3, where a two layered approach based on the idea of the innate and adaptive systems was adopted.

From a machine learning perspective, artificial immune systems are one of the few strategies that naturally incorporate both learning and evolutionary procedures of adaptation. It is possible to find, however, works in the literature addressing this issue under the perspective of the Baldwin effect. Nevertheless, AIS use a different approach. Some artificial immune network models, for example, have a network-like pattern of connectivity among cells and adapt to the environment following rules that incorporate learning with evolution in a natural way. This is usually achieved by bringing together clonal selection, argued to be of an evolutionary type, with learning strategies similar to self-organizing neural network models. In this case, we get back again to the hybrid nature and potentiality of AIS.

Finally, AIS also provide a network paradigm that is different from others established paradigms such as neural networks and Petri nets. Artificial immune networks are basically characterized by a set of cells and connections among cells. This may follow the standard of other network paradigms, but many differences are apparent, such as the meaning of the connections, the cells themselves, and the dynamics and metadynamics of the network. Cells in network models store and process information, while connections quantify cellular interactions. It is felt that the immune network approach holds a great deal of promise but, as much in AIS, still needs further investigation.

8.4.2. Some Critical Reflections about Artificial Immune Systems

As with all other computational intelligence paradigm, artificial immune systems suffer from several problems, including the non-existence of rigorous proofs of convergence, a number of user-defined parameters, and questions of how to choose the best model and initialization procedures. These practical aspects of AIS have been discussed in Chapter 6, but a little more will be said in the "future trends" section (Section 8.5).

Another aspect that might sometimes be viewed as a drawback of AIS is their lack of identity. Artificial immune systems have been applied to so many areas of research that it cannot be classified as a search or a data analysis strategy. The diversity of algorithms and application domains make them interesting for researchers in the most varied fields of research, but it in contrast make it more difficult to track and study what has been done. As a result of this intrinsic multidisciplinarity of AIS and also the presence of evolutionary and learning procedures of adaptation within the immune system, sometimes it is difficult to discern them from evolutionary algorithms or neural networks. We hope that Chapter 6 has shed some light on the distinction between the many approaches.

In many cases, AIS have shown themselves to be very effective at solving benchmark problems, but as yet, still have a long way to go to establishing themselves as a really useful tool for *real-world* applications. However, many problems faced by AIS are real world but not industrial or large scale, so AIS have already proved themselves to be useful to some degree but await further exploitation.

One last issue to consider is the accuracy of the metaphor. Those with the opinion that AIS are in some way modeling the immune system can be great critics of the field. Hopefully, this book has shown that this is not the case. Metaphors extracted from the immune system should be true to their origins in the first instance. It can be very difficult for a computer scientist to grasp the more subtle aspects of immunology and in some cases mistakes or misunderstanding can creep into the work. This is where closer collaboration between researchers developing AIS and biologists should be encouraged. Through better engagement, the field of AIS can benefit. In addition, it may be possible for AIS to feed biologists with new approaches to solving their problems.

8.5 Future Trends

As discussed in the previous section, artificial immune systems constitute an emerging computational intelligence paradigm. As such, they are expected to have a wide range of possible avenues for research and applications. To discuss some of these avenues, we are going to divide the future trends of AIS into four main streams, as summarized in Figure 8.1: 1) improvement and augmentation of the current AIS models, 2) development of new AIS, 3) novel applications, and 4) extension of the framework.

The first main stream is concerned with improving the performance of existing AIS for particular applications. The second branch for new models, in contrast, is related to the extraction of new metaphors and the development of novel algorithms by exploiting even more ideas from the immune system. Another branch is concerned with application areas. To date, a great deal of work has been done in applying AIS to established problems and domains, and research could take place for completely new areas of application in which AIS may niche themselves. The remaining branch involves the extension of the framework with which to design AIS.

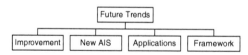

Figure 8.1. Avenues for future research on artificial immune systems.

8.5.1. Improvement and Augmentation of AIS

Well established computational intelligence techniques, such as neural networks and evolutionary algorithms, are characterized by a large number of works aimed at modifying the standard algorithms, defining new encoding schemes, improving techniques, etc. These works correspond mainly to the practical aspects of these methods presented in Sections 6.2 and 6.3, respectively. In order to improve the performance of these strategies, researchers have been using, among other approaches, ideas and metaphors extracted from the immune system (AIS). In Chapter 6 we have seen how AIS have been used as an auxiliary tool to define ANN architectures (model selection) and to initialize ANNs. In conjunction with evolutionary algorithms, AIS have been used to enhance the GA convergence, handle constraints in GAs, and maintain diversity and detect niches in GAs.

Despite all the improvements AIS have been giving to the other paradigms, very little has been done in the other way round, i.e., the use of ANNs and EAs to enhance AIS. Nevertheless, as with all computational intelligence paradigms, AIS can always be improved. Let's start the discussion by considering the necessity of reducing the number of user-defined parameters and adhoc procedures that are prevalent in most immune algorithms. For example, the positive and negative selection algorithms still require optimized strategies to generate a potential repertoire (**P**) to match the self-set (**S**). Although a new strategy was proposed to alleviate this difficulty and other works from the literature that tackle the same problem were reviewed, there is still much to be done. In the case of the clonal selection algorithm, several user-defined parameters have to be defined a-priori. As clonal selection models usually present evolutionary-like patterns of behavior, the study of model selection, initialization, convergence analysis, and parameter setting techniques of evolutionary algorithms might give insights into how to tackle these problems in AIS. Similar approaches can be suggested for artificial immune network models and neural networks. Is it feasible to apply ANN initialization strategies, model selection, convergence analysis, and automatic parameter definition of an ANN into an AIS? It might be one possible and worthy way of starting.

Slight variations and improvements of individual algorithms are important and necessary, but in many cases problem-dependent. Therefore, a detailed list of enhancements for each individual algorithm is not going to be presented. In general, the practical applications of artificial immune system present the same four aspects as those of ANNs and EAs: *model selection, initialization of free parameters, convergence and performance analysis*, and *parameter setting*, as summarized in Figure 8.2.

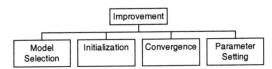

Figure 8.2. Possible avenues for improvement and augmentation of AIS.

8.5.2. New Artificial Immune Systems

Chapter 2 exposed the reader to a small amount of ideas of how the vertebrate immune system works. The topic of immunology is vast, and the immune system is fascinatingly complex. As one might imagine, there are many interesting avenues of research to be exploited in terms of new metaphors for algorithms. In Figure 8.3 we suggest two new lines of research that can be followed to develop new artificial immune systems.

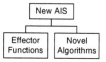

Figure 8.3. Possible (non-exhaustive) lines of research for the development of new AIS.

There is a whole and wide range of effector mechanisms used by the immune system to eliminate foreign pathogens, debris, or malfunctioning cells. Almost none of these processes have ever been modeled in AIS. For instance, those artificial immune systems used for anomaly detection and pattern recognition only incorporate immune metaphors for the detection of patterns (anomalous or not). Some of the mechanisms used by the immune system to eliminate these detected patterns could be used as sources of inspiration for the development of computational strategies also capable of eliminating patterns in a computer system. These can be useful for the elimination of computer viruses for example.

The second trend in the development of new AIS refers to the modeling of other immune parts and processes and their application to problem solving. Here, we can outline several processes of the immune system that may suggest new computing algorithms:

- *Germinal centers* (GC): areas within the lymph nodes where the B-cell clonal expansion and affinity maturation occurs. They play an important functional role during an adaptive immune response. Dasgupta and Krishnan (2000) argued that from an information processing perspective, germinal centers can be viewed as production factories where specialized cells and molecules are evolved;

- *Antigenic presentation*: antigen presenting cells have the capability of internalizing pathogens and processing them so that the major histocompatibility complex (MHC) molecules present fragments, named peptides, of these pathogens in the cell surface. The complex MHC/peptide is then recognized by other cells of the immune system, particularly T-helper cells. These processes of antigenic processing and presentation might be worth studying for the development of computational systems or algorithms capable of extracting information from (noisy) patterns;

- *Complement cascade*: the complement system has many functions such as the attraction of phagocytes into the sites of infection, the coat of an organism with proteins so as to make it palatable to phagocytes, and the cause of damage to cells, some bacteria, and viruses. As such, the complement can be used as a metaphor for the development of systems to trigger effector mechanisms or it can be the effector mechanisms itself;

- *Resource allocation*: the immune system allocates resources as required. Immune responses are localized in the sites near to the infections; cells migrate into the sites of infection so as to guarantee an effective elimination of the pathogen. In addition, there has to be a counterbalance between the number of naïve cells being generated and the memory cells appearing as a result of immunity. These processes suggest interesting mechanisms to the dynamic control of populations of distributed individuals (agents);
- *Regulation of immune response*: the study of how the different immune cells and molecules interact with one another might provide interesting ideas for the development of control systems.
- *Detection and elimination of malfunctioning cells*: in addition to anomaly detection (nonself detection), the immune system is capable of detecting malfunctioning cells. Though most researchers have been using negative selection as a metaphor for fault detection, we believe that this has more to do with the detection of malfunctioning self. This way, the study of how the immune system copes with altered self might give insights to the development of fault-detection algorithms that are different from negative selection;
- *Vaccination*: this allows the immune system to receive prior information about a given pathogen (problem); this is an interesting metaphor to be incorporated is AIS.

8.5.3. Application Areas

The survey presented in Chapter 4 demonstrates the impressive broad applicability of artificial immune systems. This is due to many reasons. One is that the immune system has a number of diverse structures, mechanisms, and processes that have been used as inspiration for the development of adaptive computational tools for problem solving. Another reason is that AIS have been hybridized with many other paradigms to improve individual performances. The multidisciplinarity of the field has also contributed for its application in diverse domains.

In Section 3.4, we presented a list containing the scope of AIS. Figure 8.4 summarizes the scope of AIS by grouping individual applications into major classes. The domain of pattern recognition embodies fault and anomaly detection, and image, speech and spectra recognition. Data analysis includes data mining and compression, classification, etc. Optimization incorporates function, multimodal, multiobjective, combinatorial, and constrained search procedures. Robotics involves autonomous navigation, coordination of collective behaviors, and walking robots. Control includes identification, synthesis, and adaptive (intelligent) control. (Note that robotics can be viewed as a branch of control.) Finally, machine learning involves the study of supervised, unsupervised and reinforcement learning systems.

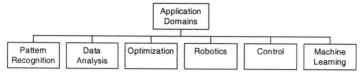

Figure 8.4. Main domains of application for AIS.

There are innumerable applications within each of these six major domains to which AIS have not been applied yet. For example, if we view the immune system as a defense system, then could we use it as an inspiration for the development of novel defense strategies? As the immune system is very good at detecting anomalies, no matter how singular they are, could we use it to detect outliers in data analysis problems? Does the immune system really present a novel perspective for combining evolution with self-organization in computational systems? As a biologically motivated computing paradigm that incorporates learning and evolutionary procedures of adaptation regulated by local rules of interactions, can we use it as another artificial life technique?

8.5.4. Extending the Framework

To design an artificial immune system, the framework introduced in Chapter 3 requires three basic steps: 1) a representation scheme for the components of the AIS, 2) one or more measure to quantify the state of the system (affinity and fitness measures), and 3) immune algorithms to govern the behavior of the system. In all of these three branches, the framework can be extended (Figure 8.5).

The representation adopted for immune cells and molecules is an extended version of the shape-space approach proposed by Perelson and Oster (1979). We suggested four main types of shape-space: Hamming, Euclidean, Integer, and Symbolic. In addition to these, other more complex shape-spaces were discussed, such as Neural, Fuzzy, and DNA shape-spaces. The shape-space is basically a formalism to represent those portions of an immune cell or molecules that are responsible to define is features that allow it to recognize or be recognized by other elements. Much research remains to be done regarding the proposal of new shape-spaces and the formalization of the existing shape-spaces. It is important to provide guidelines as to which kind of shape-space is more appropriate to which kind of application.

Evaluation functions of AIS vary in type and function. For instance, affinity and fitness measures are used to quantify different aspects of an AIS. Although there are several different affinity measures for Hamming shape-spaces, no work from the literature has been found comparing theoretically or empirically when an affinity measure would be more suited than another one. Affinity measures can be proposed to examine differently separate portions of a given string, increasing/decreasing the influence of these portions. For example, if we assume that the interactions between two molecules is stronger in the center of their shapes, then an affinity function that increases the contribution of matches in the central portions of the string could be devised. Very few studies using affinity functions in a space that is not Hamming were described, and most of the ones that were described were based upon an Euclidean distance.

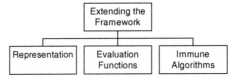

Figure 8.5. Areas to extend the AIS framework.

Four major types of algorithms were described: bone marrow models, used to generate repertoires of attribute strings; thymus models, used to perform self-nonself discrimination based on positive or negative selection; clonal selection and affinity maturation algorithms, described as evolutionary procedures of adaptation; and immune network models, divided into continuous and discrete networks. Although it might seem that the basic aspects of each of these theories have been studied and incorporated into the algorithms already, we would not be surprised if other researchers, by reading biology texts, could actually find other properties of these algorithms which were not accounted for yet. These could result in even more useful algorithms. In addition, a whole set of new algorithms and processes could be modeled and added to the proposed framework, such as the ones suggested in the section about "new artificial immune systems".

8.6   Reflective Comments

In this section we would like to present our own reflective viewpoint about this book. One of the most difficult aspects of writing a book in such a young field of research is the decision of what to cover and how to present the topics. Our approach was to introduce a text that covers a large and varied number of concepts and works from many application areas. This was primarily done as this is the first book on the topic, and we felt it appropriate to write a wider ranging text. Naturally, nobody would expect a deep analysis of all subjects presented when such a broad coverage is pursued. In light of the proposed framework, another form of writing such a book would have been to dedicate a single chapter for each of the elements of the framework. For example, one chapter to discuss shape-spaces, another one to discuss affinity measures, one chapter with the general ideas of the algorithms, and one chapter to describe each of the algorithms themselves. This by itself could have constituted (or might still constitute!) a book on AIS.

We are aware that bringing together so many subjects (from biology to computing) into a single volume is not an easy task. Nevertheless, we presented the basic ideas of artificial immune systems, including design principles and general-purpose algorithms. In addition, we are aware that we did talk in detail about biology, even though one of us is an electrical engineer and the other a computer scientist. This was supported by the belief that by doing this, it would help us to improve our understanding of the organism as a whole, the patterns of behavior of AIS, and also the possibility of creating new hybrid systems. The idea was also to bridge a gap between biology, in particular immunology and engineering, so as to show the reader that a multidisciplinary research can be very fruitful for many fields of research.

A high point in this book was Chapter 6, which deserves one book on its own (more than one actually). Again, we covered a wide range of material and presented a comparison between the several computational intelligence paradigms with AIS. This was one of the hardest chapters to write. It required a wide bibliographical search and knowledge on different fields that are constantly being improved and reshaped. Some support from the literature had to be combined with our own perspective of how these approaches compare with each other and fit together into a unified hybrid paradigm.

8.7   Final Remarks

This book shows that biology and computing have much to gain from each other. It illustrates that although these fields have different approaches and rationales, a bidirectional interaction can be fruitful. Our focus was primarily on how ideas gleaned from theoretical and practical immunology have been used in the development of computational systems. In this avenue, computer science and engineering have already greatly benefited from the science of immunology. It is now time to also try and study how AIS can aid immunologists and biologists, in the understanding of the immune system itself, and in the solving of problems in areas such as bioinformatics.

Artificial immune systems were introduced as a new computational intelligence paradigm, a framework to design and understand AIS was proposed, a broad survey of the field was presented, and it was placed in context with many biological systems and processes, together with other computational intelligence paradigms. The double-plasticity of the immune system lead to the natural development of AIS with architectures capable of adapting themselves to the problems under study. This is the current tendency of all computational intelligence paradigms: self-adapting architectures and algorithms. Therefore, AIS represent a powerful technique that already emerged embodying some of the features that took many years for other approaches to start focusing on.

Finally, this book was a joint effort between both authors in which we provided a reasonable background on biology, in an attempt to seek a middle ground that encompasses all disciplines. To us, it seems that nature, fine-tuning life for billions of years, has found a good working method to protect our bodies against infectious diseases and malfunctioning cells. This book supports the argument that it is well worth learning about biological processes, whether you want to have a better understanding of biology – in this case the immune system and how it interacts with other systems – or to develop novel computational tools to tackle problems in many different domains. The immune system offers a great deal of interest to the more "blue-sky" research oriented people, and it is possible to find a convergence with the more applied research as well. As seems to be more and more the case today, application-oriented investigations indicate that, in many situations, the best problem solving strategies available are those that nature herself has been shaping and using for many years. Nature has still much to inspire us through the use of metaphors for the development and improvement of computational intelligence systems.

References

Bonabeau, E., Dorigo, M. & Theraulaz, G. (1999), *Swarm Intelligence from Natural to Artificial Systems*, Oxford University Press.

Dasgupta, D. & Krishnan (2000), "Role of Germinal Centers: From a Computational Viewpoint", *Proc. of the Genetic and Evolutionary Computation Conference*, Workshop on Artificial Immune Systems, pp. 29-30.

Farmer, J. D., Packard, N. H. & Perelson, A. S. (1986), "The Immune System, Adaptation, and Machine Learning", *Physica 22D*, pp. 187-204.

Fogel, D. B. (2000), *Evolutionary Computation: Toward a New Philosophy of Machine Intelligence*, 2nd Ed., IEEE Press.

Kennedy, J., Eberhart, R. C. & Shi, Y. (2001), *Swarm Intelligence*, Morgan Kaufmann.

Minsky, M. & Papert, S. (1968), *Perceptrons*, MIT Press.

Perelson, A. S. & Oster, G. F. (1979), "Theoretical Studies of Clonal Selection: Minimal Antibody Repertoire Size and Reliability of Self-Nonself Discrimination", *J. Theor.Biol.*, **81**, pp. 645-670.

Rumelhart, D. E., McClelland, J. L. & The PDP Research Group, eds. (1986), *Parallel Distributed Processing*, Cambridge MIT Press.

Wolpert, D. H. & Macready, W. G. (1997), "No Free Lunch Theorem for Search", *IEEE Trans. on Evolutionary Computation*, **1**, pp. 67-82.

Appendix I

Glossary of Biological Terms

The purpose of this glossary is to provide a quick reference for biological terminology that can be found within this book, in particular Chapters 2 and 5. The main sources of reference were: Futuyma, 1979; Vander *et al.*, 1990; Barrett, 1983; Ottoson, 1983; Bullock *et al.*, 1984; Hood *et al.*, 1984; McClintic, 1985; Klein, 1990; Salomon *et al.*, 1990; Guyton, 1991; Coleman *et al.*, 1992; Krebs, 1994; Tizard, 1995; Benjamini *et al.*, 1996; Abbas *et al*, 1998; Mackenna and Callendar, 1998; Janeway *et al.*, 1999; Roitt, 1997, Paul, 1999; Lydyard *et al.*, 2000; Cancer Web Online Dictionary, and Biology Online.

A

Accessory cell: cell required to initiate an immune response. A term often used to describe antigen-presenting cells (APC).

Action potential: electric signal propagated over long distances by excitable cells, e.g., nerve and muscle; it is characterized by an all-or-none reversal of the membrane potential in which the inside of the cell temporarily becomes positive relative to the outside; has a threshold and is conducted without decrement. Also known as *nerve impulse*.

Acute Phase Protein (APP): heterogeneous group of plasma proteins important in innate defense against microbes (mostly bacteria) and in limiting tissue damage caused by infection, trauma, malignancy and other diseases. They are mainly produced in the liver, usually in response to inflammation or infection.

Adaptive immune response: immune response highly specific to antigens, including those associated with microbes. It has an associated lag time and is capable of developing a memory, i.e., to remember previously encountered antigens.

Adenine: purine base, $C_5H_5N_5$, that is the constituent involved in base pairing with thymine in DNA and with uracil in RNA.

Adrenal gland: either of two small, dissimilarly shaped endocrine glands, one located above each kidney, consisting of the cortex, which secretes several steroid hormones, and the medulla, which secretes epinephrine. It is also called suprarenal gland.

Affinity: measure or tightness of the binding between an antigen combining site and an antigenic determinant; the stronger binding, the higher the affinity. Antibodies produced in a secondary (memory) immune response usually present higher affinities than those of the primary response.

Affinity landscape: representation of the space of all possible antigen binding sites (antibodies or TCRs) along with their affinities.

Affinity maturation: the increase in antibody affinity frequently seen during a secondary immune response.

Allele: one member of a pair or series of genes that occupy a specific position (or locus) on a specific chromosome.

Allergen: a substance (antigen) that causes an allergy by inducing IgE synthesis.

Allergy: an inappropriate and harmful response of the immune system to normally harmless (nonpathogenic) substances. Used as a synonim to *hypersensitivity*.

Alternate complement pathway of activation: mechanism of complement activation that does not involve a serologic reaction (antigen-antibody complexes).

Amine: one of a class of strongly basic substances derived from ammonia by replacement of one or more hydrogen atoms by a basic atom or radical.

Amino acid: an organic compound containing an amino group, a carboxylic acid group, and any of various side groups that link together by peptide bonds to form proteins or that function as chemical messengers and as intermediataries in metabolism.

Anaphilaxys: immediate hypersensitivity response to antigenic challenge, mediated by a IgE and mast cells. It is a life-threatening allergic reaction caused by the release of pharmacologically active agents.

Androgen: general term for any male sex hormone (e.g. testosterone or androsterone) that control the development and maintenance of male sexual characteristics. Also called *androgenic hormone*.

Anergy: lack of normal immune function, either generalized or antigen specific.

Antibody (**Ab**): a soluble (serum) protein molecule produced and secreted by B-cells in response to an antigen. Antibodies are usually defined in terms of their specific binding to an antigen.

Antigen (**Ag**): any substance that when introduced into the body, is capable of inducing an immune response.

Antigen binding site: the part of an antibody molecule that binds specifically to an antigen.

Antigen presentation: process by which certain cells in the body, named antigen presenting cells – APCs, express antigen on their surfaces in a form recognizable by lymphocytes.

Antigen presenting cells (**APC**): B-cells, cells of the monocyte lineage (including macrophages as well as dendritic cells), and various other body cells that "present" antigen in a form that B- and T-cells can recognize.

Antigen processing: the conversion of an antigen into a form in which it can be recognized by lymphocytes.

Antigen receptor: specific antigen-binding site on B- and T-cells.

Apoptosis: form of programmed cell death caused by the activation of endogenous molecules leading to the fragmentation of DNA.

Autonomic nervous system: part of the vertebrate nervous system that regulates involuntary action, such as the intestines, heart, and glands. It is divided into the sympathetic nervous system and the parasympathetic nervous system.

Associative memory: also named content addressable memory (CAM) and is a kind of storage device which includes comparison with each elment of storage. A data value is broadcast to all elements of storage and compared with the values there. Those that match are flagged in some way. Subsequent operations can then work on flagged elements, e.g., read them out one at a time or write to certain positions in all of them. A CAM can thus operate as a data parallel processor.

Astrocyte (astroglia): a star-shaped cell, especially a neuroglial cell of nervous tissue that supports the neurons.

Attenuate: to weaken the effects of a pathogenic microorganism whilst retaining its viability.

Autoantibody: an antibody that reacts against a person's own tissue or components.

Autoantigen: a molecule that behaves as a self-antigen.

Autoimmune disease: a disease that arises when the immune system mistakenly attacks the body's own tissues or components. It is the result of a breakdown in self-tolerance. Factors predisposing and/or contributing to the development of autoimmune diseases include age, genetics, gender, infections and the nature of the *autoantigen*. Reumathoid arthritis and systemic lupus erythematosus are examples of autoimmune diseases.

Avidity: the summation of multiple affinities.

Axon: the usually long process of a nerve fiber that generally conducts impulses away from the body of the nerve cell.

B

Bacterium: unicellular prokaryotic microorganism of the class schizomycetes which vary in terms of morphology, oxygen and nutritional requirements, and motility. It may be free-living, saprophytic, or pathogenic in plants or animals.

Basophil: a white blood cell containing granules (*granulocyte*) that contributes to inflammatory reactions. Along with mast cells, basophils are responsible for the symptoms of allergy.

B-cell: small white blood cells expressing immunoglobulin molecules on its surface. Also known as B-lymphocytes, they are derived from the bone marrow and develop into plasma cells that are the main antibodiy secretors.

B-cell receptor (**BCR**): immunoglobulin molecule on the surface of B-cells. It is composed of four polypeptide chains: two identical heavy (H) and two identical light (L) chains.

Blood-brain barrier (**BBB**): a physiological mechanism that alters the permeability of brain capillaries, so that some substances, such as certain drugs, are prevented from entering brain tissue, while other substances are allowed to enter freely.

Bone marrow: soft tissue located in the cavity of the bones. It is the source of all blood cells.

Bony spine: the spinal column of a vertebrate.

Brain: portion of the vertebrate central nervous system that is enclosed within the cranium, continuous with the spinal cord, and composed of gray matter and white matter. It is the primary center for the regulation and control of bodily activities, receiving and interpreting sensory impulses, and transmitting information to the muscles and body organs. It is also the seat of consciousness, thought, memory, and emotion.

Brainstem: portion of the brain, consisting of the medulla oblongata, pons Varolii, and midbrain, that connects the spinal cord to the forebrain and cerebrum.

C

Cell body: the portion of a nerve cell that contains the nucleus but does not incorporate the dendrites or axon. Also called *soma*.

Cell differentiation: process by which the initially identical cells present during the earliest stages of development not only undergo anatomical alteration but also acquire specialized functional properties, e.g., the antibody production and secretion in high volumes by the plasma cells.

Cellular immunity: immune protection provided by the direct action of immune cells.

Central lymphoid organs: lymphoid organs primarily involved in the production and maturation of immune cells. They include the bone marrow and thymus.

Central nervous system: the portion of the vertebrate nervous system consisting of the brain and spinal cord.

Central tolerance: process whereby immature T- and B-cells acquire tolerance to self-antigens during maturation within the primary lymphoid organs (thymus and bone marrow, respectively). It involves the elimination of cells with receptors for self-antigens.

Cerebellum: trilobed structure of the brain lying posterior to the pons and medulla oblongata and inferior to the occipital lobes of the cerebral hemispheres. It is responsible for the regulation and coordination of complex voluntary muscular movement as well as the maintenance of posture and balance.

Cerebrum: large rounded structure of the brain occupying most of the cranial cavity, divided into two cerebral hemispheres that are joined at the bottom by the corpus callosum. It controls and integrates motor, sensory, and higher mental functions, such as thought, reason, emotion, and memory.

Chemokines: cytokines that direct cell migration and/or activate cells.

Chemotaxis: attraction of leukocytes or other cells by chemicals.

Chickenpox: acute contagious disease, primarily of children. It is caused by the varicella-zoster virus and characterized by skin eruptions, slight fever, and malaise. Also called *varicella*.

Chromosome: a threadlike linear strand of DNA and associated proteins in the nucleus of eukaryotic cells that carries the genes and functions in the transmission of hereditary information. Each human cell has 23 pairs of chromosomes.

Classical pathway of complement activation: mechanism of complement activation initiated by antigen-antibody aggregates.

Clonal deletion: the loss of lymphocytes of a particular specificity due mainly to contact with self-antigens.

Clonal selection principle: the prevalent theory stating that the specificity and diversity of an immune response are the result of selection by antigen of specifically reactive clones from a large repertoire of preformed lymphocytes, each with individual specificities.

Clone: (n.) a group of genetically identical cells or organisms descended from a single common ancestor; (v.) to reproduce multiple identical copies.

Colony stimulator factor: cytokine that drive the development, differentiation, and expansion of cells of the myeloid series.

Combinatorial joining: the joining of DNA segments to generate essentially new genetic information, as occurs with BCR and TCR genes during the development of B- and T-cells. Combinatorial joining, or assembly, allows multiple opportunities for a few sets of genes to combine in several different ways.

Complement: a complex series of blood serum proteins, which on sequential activation may mediate protection against microbial infection and contribute to the inflammatory response. They are synthesized by hapatocytes and monocytes and help (complement) antibody responses through a wide spectrum of activities, including a pivotal role in innate defense mechanisms. It might be activated by either the classical (through antibody) or alternative pathway (innate).

Complement cascade: sequence of events usually triggered by an antigen-antibody complex, in which each component of the complement system is activated in turn.

Constant region (C-region): the carboxyl-terminal portion of an immunoglobulins heavy and light chains having an amino acid sequence that does not vary within a given class or subclass of immunoglobulin.

Cortex: outer layer of gray matter that covers the surface of the cerebral hemisphere.

Co-stimulation: the delivery of a second signal from an APC to a T-cell. The second signal rescues the activated T-cell from anergy, allowing it to produce the lymphokines necessary for the growth of additional T-cells.

Cowpox: mild contagious skin disease of cattle, usually affecting the udder. It is caused by a virus and characterized by the eruption of a pustular rash. When the virus is transmitted to humans, as by vaccination, it can confer immunity to *smallpox*. Also called *vaccinia*.

Cranium: the part of the skull enclosing the brain; the braincase.

Crossover: exchange of genetic material in sexual reproduction. In each one of the parents, genes are exchanged between pairs of homologous chromosomes to form a single one.

Cross-reactivity: the ability of an antibody, specific for one antigen, to react with a slightly different antigen; a measure of relatedness between two different antigenic substances.

Cytokine: small molecule that signal between cells, inducing growth, differentiation, chemotaxis, activation, enhanced cytotoxicity and/or regulation of immunity. They are referred to as lymphokines if produced by lymphocytes, interleukines if produced by leukocytes, and monokines if produced by monocytes and macrophages.

Cytotoxic T-cell (**CTL** – *cytotoxic T lymphocyte*): a T-cell subset that can directly kill body cells infected by viruses or transformed by cancer. It is also named killer T-cell (T_K)

D

Dendrite: short fiber that conducts information toward the cell body of the neuron.

Dendritic cells: set of antigen-presenting cells (APCs) present in lymph nodes, spleen and at low levels in blood, which are particularly active in stimulating T-cells.

Determinant: part of the antigen molecule that binds to an antibody-combining site or to a receptor on a T-cell. It is also termed *epitope*.

Diploid: cell with a full set of genetic material, consisting of chromosomes in homologous pairs and thus having two copies of each autosomal genetic locus. A diploid cell has one chromosome from each parental set.

Disease: alteration in the state of the body or of some of its organs, interrupting or disturbing the performance of the vital functions, and causing or threatening pain and weakness. Also termed *malady, affection, illness* or *sickness*.

DNA: nucleic acid that carries the genetic information in the cell and is capable of self-replication and synthesis of RNA. DNA consists of two long chains of nucleotides twisted into a double helix and joined by hydrogen bonds between the complementary bases *adenine* and *thymine* or *cytosine* and *guanine*. The sequence of nucleotides determines individual hereditary characteristics.

Domain: a compact segment of an immunoglobulin or TCR chain, made up of amino acids.

Dwarfism: condition that results from the insufficient production of growth hormone by the pituitary gland. It is characterised by abnormally short stature and is also known as *nanism*.

E

Ecology: science that studies the relationship of organisms to each other and to their environment.

Ecosystem: a system formed by the interaction of a community of organisms with their physical environment.

Electroencephalogram (**EEG**): record of electrical activity of the brain obtained from scalp electrodes. Also called *encephalogram*.

Endocrine gland: any of various glands (of the endocrine system) producing hormonal secretions that pass directly into the bloodstream. The endocrine glands include the thyroid, parathyroids, anterior and posterior pituitary, pancreas, adrenals, pineal, and gonads. They are also termed *ductless gland*.

Endocrine system: the system of glands that produce endocrine secretions (hormones), which help to control bodily metabolic activity.

Endorphin: group of peptide hormones that bind to opiate receptors and are found mainly in the brain. Endorphins reduce the sensation of pain and affect emotions.

Environment: totality of the factors that influence the activities, achievements, and ultimate fate of an animal or plant.

Enzyme: any of numerous proteins or conjugated proteins produced by living organisms and functioning as biochemical catalysts.

Eosinophil: white blood cell that contains cytoplasmic granules filled with chemicals capable of damaging parasites, and enzymes that damp down inflammatory reactions.

Epigenesis: theory that development is a process of gradual increase in complexity as opposed to the preformationist view which supposed that a mere increase in size is sufficient to produce adult from embryo.

Epistemology: science (branch of philosophy) that studies the nature of knowledge, its presuppositions and foundations, and its extent and validity.

Epitope: a unique shape, or marker, carried on an antigen's surface, which triggers a corresponding antibody response.

Estrogen: steroid hormones produced chiefly by the ovaries and responsible for promoting estrus and the development and maintenance of female secondary sex characteristics.

Exocrine gland: externally secreting gland, such as a salivary gland or sweat gland that releases its secretions directly or through a duct.

Exon: sequence of DNA that codes information for protein synthesis that is transcribed to messenger RNA.

F

Fab: fragment of antibody containing one antigen-binding site; generated by cleavage of the antibody with the enzyme papain, which cuts at the hinge region N-terminally to the interheavy-chain disulfide bond and generates two Fab fragments from one antibody molecule.

Fc: fragment of antibody without antigen-binding sites, generated by cleavage with papain. The Fc fragment contains the C-terminal domains of the immunoglobulin heavy chains.

Fever: a diseased state of the system, marked by increased heat, acceleration of the pulse, and a general derangement of the functions, including usually, thirst and loss of appetite.

Fitness: extent to which an organism is adapted to, suitable, or able to produce offspring in a particular environment.

Follicular dendritic cells: a virus-trapping dendritic cell found in lymph node follicles.

Forebrain: anterior of the three principal divisions of the brain.

Fungus: general term used to denote a group of eukaryotic protists, including mushrooms, yeasts, rusts, moulds, smuts, etc., which are characterized by the absence of chlorophyll and by the presence of a rigid cell wall composed of chitin, mannans and sometimes cellulose. They are usually of simple morphological form or show some reversible cellular specialization, such as the formation of pseudoparenchymatous tissue in the fruiting body of a mushroom. The dimorphic fungi grow, according to environmental conditions, as moulds or yeasts.

G

Gamete: cell involved in sexual reproduction, which has half the gentic makeup of the parent cell.

Ganglia: general term for a group of nerve cell bodies located outside the central nervous system, occasionally applied to certain nuclear groups within the brain or spinal cord, e.g., basal ganglia.

Gel electrophoresis: electrophoresis performed in a gel. Electrophoresis is a method of separating substances, especially proteins, and analyzing molecular structure based on the rate of movement of each component in a colloidal suspension while under the influence of an electric field.

Gene: a hereditary unit consisting of a sequence of DNA that occupies a specific locus on a chromosome and determines a particular characteristic in an organism. Genes undergo mutation when their DNA sequence changes.

Genetic recombination: formation of new combination of alleles in offspring as a result of exchange of DNA sequences between molecules. It occurs naturally in the crossing over between homologous chromosomes in meiosis.

Generalization: formulation of general concepts/knowledge by abstracting/extracting common properties of known instances of a similar situation.

Genome: the complete collection of genetic material carried by an organism or cell.

Genotype: genetic constitution of an organism or cell, which is distinct from its expressed features or phenotype. In practice, it usually refers to the particular alleles present at the loci in question.

Germ line: refers to the genes in germ cells as opposed to somatic cells. In immunology it refers to the genes in their unrearranged state rather than those rearranged for production of immunoglobulin or TCR molecules.

Germinal center: areas within lymph nodes where B-cells rapidly proliferate and differentiate. They are important for the generation of memory B-cells and the maturation of the antibody affinity (immune response).

Gigantism: excessive growth of the body or any of its parts, especially as a result of oversecretion of the growth hormone by the pituitary gland. It is also called *giantism*.

Gland: organ that produces a secretion for use elsewhere in the body or in a body cavity or for elimination from the body.

Glia: sustentacular tissue that surrounds and supports neurons in the central nervous system; glial and neural cells together compose the tissue of the central nervous system. Also named *neuroglia*, glial cells do not conduct electrical impulses, unlike neurons.

Granulocyte: collective term for leukocytes with pronounced cytoplasmic granulation. The granules containing potent chemicals allow the cells to digest microorganisms, or to produce inflammatory reactions. In humans, granulocytes are also classified as *polymorphonuclear leucocytes* and are subdivided according to the staining properties of the granules into *eosinophils, basophils* and *neutrophils*.

H

Haploid: nucleus, cell or organism possessing a single set of unpaired chromosomes.

Hapten: small molecule that reacts with a specific antibody but cannot induce the formation of antibodies unless bound to a carrier protein or other large antigenic molecule.

Heavy chain: the larger of the two types of polypeptide chains that comprise a normal immunoglobulin or antibody molecule. It consists of an antigen-binding portion having a variable amino acid sequence and a constant region that defines the antibody class.

Helper T-cells: a subset of T-cells that when stimulated by a specific antigen release lymphokines that promote the activation and function of B-cells and killer T-cells. Also called T-helper cell.

Histamin: physiologically active amine, $C_5H_9N_3$, found in plant and animal tissue and released from mast cells as part of an allergic reaction in humans. It stimulates gastric secretion and causes dilation of capillaries, constriction of bronchial smooth muscle, and decreased blood pressure.

Histocompatibility: if tissues of two organisms are histocompatible, then grafts between the organisms will not be rejected. If however, major histocompatibility antigens are different, then an immune response will be mounted against the foreign tissue.

Homeostasis: tendency to stability in the normal body states (internal environment) of the organism. It is basically achieved by a system of feedback regulatory (control) mechanisms.

Hormone: naturally occuring substance secreted by specialized cells which affect the metabolism or behavior of other cells possessing functional receptors for the hormone. Hormones may be hydrophilic like insulin, in which case the receptors are on the cell surface or lipophilic, like the steroids, where the receptor can be intracellular.

Humoral: pertaining to the extracellular fluids, including the serum and lymph.

Humoral immunity: immune reaction provided with immune fluids, i.e., soluble factors such as antibodies, which circulate in the body's fluids or "humors", primarily serum and lymph.

Hypersensitivity: state of reactivity to antigen that is greater than normal for the antigenic challenge. It is the same as *allergy* and denotes a deleterious outcome rather than a protective one.

Hypothalamus: part of the brain that lies below the thalamus and functioning to regulate bodily temperature, certain metabolic processes, and other autonomic activities.

I

Idiotope: antigenic determinant (*epitope*) unique to a single clone of cells and located in the variable region of the immunoglobulin product of that clone. The idiotope forms part of the antigen-binding site. Any single immunoglobulin may have more than one idiotope.

Idiotype: the antigenic specificites defined by the unique sequences (idiotopes) of the antigen-combining site. Thus, anti-idiotype antibodies combined with those specific sequences may block immunological reactions and may resemble the epitope to which the first antibody reacts.

Immune response: alteration in the reactivity of an organisms' immune system in response to an antigen. In vertebrates, this may involve antibody production, induction of cell-mediated immunity, complement activation, or development of immunological tolerance.

Immune system: integrated body system of organs, tissues, cells, and cell products such as antibodies that differentiates self from nonself and neutralizes potentially pathogenic microorganisms or substances.

Immunity: condition of being resistant to an infection.

Immunization: process that increases the reaction of the organisms to a given antigen and therefore improves its ability to resist or overcome infection. The term immunization also describes a technique used to induce immune resistance to a specific disease by exposing the individual to a weakened or died antigen in order to raise antibodies to that antigen.

Immunocompetent: capable of recognizing and acting against an antigen.

Immunogen: a substance capable of inducing an immune response, as well as reacting with the products of an immune response. See *antigen*.

Immunoglobulin: general term for all antibody molecules. See *antibody*.

Immunology: science concerned mainly with the study of the structure and function of the immune system, innate and acquired immunity, the bodily distinction of self from nonself, and laboratory techniques involving the interaction of antigens with specific antibodies.

Infection: invasion and multiplication of microorganisms in body tissues, which may be not clinically apparent or may result in local cellular injury due to competitive metabolism, toxins, intracellular replication or antigen-antibody response. The infection may remain localized, subclinical, and temporary if the body's defensive mechanisms are effective. A local infection may persist and spread by extension to become an acute, subacute or chronic clinical infection or disease state. A local infection may also become systemic when the microorganisms gain access to the lymphatic or vascular system.

Inflammatory response: a localised protective response elicited by injury or destruction of tissues, which serves to destroy, dilute or wall off (sequester) both the injurious agent and the injured tissue. It is characterized in the acute form by the classical signs of pain (dolor), heat (calor), redness (rubor), swelling (tumour) and loss of function (functio laesa). Histologically, it involves a complex series of events, including dilatation of arterioles, capillaries and venules, with increased permeability and blood flow, exudation of fluids, including plasma proteins and leucocytic migration into the inflammatory focus.

Innate immune response: first immune response against infections. It works rapidly, gives rise to the acute inflammatory response, and has some specificity for microbes.

Inoculation: act or instance of inoculating, especially the introduction of an antigenic substance or vaccine into the body in order to produce immunity to a specific disease.

Interferon (**INF**): cytokine involved in defense against viral infection and in activation and modulation of immunity.

Interleukine (**IL**): glycoproteins secreted by a variety of leukocytes that have effects on other leukocytes.

Internal image: spatial configuration of the combining site of an anti-idiotype antibody that resembles the epitope to which the idiotype is directed.

Intron: segment of DNA that does not code for protein. The intervening sequence of nucleotides between coding sequences or *exons*.

K

Killer T-cell: T-cell subset that can directly kill body cells infected by viruses or transformed by cancer. Also called *cytotoxic T-cell*.

L

Learning: act, process, or experience of gaining knowledge or skill; behavioral modification especially through experience or conditioning.

Lesion: any pathological or traumatic discontinuity of tissue or loss of function of a part.

Leukocyte: any of various blood cells that have a nucleus and cytoplasm, separate into a thin white layer when whole blood is centrifuged, and help protect the body from infection and disease. Include *neutrophils*, *eosinophils*, *basophils*, *lymphocytes*, and *monocytes*. Also called *white blood cells*.

Ligand: linking (or binding) molecule.

Light chain: the smaller of the two types of polypeptide chains in immunoglobulins, consisting of an antigen-binding portion with a variable amino acid sequence, and a constant region with an amino acid sequence that is relatively unchanging.

Lipopolysaccharide: any of a group of polysaccharides in which a lipid constitutes a portion of the molecule. The major constituents of the cell walls of gram-negative bacteria. Highly immunogenic and stimulates the production of endogenous pyrogen interleukin-1 and tumour necrosis factor.

Locus: position on a chromosome at which a particular gene is found.

Lymph: clear, watery, sometimes faintly yellowish fluid derived from body tissues that contains white blood cells and circulates throughout the lymphatic system, returning to the venous bloodstream through the thoracic duct. Lymph acts to remove bacteria and certain proteins from the tissues, transport fat from the small intestine, and supply mature lymphocytes to the blood.

Lymph nodes: small bean-shaped organs of the immune system, widely distributed throughout the body and linked by lymphatic vessels. The lymph nodes store special cells that can trap cancer cells or bacteria that are traveling through the body in lymph. Also called *lymph glands*.

Lymphatic vessels: a bodywide network of channels, similar to the blood vessels, which remove cellular waste from the body by filtering through lymph nodes and eventually emptying into the blood stream. They carry the *lymph* and are also named *lymphatics*.

Lymphocyte: small white blood cell with virtually no cytoplasm, found in blood, tissue, and in lymphoid organs such as lymph nodes, spleen and Peyer's patches; bears antigen-specific receptors.

Lymphoid organs: the organs of the immune system where lymphocytes develop and congregate. They include the bone marrow, thymus, lymph nodes, spleen and various other clusters of lymphoid tissue. The blood vessels and lymphatic vessels can also be considered lymphoid organs.

Lymphokines: generic term for molecules other than antibodies that are involved in signalling between cells of the immune system and are produced by lymphocytes. These soluble molecules help and regulate the immune responses.

Lysis: dissolution or destruction of cells, such as blood cells or bacteria, as by the action of a specific lysin that disrupts the cell membrane and causes the loss of cytoplasm.

M

Macrophage: a large and versatile immune cell derived from monocytes, which acts as a microbe-devouring phagocyte. It is also an antigen-presenting cell and an important source of immune secretions.

Major histocompatibility complex (**MHC**): a group of genes encoding polymorphic cell-surface molecules (MHC class I and II) that are involved in controlling several aspects of the immune response. MHC genes code for self-markers on all body cells and play a major role in transplantation rejection. Several other proteins are encoded in this region.

Maturation of the immune response: process by which the B-cell receptors (antibodies) increase their affinity in relation to the selective antigenic stimulus. It occurs through a combination of mutational and selective events.

Medulla: the inner portion of an organ.

Meiosis: process of cell division in sexually reproducing organisms that reduces the number of chromosomes in reproductive cells from diploid to haploid, leading to the production of gametes in animals and spores in plants.

Memory: faculty of retaining and recalling past experience.

Memory cell: cell that presents an active state of immunity to a specific antigen, such that a second encounter with that antigen leads to an enhanced and faster response.

Metabolism: act or process, by which living tissues or cells take up and convert into their own proper substance the nutritive material brought to them by the blood, or by which they transform their cell protoplasm into simpler substances, which are fitted either for excretion or for some special purpose, as in the manufacture of the digestive ferments. Hence, metabolism may be either constructive (*anabolism*), or destructive (*katabolism*).

MHC class I molecule: molecule encoded by the genes of the MHC that participates in antigenic presentation to cytotoxic T-cells.

MHC class II molecule: molecule encoded by the genes of the MHC that participates in antigenic presentation to helper T-cells.

Microbes: microscopic living organisms. The term is particularly applied to pathogenic organisms, such as bacteria, viruses, fungi and protozoa. Also named *microorganism*.

Microorganism: microscopic organism. It usually refers to disease causing organisms, such as viruses, bacteria and fungi.

Midbrain: portion of the vertebrate brain that develops from the middle section of the embryonic brain. It is usually involved in unconscious body function.

Mitogen: substance that stimulates the mitosis of certain cells.

Mitosis: process in cell division by which the nucleus divides, typically consisting of four stages, prophase, metaphase, anaphase, and telophase, and normally resulting in two new nuclei, each of which contains a complete copy of the parental chromosomes. Also called karyokinesis.

Molecule: smallest particle of a substance that retains its chemical and physical properties.

Monoclonal: literally, coming from a single clone. In immunology, monoclonal usually describes a preparation of antibody or T-cells that are homogenous; derived from a clone of cells with the same specificity toward an epitope.

Monocyte: large, circulating, phagocytic white blood cell, having a single well-defined nucleus and very fine granulation in the cytoplasm. They emigrate into tissue and differentiate into a *macrophage*.

Monokine: soluble factor secreted by monocytes and macrophages that act on other cells and help to direct and regulate the immune response.

Monospecificity: of single specificity. Refers to cells whose receptors present the capability of recognizing a single antigenic pattern.

Multispecificity: of multiple specificity. Refers to cells whose receptors present the capability of recognizing different antigenic patterns, as far as a minimal amount of interactions occur.

Mutation: change of the DNA sequence within a gene or chromosome of an organism resulting in the creation of a new character or trait not found in the parental type. Also an individual exhibiting such a change.

Myelin sheath: insulating envelope of myelin that surrounds the core of a nerve fiber or axon and facilitates the transmission of nerve impulses. In the peripheral nervous system, the sheath is formed from the cell membrane of the Schwann cell and in the central nervous system, from oligodendrocytes. Also called *medullary sheath*.

N

Naïve lymphocyte: lymphocyte that has not been involved in an immune response.

Natural antibody: antibody that is present in the serum of an individual who has never been immunized or clinically exposed to the antigen to which it reacts.

Natural killer cells (**NK**): large granule-filled lymphocytes that take on tumor cells and infected body cells. They are known as "natural" killer because they do not present antigenic specificity, i.e., they attack without first having to recognize specific antigens. Their number does not increase by immunization.

Natural selection: process in nature by which, according to Darwin's theory of evolution, only the organisms most adapted to their environment tend to survive and transmit their genetic characteristics (material) in increasing numbers to succeeding generations while those less adapted tend to be eliminated.

Negative selection: process that prevents self-specific lymphocytes from becoming auto-aggressive.

Nerve impulse: see *action potential*.

Nervous system: the specialized coordinating system of cells, tissues and organs that endows animals with sensation and volition. In vertebrates, it is often divided into two systems: the central (brain and spinal cord), and the peripheral (somatic and autonomic nervous system).

Neuroglia: network of branched cells and fibers that supports the tissue of the central nervous system. It is also called *glia*.

Neuron: impulse-conducting cells that constitute the brain, spinal column, and nerves, consisting of a nucleated cell body with one or more dendrites and a single axon. Also known as *nerve cell*.

Neurotransmitters: any of a group of substances that are released on excitation from the axon terminal of a presynaptic neuron of the central or peripheral nervous system and travel across the synaptic cleft to either excite or inhibit the target cell. Among the many substances that have the properties of a neurotransmitter are acetylcholine, noradrenaline, adrenaline, dopamine, glycine, glutamic acid, enkephalins, endorphins and serotonin.

Neutrophil: especially an abundant type of granular white blood cell that is highly destructive of microorganisms and important in phagocytosis.

Nucleotide: the basic structural unit of nucleic acids (DNA or RNA).

Nucleus: large, membrane-bound, usually spherical protoplasmic structure within a living cell, containing the hereditary material of the cell and controlling its metabolism, growth, and reproduction.

O

Offspring: progeny or descendants.

Ontogeny: origin and development of an individual organism from embryo to adult; history of the individual development of an organism, or of the evolution of the germ. Also called *ontogenesis*.

Opsonin: substance, usually antibody or complement component, which coats a particle such as a bacterium and enhances phagocytosis.

Opsonize: literally means "prepare to eat". The coat of an organism with antibodies or a complement protein so as to make it palatable to phagocytes.

Organ: combination of different types of tissues.

Organism: individual form of life, such as a plant, animal, bacterium, protist, or fungus; a body made up of organs, organelles, or other parts that work together to carry on the various processes of life.

Ovaries: the usually paired female or hermaphroditic reproductive organ that produces ova and, in vertebrates, secrete female hormones estrogen, which develops and maintains female characteristics, and progesterone, which prepares the uterus for pregnancy.

P

Pancreas: gland connected with the intestine of nearly all vertebrates. It is usually elongated and light-colored, and its secretion, called the pancreatic juice, is discharged, often together with the bile, into the upper part of the intestines, and is a powerful aid in digestion.

Parasite: organism that grows, feeds, and is sheltered on or in a different organism while contributing nothing to the survival of its host.

Parathyroid gland: any of four small kidney-shaped glands located in the neck, near the thyroid gland. They produce parathormone that controls calcium and phosphorus metabolism.

Paratope: an antibody-combining site that is complementary to an epitope.

Pathogen: a microorganism that causes disease.

Pathology: (study of) the nature of disease and its causes, processes, development, and consequences; anatomic or functional manifestation of a disease.

Peptide: any of various natural or synthetic compounds containing two or more amino acids linked by the carboxyl group of one amino acid to the amino group of another.

Peyer's patches: lymphoid organs located in the sub mucosal tissue of the mammalian gut containing very high proportions of cells capable of secreting a specific type of antibody. The patches have B- and T-dependent regions and germinal centers. A specialized epithelium lies between the patch and the intestine. It is involved in gut associated immunity.

Phagocyte: large white blood cells that contribute to the immune defenses by ingesting and digesting waste material, microbes or other cells and foreign particles.

Phagocytosis: process by which cells engulf material and enclose it within a vacuole (phagosome) in the cytoplasm.

Phenotype: the physical or biochemical expression of an indivduals' genotype; observable expressed traits, such as eye and skin color.

Physiology: (study of) the functions of living organisms and their parts

Pineal gland: small, cone-shaped gland in the brain of most vertebrates that secretes melatonin, a hormone involved with daily biological rhythms. Also called *epiphysis*, *pineal body* or *pineal organ*.

Pituitary gland: small oval endocrine gland attached to the base of the vertebrate brain and consisting of an anterior and a posterior lobe, the secretions of which control the other endocrine glands (thyroid, adrenal, testicles and ovaries) and influence growth, metabolism, and reproduction. Also called hypophysis, pituitary body.

Plasma cells: terminally differentiated antibody-producing cells that develop from B-cells.

Platelets: cytoplasmic fragments of a parent cell found within the bone marrow. They have a diameter less than half of an erythrocyte.

Polymorfonuclear lymphocyte: collective term for leukocytes with pronounced cytoplasmic granulation. The granules containing potent chemicals allow the cells to digest microorganisms, or to produce inflammatory reactions. In humans, polymorphonuclear leucocytes are also classified as *granulocytes* and are subdivided according to the staining properties of the granules into *eosinophils*, *basophils* and *neutrophils*.

Polypeptide: a peptide, such as a small protein, containing many molecules of amino acids.

Pons: band of nerve fibers on the ventral surface of the brain stem that links the medulla oblongata and the cerebellum with upper portions of the brain. It is also called *pons Varolii*.

Positive selection: serves the purpose of avoiding the accumulation of useless lymphocytes with either no receptor at all or with receptors that are unproductive for the organism.

Primary lymphoid organs: organs mainly responsible for the production and maturation of lymphocytes.

Primary response: immune response as a consequence of the first encounter with a given antigen. It is generally weak, has a long lag phase and generates immune memory.

Progestin: any of a group of steroid hormones that exhibit progesterone-like activity, i.e. prepare the uterus for egg implantation and pregnancy.

Proteins: organic compounds made up of amino acids, which are one of the major constituents of plants and animal cells.

R

Receptor: cell surface molecule that binds specifically to particular proteins or peptides.

Receptor editing: process through which some B-cells delete their receptors and develop entirely new receptors by V(D)J recombination.

Recognition: process by which an immune cell or molecule specifically identifies and matches (bind) with a given antigen.

Red blood cell: cell in the blood of vertebrates that transports oxygen and carbon dioxide to and from the tissues. In mammals, the red blood cell is disk-shaped and biconcave, contains haemoglobin, and lacks a nucleus. Also called *erythrocyte, red cell, red corpuscle*.

Reflex: involuntary action or response, such as a sneeze, blink, or hiccup. It is also used to describe muscle responses.

Repertoire: set of cells or molecules in the immune system. Used as a synonym to *population*.

Resilience: for what disturbance the system might flip out of it stability domain; the better the resilience the larger the disturbance required to get the system out of its stability domain.

S

Scavenger cells: any of a diverse group of cells that have the capacity to engulf and destroy foreign material, dead tissues or other cells.

Second signal: the delivery of a co-stimulatory signal from an APC to a T-cell. The co-stimulatory signal rescues the activated T-cell from anergy, allowing it to produce the lymphokines necessary for the growth of additional T-cells.

Secondary lymphoid organs: organs where the immune cells interact with the antigenic stimuli, thus initiating adaptive immune responses.

Secondary response: immune response that follows a second or subsequent encounter with a particular antigen.

Serum: the clear fluid that is obtained upon separating whole blood into its solid and liquid components after it has been allowed to clot. Blood serum from the tissues of immunized animals contains antibodies that are used to transfer immunity to another individual.

Skull: bony or cartilaginous framework of the head of vertebrates made up of the bones of the braincase and face. It is also named *cranium*.

Smallpox: acute, highly infectious, often fatal disease caused by a poxvirus and characterized by high fever and aches with subsequent widespread eruption of pimples that blister, produce pus, and form pockmarks; officially announced as globally eradicated in 1979. It is also called *variola*.

Soma: the neuron cell body that contains the nucleus.

Somatic mutation: process occurring during B-cell clonal expansion and affecting the antibody gene region, which, together with selection, permits refinement of the antibody specificity with relation to the selective antigen.

Spinal cord: thick, whitish cord of nerve tissue that extends from the medulla oblongata down through the spinal column and from which the spinal nerves branch off to various parts of the body.

Spleen: large, highly vascular lymphoid organ, lying in the human body to the left of the stomach below the diaphragm, serving to store blood, disintegrate old blood cells and filter foreign substances from the blood.

Splicing: to join together or insert (segments of DNA or RNA) so as to form new genetic combinations or alter a genetic structure.

Stem cell: cell that gives rise to a lineage of cells. Particularly used to describe the most primitive cells in the bone marrow from which all the various types of blood cells are derived.

Steroid: group name for lipids that contain a hydrogenated ring system, include progesterone, adrenocortical hormones, gonadal hormones, bile acids and sterols.

Stimulus: a factor that can be detected by a receptor, which in turn produces a response.

Supression: mechanism for producing a specific state of immunologic unresponsiveness by which one cell or its products act on another cell.

Suppressor T-cells: subpopulation of T-cells that acts to reduce the immune responses of other T-cells or B-cells. Suppression may be antigen-specific, idiotype-specific, or nonspecific in different circumstances.

Synapse: junction across which a nerve impulse passes from an axon terminal to a neuron, muscle cell, or gland cell.

Synaptic cleft: narrow space between the presynaptic cell and the postsynaptic cell in a chemical synapse, across which the neurotransmitter diffuses.

T

T-cell: small white blood cell that orchestrate and/or directly participate in the immune defenses. Also known as T lymphocyte, it maturates in the thymus and secretes lymphokines.

Template: structure in some direct physical process can cause the patterning of a second structure, usually complementary to it in some sense.

Thalamus: large ovoid mass of grey matter situated in the posterior part of the forebrain that relays sensory and motor impulses to the cerebral cortex.

Thymectomy: the excision of the thymus by surgery, radiation or chemical means.

Thymocyte: lymphocyte that derives from the thymus and is the precursor of a T-cell; immature T-cell.

Thymus: small glandular primary lymphoid organ situated behind the top of the breastbone; site where T-cells proliferate and maturate. It is also considered to be an endocrine organ.

Thyroid: butterfly-shaped endocrine gland in the neck that is found on both sides of the traches. It secretes the hormone thyroxine that controls the rate of metabolism and blood calcium levels.

Tissue: organization of differentiated cells of of a similar type. There are four basic types of tissue: muscle, nerve, epidermal, and connective

Tolerance: a state of non-responsiveness to a particular antigen or group of antigens.

Tonsils and adenoids: prominent oval masses of lymphoid tissues on either sides of the throat. They are primarily associated with the protection of the respiratory system.

Toxins: poisonous substance, especially a protein, produced by living cells or organisms, normally very damaging to mammalian cells, that can be delivered directly to target cells by linking them to antibodies or lymphokines. They are different from the simple chemical poisons by their high molecular weight and antigenicity.

Trait: genetically determined characteristic or condition.

Transcription: process by which messenger RNA is synthesized from a DNA template resulting in the transfer of genetic information from the DNA molecule to the messenger RNA.

Translation: process by which messenger RNA directs the amino acid sequence of a growing polypeptide during protein synthesis.

Tumor: abnormal growth of tissue resulting from uncontrolled, progressive multiplication of cells and serving no physiological function; may be benign (not cancerous) or malignant. It is also called a *neoplasm*.

Tumor necrosis factor (**TNF**): protein produced by macrophages in the presence of an endotoxin and shown experimentally to be capable of attacking and destroying cancerous tumors.

U

Unresponsiveness: inability to respond to an antigenic stimulus. It may be specific for a particular antigen (see *tolerance*), or broadly nonspecific as a result of damage to the entire immune system, e.g., after whole-body irradiation.

V

Vaccine: preparation of a weakened or killed pathogen, such as a bacterium or virus, or of a portion of the pathogen's structure that upon administration stimulates antibody production or cellular immunity against the pathogen but is incapable of causing severe infection. By stimulating an immune response (but not disease), it protects against subsequent infection by that organism.

Vaccination: process of inoculating an individual with a vaccine in order to protect against a particular disease.

Vaccinia: mild contagious skin disease of cattle, usually affecting the udder, that is caused by a virus and characterized by the eruption of a pustular rash. When the virus is transmitted to humans, as by vaccination, it can confer immunity to *smallpox*. Also called *cowpox*.

Variable region (V-region): that part of an antibody's structure responsible for the antigenic recognition and that contains particular variable sub-regions whose composition might be a consequence of the contact with an antigen. These sub-regions are usually named *complementary determining regions* (CDR).

Vertebrates: animals having a vertebral column, members of the phylum chordata, subphylum vertebrata comprising mammals, birds, reptiles, amphibians and fishes.

Virus: obligate intracellular parasite that often causes disease and that consist essentially of a core of RNA or DNA surrounded by a protein coat.

Viscera: soft internal organs of the body, especially those contained within the abdominal and thoracic cavities.

W

Watson-Crick Complementarity: Process in DNA bonding where the nucleotide A bonds with T and G bonds with C.

White blood cell: any of various blood cells that have a nucleus and cytoplasm, separate into a thin white layer when whole blood is centrifuged, and help protect the body from infection and disease. White blood cells include *neutrophils, eosinophils, basophils, lymphocytes,* and *monocytes*. It is also called *leukocytes, white cells* and *white corpuscles*.

References

Abbas, A. K., Lichtman, A. H. & Pober, J. S. (1998), *Cellular and Molecular Immunology*, W. B. Saunders Company.

Barret, J. T. (1983), *Textbook of Immunology An Introduction to Immunochemistry and Immunobiology*, 4th Ed., The C. V. Mosby Company.

Benjamini, E., Sunshine, G. & Leskowitz, S. (1996), *Immunology A Short Course*, 3rd Ed., Wiley-Liss.

Biology Online: *Information in the Biological Sciences*, [On Line] http://www. biology-online.org/default.htm

Bullock, J., Boyle, J. & Wang, M. B. (1984), *Physiology*, New York: J. Wiley, Pennsylvania: Harwal Pub.

Cancer WEB Online Dictionary: *On-line Medical Dictionary*, © 1997-98 Academic Medical Publishing & CancerWEB [On Line] http://cancerweb.ncl.ac.uk/.

Coleman, R. M., Lombard, M. F. & Sicard, R. E. (1992), *Fundamental Immunology*, 2nd Ed., Wm. C. Brown Publishers.

Futuyma, D. J., (1979), *Evolutionary Biology*, Sinauer Associates, Inc.

Guyton, A. C. (1991), *Textbook of Medical Physiology*, 8th Ed., W. B. Saunders Company.

Hood, L. E., Weissman, I. L., Wood, W. B. & Wilson, J. H. (1984), *Immunology*, 2nd Ed., The Benjamin/Cummings Publishing Company, Inc.

Janeway, C. A., P. Travers, Walport, M. & Capra, J. D. (1999), "Immunobiology: The Immune System in Health and Disease", 4th Ed., Garland Publishing.

Klein, J. (1990), *Immunology*, Blackwell Scientific Publications.

Krebs, C. J. (1994), *Ecology The Experimental Analysis of Distribution and Abundance*, 4th Ed., Harper Collins College Publishers.

Lydyard, P. M., Whelan, A. & Fanger, M. W. (2000), *Instant Notes in Immunology*, BIOS Scientific Publishers Limited.

Mackenna, B. R. & Callander, R. (1998), *Illustrated Physiology*, Churchill Livingstone.

McClintic, J. R. (1985), *Physiology of the Human Body*, 3rd Ed., John Wiley & Sons.

Ottoson, S. D. (1983), *Physiology of the Nervous System*, New York: Oxford University Press.

Paul, W. E. (ed.) (1999), *Fundamental Immunology*, 4th Ed., Lippincott-Raven Publishers.

Roitt, I. (1997), *Essential Immunology*, 9th Ed., Blackwell Science.

Solomon, E. P., Schmidt, R. R. & Adragna, P. J. (1990), *Human Anatomy & Physiology*, Saunders College Publishing.

Tizard, I. R. (1995), *Immunology An Introduction*, 4th Ed, Saunders College Publishing.

Vander, A. J., Sherman, J. H. & Luciano, D. S. (1990), *Human Physiology The Mechanisms of Body Function*, 5th Ed., McGraw-Hill Book Company.

Appendix II

Pseudocode for Immune Algorithms

The aim of this appendix is to provide the reader with pseudocode for the immune algorithms described in this book. The pseudocode provided are for the following algorithms: positive selection, negative selection, clonal selection, RAIN, and aiNet. To simplify the presentation of each pseudocode, a set of general functions will be provided, together with their input and output arguments, and a brief description.

General Functions

1. $A \leftarrow \textbf{rand}(N, L)$
    The function $\textbf{rand}(\cdot,\cdot)$ randomly generates a set A with N attribute strings of length L each.

2. $v \leftarrow \textbf{affinity}(B, C, r)$
    Function $\textbf{rand}(\cdot,\cdot,\cdot)$ determines the vector v of affinities between the elements of C in relation to the elements of B, assuming a cross-reactivity threshold r. In cases r is not input to the algorithm, no cross-reactivity threshold is accounted for in the algorithm.

3. $v \leftarrow \textbf{stim}(B, s, h)$
    The function $\textbf{stim}(\cdot,\cdot,\cdot)$ returns the vector v containing the stimulation level of each individual b of B, based on Equation 3.21, where s is the antigenic pattern and h its neighbohood, i.e., the connected individuals.

4. $A \leftarrow \textbf{insert}(B, C)$
    Function $\textbf{insert}(\cdot,\cdot)$ returns a matrix A with the elements of C concatenated into B.

5. $B \leftarrow \textbf{sort}(B, v)$
    Function $\textbf{sort}(\cdot,\cdot)$ returns the matrix B with its elements sorted in ascending order as defined by v.

6. $A \leftarrow \textbf{select}(B, n)$
    Function $\textbf{select}(\cdot,\cdot)$ returns a matrix A containing the n first individuals of B. (This function assumes that the individuals of B are sorted in ascending order, so that the best elements are selected.)

7. $B \leftarrow$ **hypermut**(B, v)

    The function **hypermut**$(\cdot, \cdot)$ returns a matrix B with its elements mutated in proportion to v.

8. $B \leftarrow$ **replace**(B, C, n)

    In function **replace**$(\cdot, \cdot, \cdot)$, n elements of B are replaced by C (the length of C is equal to n).

9. $B \leftarrow$ **remove**(B, b)

    Function **remove**$(\cdot, \cdot)$ removes the element b from B.

10. $e \leftarrow$ **resources**(b, v)

    Function **resources**$(\cdot, \cdot)$ returns a number e of resources allocated to an individual b based on the value v.

11. $A \leftarrow$ **randSelect**(B, n)

    Function **randSelect**$(\cdot, \cdot)$ returns a set A of n elements randomly selected (without replacement) from the set B.

Positive Selection Algorithm

function Positive_Selection *(S, r, n)* **returns** a detector set *A*

inputs: *S*   set of strings that define the self
          r   cross-reactivity threshold
          n   number of detectors required

---

begin
   j ← 0
   while *j* <= *n* **do**
       m ← rand(1,*L*)   // *Initialization*
       for every *s* of *S* **do**
           aff ← affinity(*m*, *s*, *r*)   // *Affinity evaluation*
           if *aff* >= *r* **then**   // *Generation of the available repertoire*
               A ← insert(*A*, *m*)
           endIf
       endFor
       j ← *j* + 1
   endWhile
   return *A*
end

Negative Selection Algorithm

function Negative_Selection (S, r, n) **returns** a detector set A

inputs: S set of strings that define the self
           r cross-reactivity threshold
           n number of detectors required

---

begin
    $j \leftarrow 0$
    while $j <= n$ **do**
        $m \leftarrow \text{rand}(1, L)$ // *Initialization*
        for every s of S **do**
            $aff \leftarrow \text{affinity}(m, s, r)$ // *Affinity evaluation*
            if $aff <= r$ **then**   // *Generation of the available repertoire*
                $A \leftarrow \text{insert}(A, m)$
            endIf
        endFor
        $j \leftarrow j + 1$
    endWhile
    return A
end

Clonal Selection Algorithm

function CLONALG (S, g, N, n_1, n_2) **returns** set of memory individuals M

inputs:	S	patterns to be recognized
	g	number of iterations
	N	size of the population
	n_1	number of high affinity elements to be selected for cloning
	n_2	number of low affinity elements to be replaced at end of iteration

---

begin

    $j \leftarrow 0$

    $P \leftarrow \text{rand}(N, L)$ // *Initialization*

    while $j < g$ **do**

        for each s *of* S **do**   // *Antigenic presentation*

            for each p of P **do**   //*Affinity evaluation*

                $aff(p) \leftarrow \text{match}(s, p);$

            endFor

            $P \leftarrow \text{sort}(P, aff)$ // *Clonal selection*

            $P1 \leftarrow \text{select}(P, n_1)$

            for $i < n_1$ **do**   // *Clonal expansion*

                $C \leftarrow clone(P1, aff(P1))$

            endFor

            for every c of C **do**   // *Affinity maturation*

               $C1 \leftarrow \text{hypermut}(c, aff(P1))$

            endFor

            for each $c1$ of $C1$ **do**

                $aff(c1) \leftarrow \text{affinity}(c1, s)$

            endFor

            $M1 \leftarrow \text{sort}(aff(C1))$

            $M(s) \leftarrow select(M1, 1)$

            $m \leftarrow \text{rand}(n_2, L)$ // *Metadynamics*

            $P \leftarrow \text{replace}(P, m, n_2)$

        endFor

        $j \leftarrow j + 1$

    endWhile

    return M

end

Discrete Immune Network: aiNet

function aiNet $(S, g, n_1, n_2, n_3, \alpha, \beta)$ **returns** set of memory individuals M

inputs:	S	patterns to be recognized
	g	number of iterations
	n_1	number of high affinity elements to be selected for cloning
	n_2	number of high affinity clones to be places into the memory set
	n_3	number of elements to be introduced
	α	threshold for clonal suppression (suppression threshold)
	β	affinity threshold

```
begin
    j ← 0
    P ← rand(N, L)                                  // Initialization
    while j < g do
        for each s of S do                          // Antigenic presentation
            for each p of P do                      //Affinity evaluation
                aff (p) ← affinity(s, p);
            endFor
            P ← sort(P, aff)                        // Clonal selection
            P1 ← select(P, n₁)
            for i < n₁ do                           // Clonal expansion
                C ← clone(P1, aff (P1))
            endFor
            for every c of C do                     // Affinity maturation
                C1 ← hypermut(c, aff (P1))
            endFor
            for each c1 of C1 do
                aff (c1) ← affinity(c1, s)
            endFor
            M1 ← sort(aff (C1))
            M2 ← select(M1, n₂)
            for each m of M2 do
                if aff (m) < β then                 // Metadynamics
                    M2 ← remove(M2, m)
                endIf
                clonal_aff (m) ← affinity(M2, m)    // Clonal interactions
                if clonal_aff (m) < α then          // Clonal suppression
                    M2 ← remove(M2, m)
                endIf
            endFor
            M ← insert(P, M2)                       // Network construction
        endFor                                      // End For antigenic presentation
```

```
        for each m of M do                      // Network interactions
            aff (m) ← affinity(M, m);
            if aff (m) < β then                  // Network suppression
                M ← remove(M, m)
            endIf
        endFor
        R ← rand(n₃, L)                          // Diversity
        P ← insert(M, R)
        j ← j + 1
    endWhile
    return M
end
```

Discrete Immune Network: RAIN

function RAIN (S, n, k, r, t, c, g) **returns** a set of antibodies P

inputs:

S	set of patterns to be recognized
n	network affinity threshold
k	network affinity threshold scalar
r	mutation rate
t	maximum number of resources (B-cells) in system
c	maximum number of clones produced by ARBs
g	number of iterations

---

begin
    $P \leftarrow$ randSelect(S, i) // *Initialization*
    $j \leftarrow 0$
    $n \leftarrow n * k$
    for each p of P **do**
        a $\leftarrow$ affinity(p, p', i)
            if $a < n$ **then**
            neighbourhood_value$(p) \leftarrow a$
        endIf
    endFor
    while $j < g$ **do**
        for each s of S **do**   // *Antigenic presentation*
            for each p of P **do**   // *Affinity evaluation*
                $a \leftarrow$ affinity(p, s, i)
                if $a < n$ **then**
                    aff$(p) \leftarrow a$
                endif
            endFor
        endFor
        for every p of P **do**   // *Clonal selection...*
            p$(s) \leftarrow$ stim(p) // *...and network interactions*
        endFor   // *See Equation 3.21*
        for every p of P **do**   // *Metadynamics*
            $p(r) \leftarrow$ resources(p, l)
            $q \leftarrow \Sigma$ p(r)
            if $q > t$ **then**
                $z \leftarrow q - t$
                $P \leftarrow$ sort$(P, p(r))$
                while $z > 0$ **do**
                    remove z resources from p

```
                              if p(r) == 0 then
                                  P ← remove(P, p)
                                  z ← z - p(r)
                              endIf
                        endWhile
                    endIf
                endFor
                for every p of P do                    // Clonal expansion
                    C ← clone(P, aff(P))
                endFor
                for every c of C do                    // Somatic hypermutation
                    C1 ← hypermut(c, aff (C1))
                endFor
                for every c of C1  do                  // Network construction
                        a ← affinity(c, C1)
                        if a < n then
                            neighbourhood_value(c) ← a
                        endIf
                endFor
                P ← insert(P, C1)
                j ← j + 1
                endWhile
                return P
        end
```

Appendix III

Web Resources on Artificial Immune Systems

There are several research schools, people and organizations doing research on artificial immune systems. This Appendix lists web addresses for individual and organizations home pages. The main research interest on AIS of each author is given based upon their reviewed works discussed on Chapters 4, 6 and 7. The last access to all the web sites listed was done on 5th April 2002. The list contains a few theoretical immunologists particularly important for the development of AIS.

Personal Home Pages

- **Akio Ishiguro**
  Robotics
  http://www.cmplx.cse.nagoya-u.ac.jp/member/ishiguro/

- **Alan S. Perelson**
  Theoretical immunology
  http://www.t10.lanl.gov/profiles/perelson.html

- **Alessio Gaspar**
  Time dependent optimization
  http://www.essi.fr/~gaspar

- **Andrew M. Tyrrell**
  Hardware fault tolerance
  http://www.elec.york.ac.uk/staff/academic/amt.html

- **Derek J. Smith**
  Theoretical immunology
  http://www.santafe.edu/~dsmith

- **Dipankar Dasgupta**
  Computer network security, spectra recognition, theory and survey of AIS
  http://www.msci.memphis.edu/~dasgupta

- **Emma Hart**
  Job-Shop Scheduling
  http://www.dcs.napier.ac.uk/~emmah/

- **Fernando J. Von Zuben**
  Engineering applications
  http://www.dca.fee.unicamp.br/~vonzuben

- **Jon Timmis**
  Data mining, immunised fault tolerance, theory of AIS
  http://www.cs.ukc.ac.uk/people/staff/jt6

- **Jungwon Kim**
  Computer network security
  http://www.dcs.kcl.ac.uk/staff/jungwon/

- **Peter Bentley**
  Computer network security
  http://www.cs.ucl.ac.uk/staff/P.Bentley/

- **Junichi Suzuki**
  Webserver coordination
  http://www.yy.cs.keio.ac.jp/~suzuki/project/immunity/index.html

- **Leandro N. de Castro**
  Engineering applications, theory and survey of AIS
  http://www.dca.fee.unicamp.br/~lnunes

- **Mark Burgess**
  Computer security
  http://www.iu.hio.no/~mark/

- **Mihaela Oprea**
  Theoretical immunology
  http://genomes.rockefeller.edu/mihaela/mihaela.shtml

- **Nikolai Nikolaev**
  Inductive problem solving, genetic programming
  http://homepages.gold.ac.uk/nikolaev/

- **Patrik D'haeseleer**
  Negative selection
  http://www.cs.unm.edu/~patrik

- **Prabhat Hajela**
  Constrained structural optimization
  http://www.rpi.edu/~hajela

- **Stephanie Forrest**
  Computer network security, evolution of gene libraries, pattern recognition
  http://www.cs.unm.edu/~forrest

- **Steven A. Hofmeyr**
  Computer network security
  http://www.cs.unm.edu/~steveah

- **Yuji Watanabe**
  Robotics
  http://www.sys.tutkie.tut.ac.jp/~watanabe/

- **Yoshitero Ishida**
  Fault diagnosis, noise neutralization, computer virus detection, survey and theory of AIS
  http://www.sys.tutkie.tut.ac.jp/~ishida

Organizations

- **CytoCom Network**
  Cytocomputational systems
  http://www.csc.liv.ac.uk/~cytocom/index.html

- **Bio-Inspired Engineering**
  Fault tolerance
  http://www.elec.york.ac.uk/bio/bioIns/main.html

- **IBM Antivirus Research**
  Computer virus detection and elimination
  http://www.research.ibm.com/antivirus.

- **Starlab**
  Immune Networks
  http://users.pandora.be/richard.wheeler1/ais/inn.html.

Subject Index